Irish Doctors
— in the —
Second World War

IRISH DOCTORS
IN THE
SECOND WORLD WAR

P.J. CASEY, K.T. CULLEN & J.P. DUIGNAN

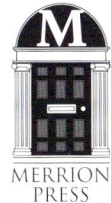

MERRION PRESS

First published in 2024 by
Merrion Press
10 George's Street
Newbridge
Co. Kildare
Ireland
www.merrionpress.ie

© P.J. Casey, K.T. Cullen & J.P. Duignan 2024

978 1 78537 514 9 (Hardback)

A CIP catalogue record for this book is available from the British Library.
All rights reserved. No part of this publication may be reproduced, stored in a retrieval system, or transmitted, in any form or by any means (electronic, mechanical, photocopying, recording or otherwise), without the prior written permission of both the copyright owner and the publisher of this book.

Typeset in Minion Pro 11/16

Design: Eamon Sinnott & Partners, Naas

Front cover images: *(top)* A patient wounded in the leg is given a blood transfusion. © IWM (TR 2410); *(bottom)* Normandy medical evacuation (public domain)
Back cover image: A Field Dressing Station in the Western Desert, June 1942. © IWM (E 13325)

Merrion Press is a member of Publishing Ireland.

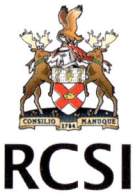

Contents

PART ONE: THE IRISH DOCTORS

Foreword — vii
Introduction — 1
Representation of Irish Medical Colleges in the Second World War — 6
Advances in the Machines of War — 8
Advances in Medical Care — 9

1. **Timeline for the Second World War** — 13

2. **Medals and Awards** — 21
   Medals for Gallantry in Action — 23
   War Campaign Medals — 25

3. **Irish Doctors in Europe and North Africa, 1939–45** — 31
   The Battle for Europe — 32
   Greece, the Balkans and Crete — 40
   North Africa and Italy — 43
   Reinvasion of Europe — 49
   The War at Sea — 50
   The Eastern Front — 54
   The End of the Second World War in Europe — 57

4. **Irish Doctors in the Far East** — 61

5. **Irish Doctors as Prisoners of War** — 71
   Major Francis O'Meara — 75
   Ion Thomas Ferguson — 77
   Alexander Draffin — 80
   Frank Murray — 81
   Aidan MacCarthy — 87

6.	**Profiles in Gallantry and Professionalism by Irish Doctors**	93
	Leslie Samuels	93
	Julius Summ	94
	Aiden Byrne	94
	Kevin Patton	94
	Terence Wilson	95
	John Martin	95
	Peter May	96
	Stephen Conway	96
	Arthur Odbert	96
	Florence Joseph O'Driscoll	97
	Theobald Phelan	97
	Robert Walker	98
	Stanley Walsh	98

Abbreviations and Acronyms	99
Select Bibliography	106
List of Illustrations	107

PART TWO: ROLL OF HONOUR OF IRISH DOCTORS WHO SERVED IN THE SECOND WORLD WAR	111

Acknowledgements	305
Index	306

Foreword

One of the advantages of coming from a relatively small country is the rewarding intensity of interconnections that often unexpectedly link today's living with yesterday's dead. Randomly searching through this enthralling exploration of the Irish who served in the Second World War, I came across RAMC General Arthur Joseph Beveridge MC, the son of the town clerk of Dublin and a Belvedere College boy with a very distinguished military career, which saw him serving in West Africa in 1942. There he would have been the commanding officer of Captain Kevin Teevan, RAMC, similarly a Belvedere boy but a generation younger, who died on active service in November 1942, and whom Beveridge almost certainly would have treated on his deathbed. Beveridge was raised in 33 Belvedere Square, Rathmines, where, many years later, I had a flat, and that young Kevin Teevan whom he treated was my uncle, after whom I have the honour to be named.

At times, these links can have almost sinister personal resonances. Kevin Patton from Meath truly was an exceptional war hero. As this extraordinary analysis reveals in its austere, yet factually rich style, he served with the RAMC in North Africa, Palestine and East Africa, where he was present for the capture of Amba Alagi. However, after his position was overrun in an Italian counterattack, he managed to escape, taking with him, as we read here, some forty wounded. Heroism is at its most beguiling when its accountancy is at its most terse. In 1942, while serving with a cavalry unit in the desert, we read that he performed a live-saving operation – probably a tracheotomy – with a blue Gillette razor blade. In an engagement at Tegna Gap he suffered severe leg injuries, after which he spent *fifteen months* in hospital, though even that failed to provide him with all the action that his life story demanded. On 27 March 1943, near El Hanna, his armoured column was attacked by enemy tanks, yet, despite having broken his ankle and being in considerable agony, he managed to treat and evacuate all his wounded from the battlefield.

For this, Patton was awarded a much-deserved Military Cross. He did not long survive the war, dying almost to the very day, on the third anniversary of his heroic feats at El Hanna. His death was recorded in very same edition of *The Irish Times* that recorded my birth, which in one sense is beside the point, yet in another, it is the very point: this was a small society whose many contributions to the world merit the kind of meticulous but spare attention that the authors have exhibited here.

Some things must inevitably escape any public record, such as the courage of Martin James Murphy, RAMC, grandfather of the well-known actors Jason O'Mara and his sister Rebecca, whose name is recorded in these pages, but not his heroism, because he refused to accept the Military Cross which he had earned in Italy. His refusal was based on his belief that others around him were more deserving, most especially his Irish commanding officer, Lt Colonel Florence Robert O'Driscoll, a legendary warrior against a foe more deadly than steel or cordite: malaria. However, Murphy was awarded, and accepted, a Polish gallantry award, perhaps because another of his Irish colleagues (with whom he retained a lifelong friendship), Samuel Lytle from Belfast, was at the same time similarly decorated. All these men are honoured here.

It is almost impossible to see one aspect of Irish history without other strands of our past inevitably leading to others. Daniel Mortimer Kelleher from Cork had a most distinguished military record, both during the war and afterwards, having served in Palestine, Egypt, Germany, Korea and Kuala Lumpur, before being made brigadier and crowning his career with his appointment as Physician to the Queen in 1966. He retired in 1968 to Surrey, where he died in 2006 at the magnificent age of 98, earning a generous obituary in *The Daily Telegraph*.

However, other tragedies lie beyond these raw details. Mortimer's father had been the dispensary doctor at Macroom in 1920, and upon him fell the melancholy duty of performing post-mortems for the seventeen RIC Auxiliaries slaughtered at Kilmichael in November that year. Mortimer's older brother Philip had won an MC with the Leinsters in the First World War and later, aged just twenty-three, was appointed as a very youthful district inspector of the RIC. Soon after that, and just before the Kilmichael massacre, he was murdered by the IRA as he sat in Kiernan's Hotel, Granard, County Longford, a crime for which Michael Collins' betrothed, Kitty Kiernan, whose family owned the hotel, was briefly arrested but later released. Hollywood fictions can never capture the intimate tragedies of Irish life.

Perhaps the experiences of no Irish doctor compared with those of Aidan MacCarthy, the Clongowes boy who was captured at Singapore, whose Japan-bound POW ship was later sunk by a US submarine, and who survived to be transferred to a camp near Nagasaki, where he witnessed the atom-bomb attack in 1945.

However, as he was later to attest, his most unusual wartime experience was when he was asked to examine fifty young female recruits for the British Army, whose enthusiastic (female) commanding officer had already prepared them. All fifty were standing smartly to attention in an aircraft hangar awaiting examination, and all were completely naked.

Beyond the scope of a work such as this, and probably beyond all reasonable analysis, are the motives of the men who became army doctors, for the impulses that drive most people are invariably too complex for simple analysis. But, nonetheless, we can make rough assessments. One reason for Irish doctors enlisting was economic necessity, especially for those of a Protestant background from the Free State. Career possibilities within public dispensaries were limited by the practice of the Department of Health of allocating such dispensaries to Catholics, apart from those in Dun Laoghaire and the Free State's Ulster counties. Furthermore, Ireland was producing far too many doctors of any religion for them to find work in their homeland, so emigration for many was inevitable. That certainty, allied with the longstanding traditions of Irishmen serving as doctors with the British military, would help explain why the RAMC was so very Irish by the start of the war. Then, of course, came the war-time recruits, such as Kevin Teevan, whose brief time as an army doctor began because of a strong sense of duty to fight Nazism, ending in that disease-ridden, pestilential hole known as Sierre Leone. Finally, there were those Irish Jewish doctors, such as Michael Cohen, Moses Isaac Elliott, Elliot Isaacson and Isidore Isaacson, whose motivation for enlisting requires no complex analysis whatsoever.

In one sense, all of history is an archaeological excavation. This volume, the compilation of which clearly required an unimaginable amount of hard work and statistical diligence, is one such excavation, initially providing a unique and invaluable insight into the Irish involvement in the Second World War. However, it is also the basis for vast amounts of further research using the otherwise unavailable information here contained. Not merely has one layer of history been peeled back, others await discovery from within these pages. Our gratitude to the authors is enormous, as it must also be to those of whom they have written. The world was made far better by such men.

Kevin Myers
May 2024

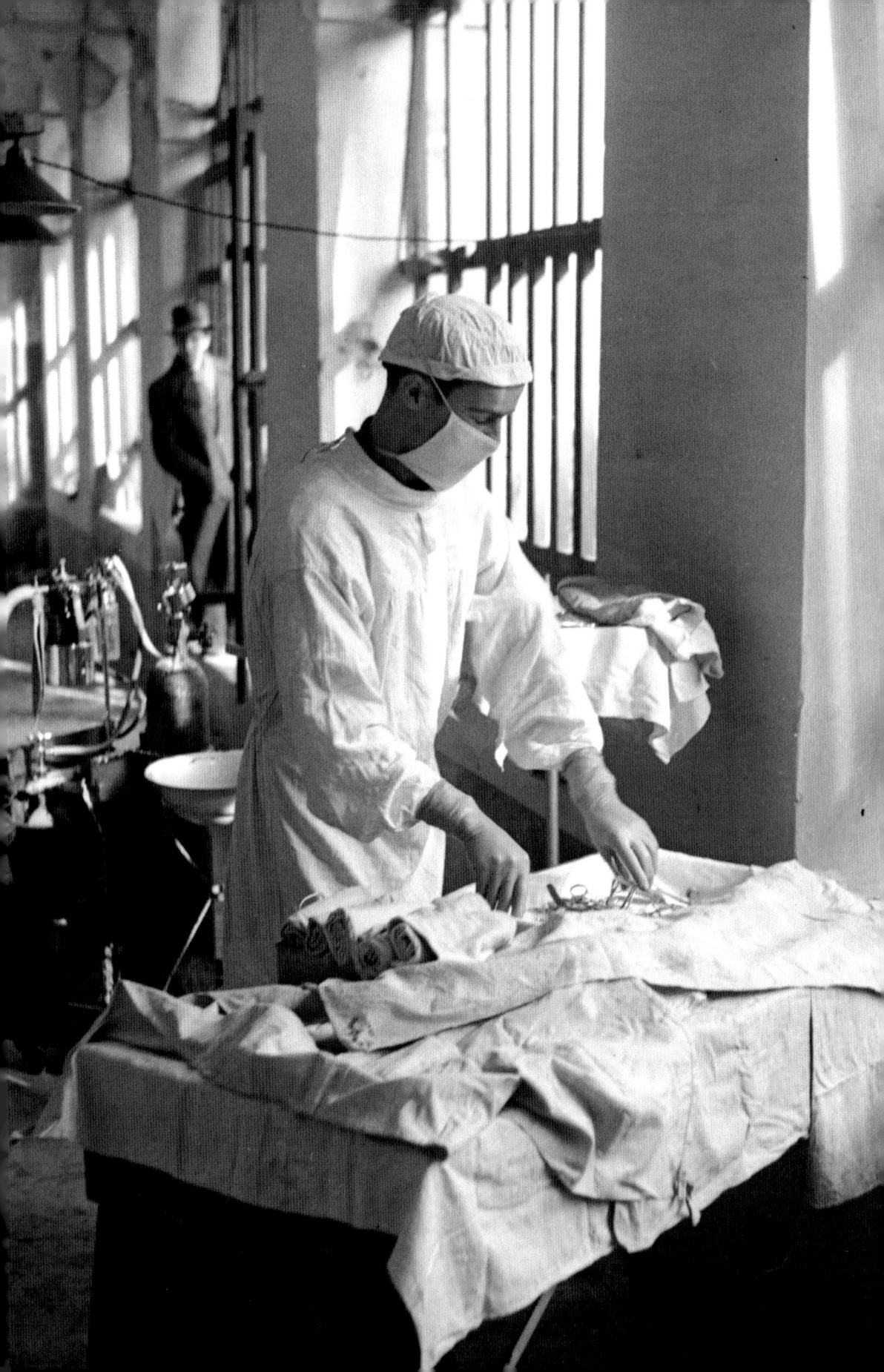

INTRODUCTION

When the hostilities of the First World War ceased in November 1918, the British government moved swiftly to reduce the size of its armed forces, which had become a significant financial burden over the four years of the conflict with Germany and her allies. A general demobilisation was initiated immediately and this included the medical wings of the Royal Navy (RN), the Royal Air Force (RAF) and the Royal Army Medical Corps (RAMC).

While the return to civilian medical duties was welcomed by most doctors, others – particularly those who held permanent commissions – decided to remain with the armed forces. These experienced surgeons and doctors served the military's need for medical personnel throughout the British Empire, for example with the Indian Medical Service (IMS) and the Malayan Medical Service (MMS) up to and including the Second World War. For those who were demobilised their experiences of returning to civilian life varied, depending on the ease with which they found employment. The lucky ones returned to hospital posts which had been kept open during their absence awaiting their return, while others were appointed to newly formed positions to cater for the large number of repatriated injured military personnel. The civilian authorities in both Britain and Ireland also had an urgent need for additional medical support as they tried to contain and manage the 1918–19 influenza epidemic.

For those who returned to Ireland, their surgical experience gained abroad and their association with the RAMC helped in their search for employment in posts related to British Army medical work. Most demobbed doctors returning to Ireland found that the number of those applying for positions outstripped the availability of hospital and Poor Law medical posts. Those who had left their medical practices to join up or those who had enlisted on graduation found the medical profession in 1919 much more overcrowded than it had been prior to 1914. According to the Medical Directory of 1920, the number of registered doctors in Ireland had increased from 2,897 in 1914 to 3,322 in 1918. This was the largest percentage increase, i.e. 15 per cent, in the number of registered doctors across any of the regions covered by the Medical Directory and was partly caused by the large number of graduations from Irish medical colleges, particularly in the latter years of the conflict.

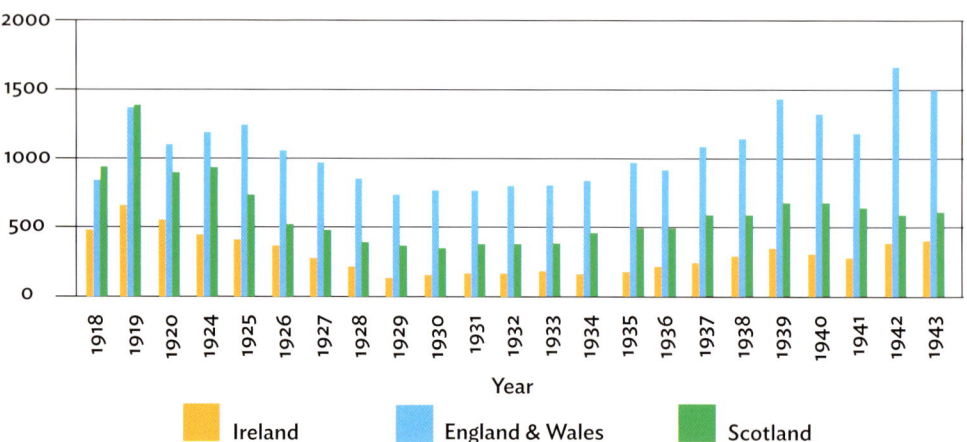

The returning military doctors also found a changed political landscape that would eventually result in the establishment of the Irish National Army Medical Corps (NAMC) following the withdrawal of the British forces from the Irish Free State in 1922. Initially a number of former RAMC officers found employment with the NAMC. However, with hospital posts filled again and with private practice opportunities limited in rural Ireland, the search for employment by the returned military medical personnel and the medical graduates reverted to the well-travelled road of emigration to Britain and further afield.

Over the next couple of years the Irish medical colleges were once again providing large numbers of medical graduates who would ultimately settle and practise in Great Britain or in the British colonies in India and the Far East.

Many would once again volunteer to join in the defence of the United Kingdom, Europe and the British Empire when called to do so at the outbreak of the Second World

War in September 1939. By the end of the Second World War some 2,000 Irish doctors served with the Allied armed forces across all the theatres of war on land and sea and in the air.

Independent Ireland remained neutral during the Second World War. However, it is estimated that in excess of 70,000 people from the island of Ireland joined the British Army between 1939 and 1945, half of whom came from the independent State.

Many of these men had already been serving in the British Army or were working in Britain and so were called up during the periods of conscription, and some had left Ireland to enlist and fight against Nazi Germany. Some 5,000 non-commissioned officers and men of the Irish Defence Forces deserted to enlist with the Allied forces during the course of the Second World War.

Conscription was not introduced into Northern Ireland despite the repeated calls for it from the government of Northern Ireland. The 38,000 who left Northern Ireland to serve during the Second World War did so as volunteers, in the same way as their fellow Irishmen and women did south of the border in the Irish Free State.

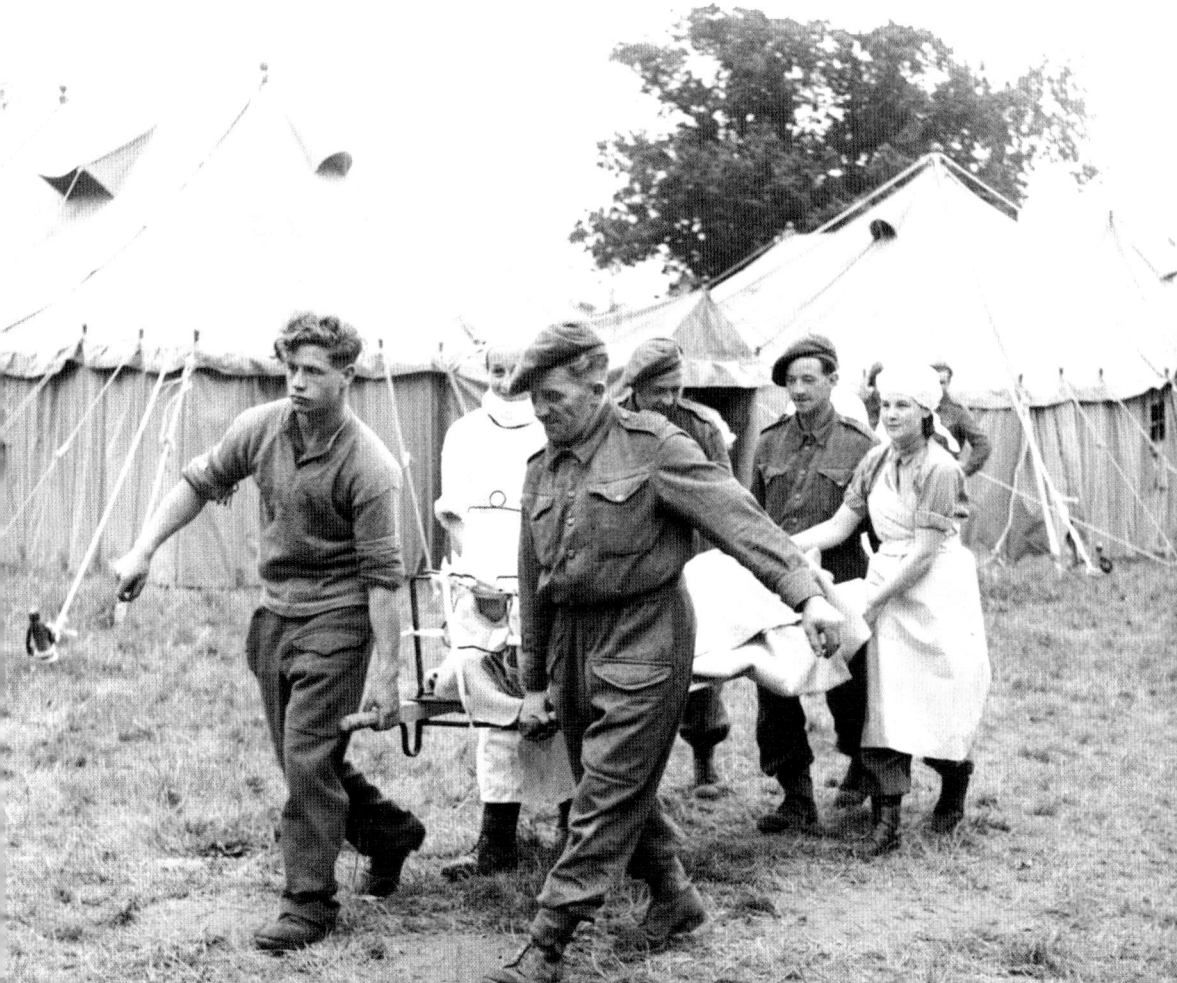

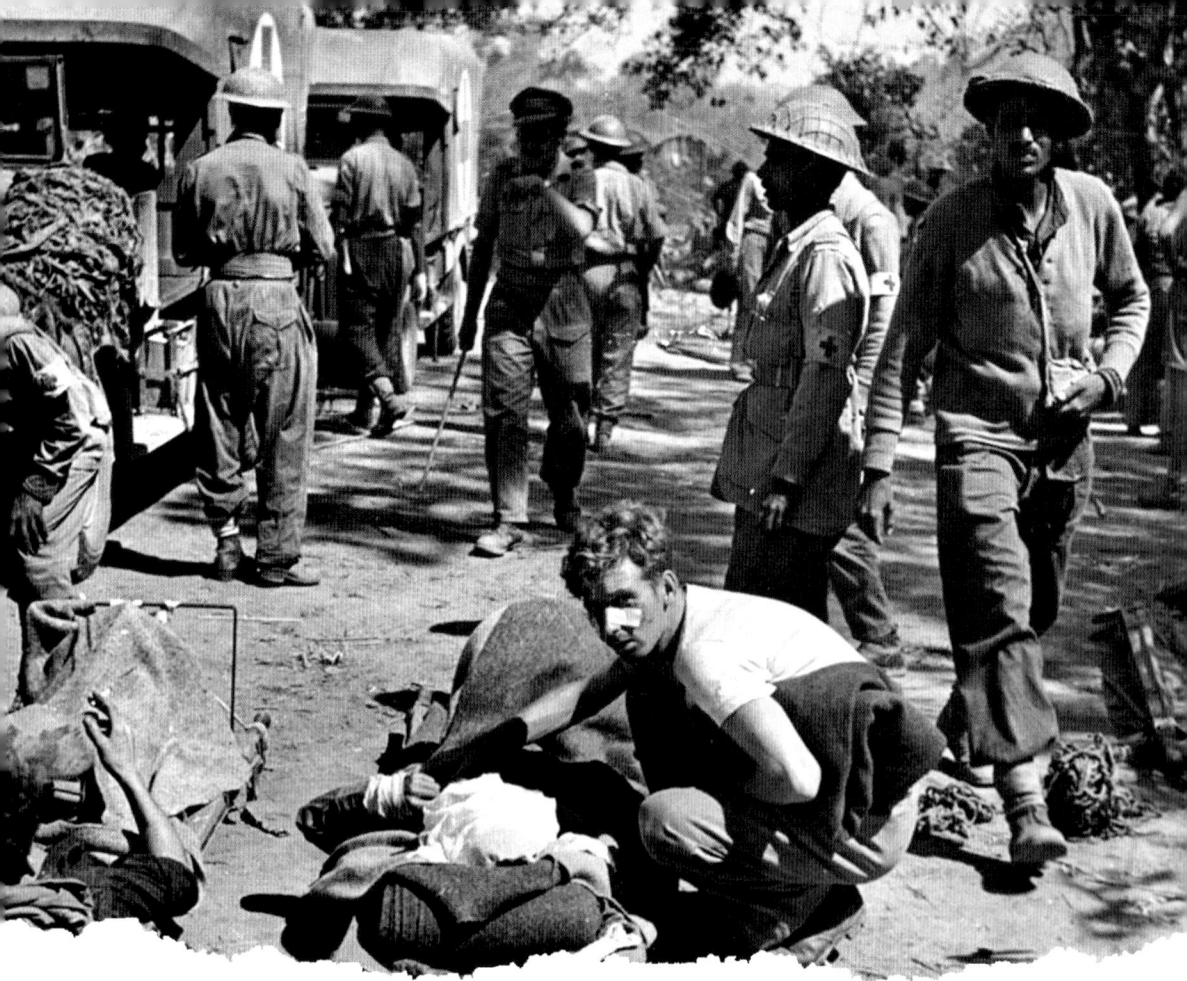

Many of these Irish volunteers became casualties and did not return home, as did some seventy Irish doctors, along with some twenty-three medical students from Queen's University Belfast (QUB) who served during the Second World War.

The medical services of the British armed forces had for a century and more provided graduates from the Irish medical colleges with much-needed employment opportunities. In fact, the Irish medical colleges produced many more graduates than could be absorbed within the Irish health system and so provided a favourable recruiting ground for naval, military and later air force medical staff to serve the British Empire at home and abroad. For those Irish medical graduates who did not wish to serve in the military, emigration to Britain and its colonies was often the only option in their search for employment. The creation of an Officer Training Corps in some of the medical colleges from 1908 provided basic military training for the undergraduates and a direct path for graduates into the officer ranks on enlistment.

By 1939 Ireland was no longer under British rule, while Northern Ireland remained within the United Kingdom. When war broke out with Germany in September 1939 the Irish doctors who were already part of the medical services of the British military were soon joined by Irish civilian doctors then working in Britain and in the colonies and by recent graduates from the Irish medical colleges. This pattern continued for the duration of the war.

While over 100 medical students from QUB would enlist during the course of the Second World War, few medical undergraduates from Ireland would see military service ahead of their graduation, instead enlisting immediately on qualifying as doctors. Table 1 shows how Irish doctors were represented in the medical services and wings of the British armed forces during the Second World War.

While the island of Ireland was to some extent physically isolated from the principal theatres of war, it was not to escape completely the loss of innocent lives, but on a much-reduced scale compared to other war zones. Belfast was to endure three bombing raids by the German Luftwaffe in April and May 1941. In the air raids of 7 and 15 April, the German bombers concentrated on damaging the ship and aircraft building industries around Belfast port, with the Harland & Wolff works being bombed extensively. Some 889 people were killed in the bombing raids. Around 700 were killed on the evening of Easter Tuesday, 15 April 1941, with a further 420 injured. The damage to civilian life in Belfast was significant, with 70,000 receiving assistance in emergency centres after the raid on Easter Tuesday.

Dublin, despite being a neutral city, was not to escape. The first bombing occurred early in January 1941, when German bombs were dropped on Terenure and South Circular Road in the south of the city. A number of people were injured, but no one was killed in these bombings. Later that year, on 31 May 1941, four German bombs fell in the North Strand area of Dublin, killing twenty-eight people.

As Ireland remained neutral during the Second World War, its ports along the Atlantic seaboard remained blocked to the Allied navies. To alleviate this situation the port of Derry or Londonderry was extensively developed as a safe harbour for the Allied fleet protecting the convoys from the United States and Canada. Following the Japanese attack on Pearl Harbour on 7 December 1941, American troops were deployed to Northern Ireland and from there saw action firstly in North Africa in late 1942 and later in the Normandy landings in June 1944.

The government of Ireland was opposed to the stationing of American troops in Northern Ireland, believing that their presence would increase the likelihood of the country becoming a target of Nazi aggression. Despite this stance, the Irish government entered into an agreement with the Allies that allowed Catalina aircraft to access Lough Erne in County Fermanagh along the Donegal Corridor.

Representation of Irish Medical Colleges in the Second World War

During and following the First World War the Irish medical colleges published the names of graduates who had enlisted in the British and Commonwealth forces in their annual reports and rolls of honour. The availability of these records allowed for the identification of some 3,000 Irish doctors who had served in the 1914–18 conflict and these are collated in our 2015 publication entitled *Irish Doctors in the First World War*. With the establishment of the Irish Free State in 1922, the medical colleges in Dublin, Cork and Galway were no longer directly controlled by the British government and its governing medical institutions. In January 1936 the Irish Medical Association merged with the Irish branch of the British Medical Association to form the Irish Free State Medical Union. In keeping with the political partitioning of Ireland in 1922, the Northern Ireland medical practitioners continued to be represented by the Northern Ireland branch of the British Medical Association.

The separation of the Irish medical colleges from British influence from 1922 onwards is reflected in the absence of formal records of medical graduates who served during the Second World War in the records at University College Dublin (UCD), University College Cork (UCC), University College Galway (UCG), the Royal College of Surgeons in Ireland (RCSI) and the Royal College of Physicians in Ireland (RCPI). In contrast, Trinity College Dublin (TCD) produced a roll of honour for those graduates who served during the 1939–45 conflict, as did QUB.

These invaluable records, along with the Kirkpatrick Archive held by the RCPI and the matching of military commissions published in *The Gazette* (the official record of commissions in the British armed forces) against the list of graduates from the remaining Irish medical schools, has allowed for the identification of over 2,000 Irish doctors who served in the Second World War. It is highly likely that this number does not fully reflect the full contribution of the Irish medical body to the Allied effort against Nazi Germany and Imperial Japan in all the theatres of war, including Europe, North Africa, the Far East and the War at Sea.

Irish doctors served with a number of British forces, including the Royal Army Corps, the RAF and the RN, in addition to the voluntary reserves (VR) of these forces and the Merchant Navy (MN) as shown in Table 1. A number of overseas wings of the British services are also represented, including the IMS, the MMS, the South African Medical Corps (SAMC) and the United States Medical Corps (USMC).

Service	Queen's University Belfast (QUB)	Trinity College Dublin (TCD)	Royal College of Surgeons (RCSI)	University College Dublin (UCD)	University College Cork (UCC)	University College Galway (UCG)	Edinburgh University (EU)	Other	Total
RAMC	425	357	80	133	81	30	12	29	1,147
RAF & RAFVR	176	88	51	38	41	12	1	0	407
RN & RNVR	98	97	32	10	5	4	1	6	253
IMS	19	31	9	14	7	1	1	3	85
MMS	5	7	0	0	1	0	0	0	13
MN	3	1	1	0	0	0	1	1	7
SAMC	0	10	0	0	0	0	0	0	10
USMC	0	5	0	0	0	0	0	0	5
Other	10	41	15	3	6	1	0	0	76
TOTAL	736	637	188	198	141	48	16	39	2,003

Table 1: Representation of Irish Doctors in the Allied Forces and Medical Services During the War

Of the doctors who died, twenty-two in the RAMC were killed and eighteen died in service. Six were killed in action in the RAF and three died on service, whereas eleven were killed in the RN and six died on service. Three died in the IMS, two of whom were killed in action, and the remaining three died in other services.

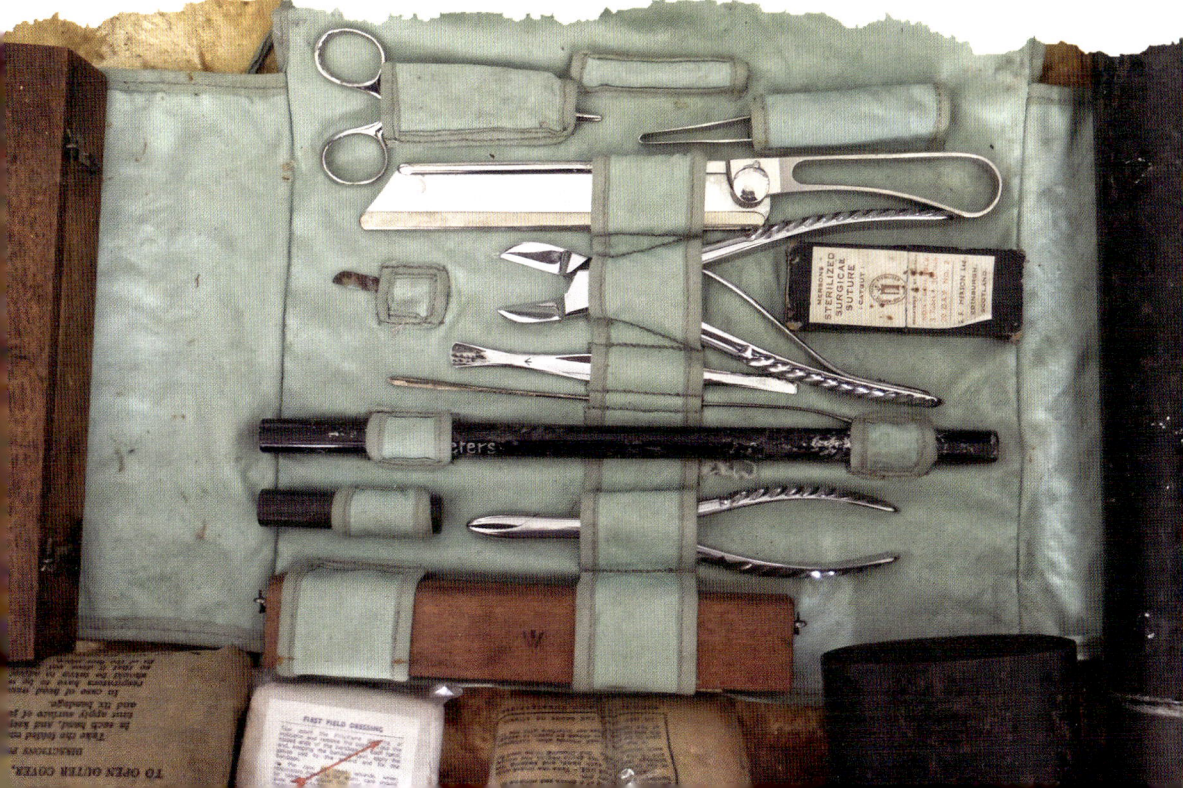

Advances in the Machines of War

The Second World War was the most destructive conflict in human history. It resulted in the spectacular development of aviation and motorised warfare, especially tanks. Submarines established themselves as potentially war-winning machines. The pressure of war generated a search for 'wonder weapons'. The jet aircraft, V-1 flying bomb and V-2 ballistic missile were all introduced by Germany late in the war. However, the atomic bomb, developed by the United States, truly heralded in a new era of warfare.

The German Luftwaffe blitzkrieg attack on Poland in 1939 and the rapid advance of German tank divisions through the Low Countries and France in 1940 announced that the pace of military warfare had changed for ever. In the air, bomber and fighter aircraft were used to attack industrial cities, land forces and shipping, both in harbour and at sea. Aircraft names such as the Spitfire, Messerschmitt, Mustang, Heinkel and Lancaster entered into the everyday wartime vocabulary.

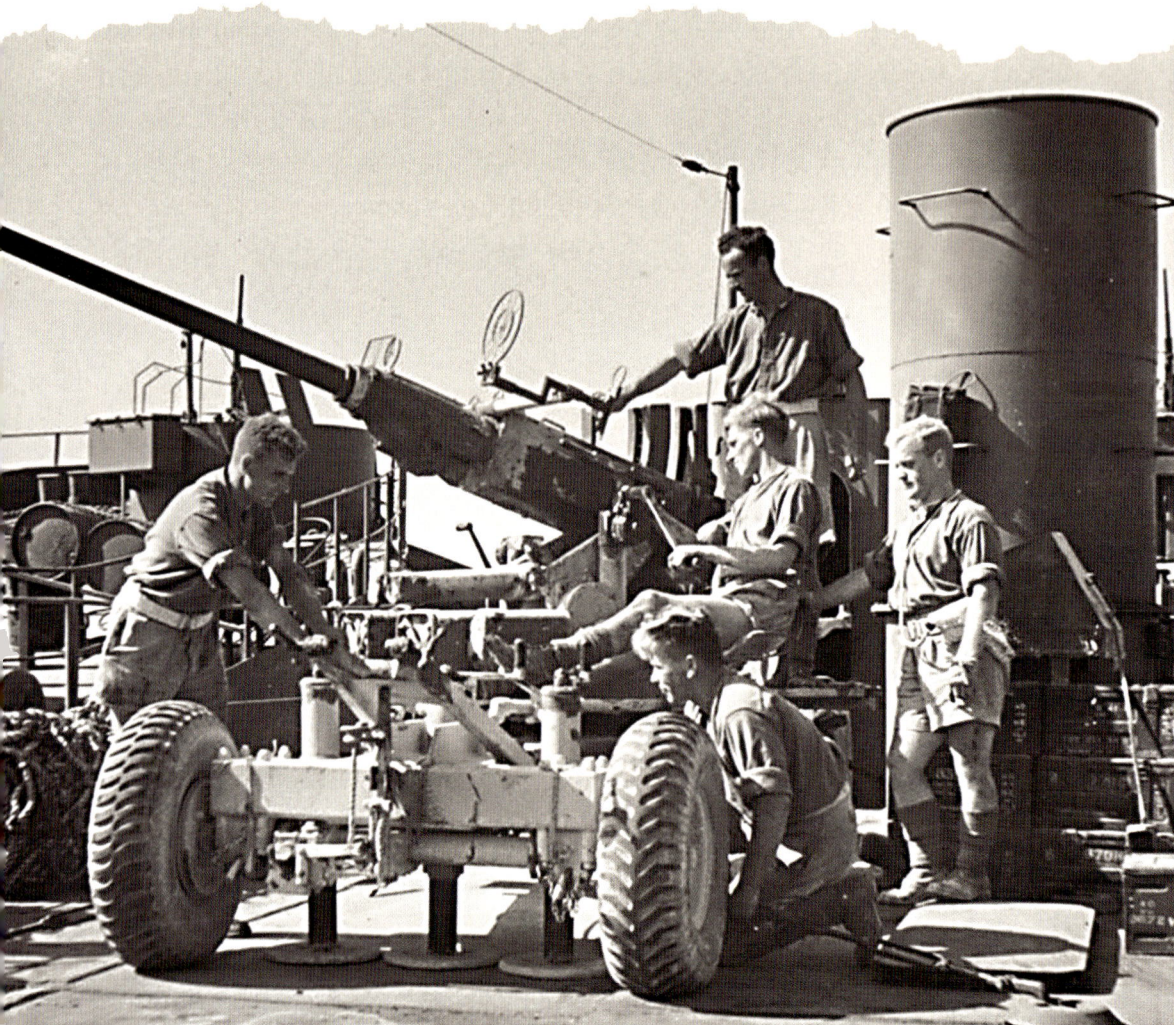

On the ground the success of 1940 German tank advances led to changes in Allied tank design to provide faster, heavier tanks with more firepower than those used by the Axis forces. As land fighting continued with the North African campaign and the invasion of Russia in 1941, tank technology evolved so much that by the end of the war, tanks provided the kind of firepower, protection and reliability that would have been undreamed of in 1939. Tank names such as the German Tiger 1 still inspire a fearsome reputation, while the American Sherman, the British Churchill and the Russian T-34 have populated media reports of battles fought across the globe.

Along with major changes on land and in the air, naval forces also experienced major innovation as the war progressed in response to technological advances in boat design and firepower. In the early stages of the war the pride-of-place large cruisers and destroyers had become vulnerable to both long-range missile and air attack as evidenced by the loss of Britain's HMS *Hood* and shortly afterwards the German *Bismarck*. Submarine U-boats provided the German Navy with its victories in the early years of the war, coming close to bringing Britain to its knees. As a consequence, both Britain's RN and the US Navy were forced to invest in measures to combat the submarine menace, which eventually led to the Allied victory in the Battle of the Atlantic.

While advances in the ground, air and naval machines of war caused destruction on a massive scale, it ultimately fell to soldiers on the ground to defend military positions and ultimately enforce a final victory, often in street-by-street fighting. Soldiers had the killing power of the self-loading rifle, which was capable of switching between semi-automatic and fully automatic modes. In addition, the lightweight sub-machine gun was capable of delivering a massive amount of firepower and was the weapon of choice for troops operating in cramped and enclosed surroundings.

Advances in Medical Care

Over the inter-war years and certainly by 1939, many advances had been incorporated into military medical care. Blood and plasma transfusions, the extensive use of intravenous fluids, the use of antibiotics (though limited to sulphonamides initially and penicillin), endotracheal intubation, thoracic and vascular surgery, and the care of burn wounds had made medical care of wounded soldiers and civilians unrecognisable compared to during the First World War.

The experience of a battle casualty in the Second World War was not radically different to that of an injured soldier in the First World War. Bullets and artillery shells were still the main causes of common injuries, and casualties were evacuated through a similar chain of medical aid posts, dressing stations and hospitals.

But at the fighting front a Second World War casualty received specialist treatment more quickly. Specialist surgical facilities were closer to the front line and transport was by motor vehicle and sometimes even by plane.

Blood transfusion services had expanded across the globe and supplied countless units of blood, which were a vital component of trauma treatment. Blood transfusion services were a major component of early care of the wounded so that those with major injuries did not die from shock. Allied to blood transfusion was the increased use of fluids such as normal saline and Ringer's lactate, which kept the blood pressure up to a reasonable level until blood was available.

Primary suture, or stitching a wound closed, was another big advance. At the outset of the Second World War most wounds were left open because of the risk of serious infection, but it soon became clear that the risk was, in fact, fairly minimal due to advances in wound cleaning and antimicrobials. It was penicillin, first identified in 1928, which was the game changer. Penicillin was not produced in realistic quantities until 1942, but even before that the primary suture was the mainstay of managing many wounds. It was clear from early on that cleaning the wound and debriding the dead tissue were the most important steps, without which the newly found antibiotics were of limited value.

In orthopaedics, another significant advance was the use of metal plates to help heal fractures. The technique of intramedullary nailing (inserting a nail into the bone marrow) for certain fractures of the femur was developed by the German military services. This was discovered by the Allies when examining captured German prisoners who had required X-rays. To the surprise of the Allied surgeons, the German patients with implants recovered in half the time.

Neurosurgery was another area where advances were made. The concept of a mobile neurosurgical unit was a major component of improved care, together with the specialised personnel. Neurosurgical units were usually attached to Casualty Clearing Stations (CCS) on the Western Front, but elsewhere, in Africa and the Far East, mobile units were used by converting buses to operating theatres. At the CCSs, head injury patients were triaged to the neurosurgical unit on admission, which allowed rapid assessment and treatment to begin.

The evacuation procedures were broadly the same in both the First and Second World Wars, the principal differences being the increased distances involved and the

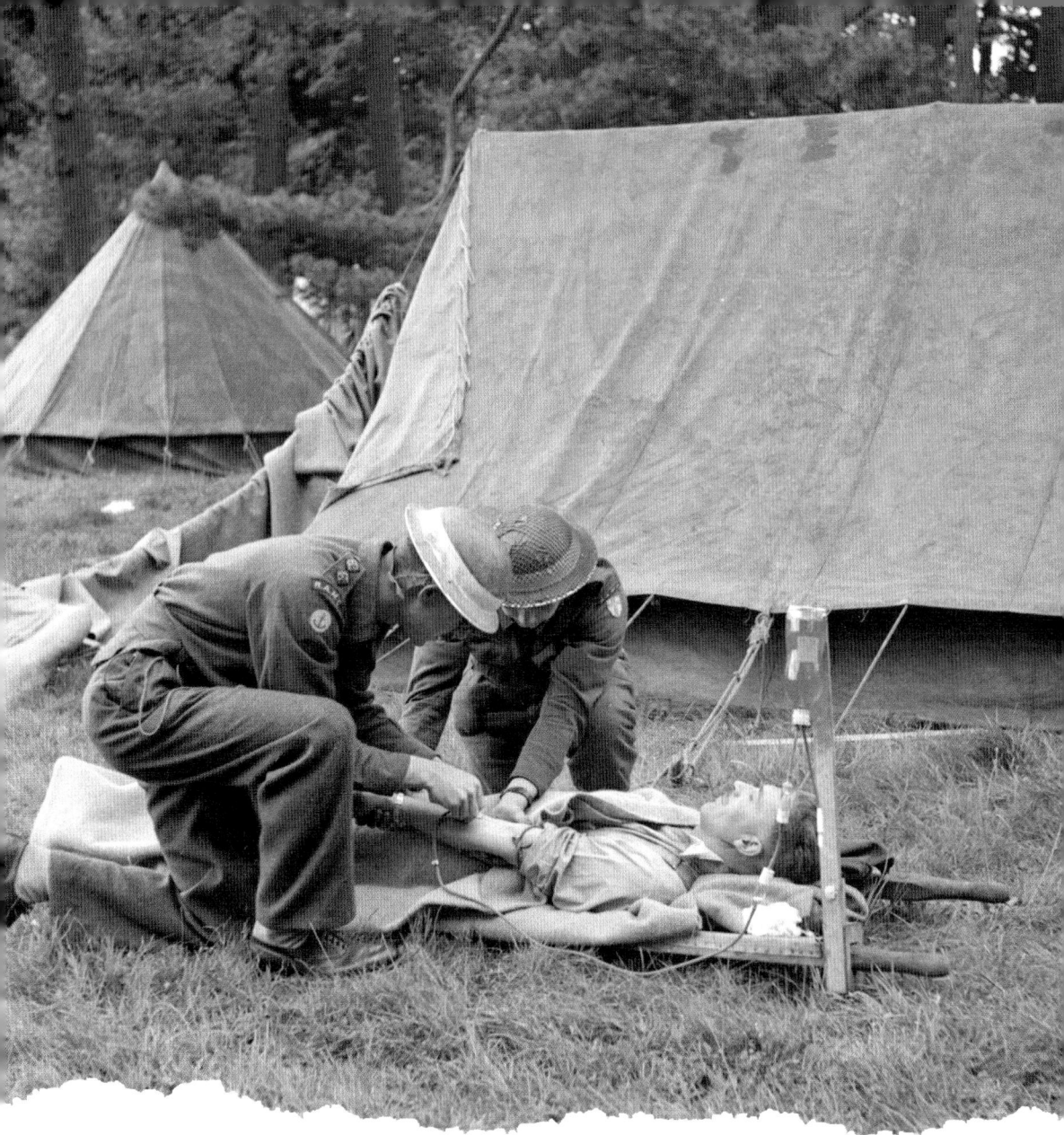

use of aircraft in the repatriation of casualties in the 1939–45 conflict. The evacuation pathway was divided into three zones: i) the collection zone containing the regimental medical infrastructures, field ambulances and ambulance convoys; ii) the evacuation zone containing the CCS and ambulance trains; iii) the distribution zone, including general hospitals, convalescent camps, hospital ships and returning military aircraft.

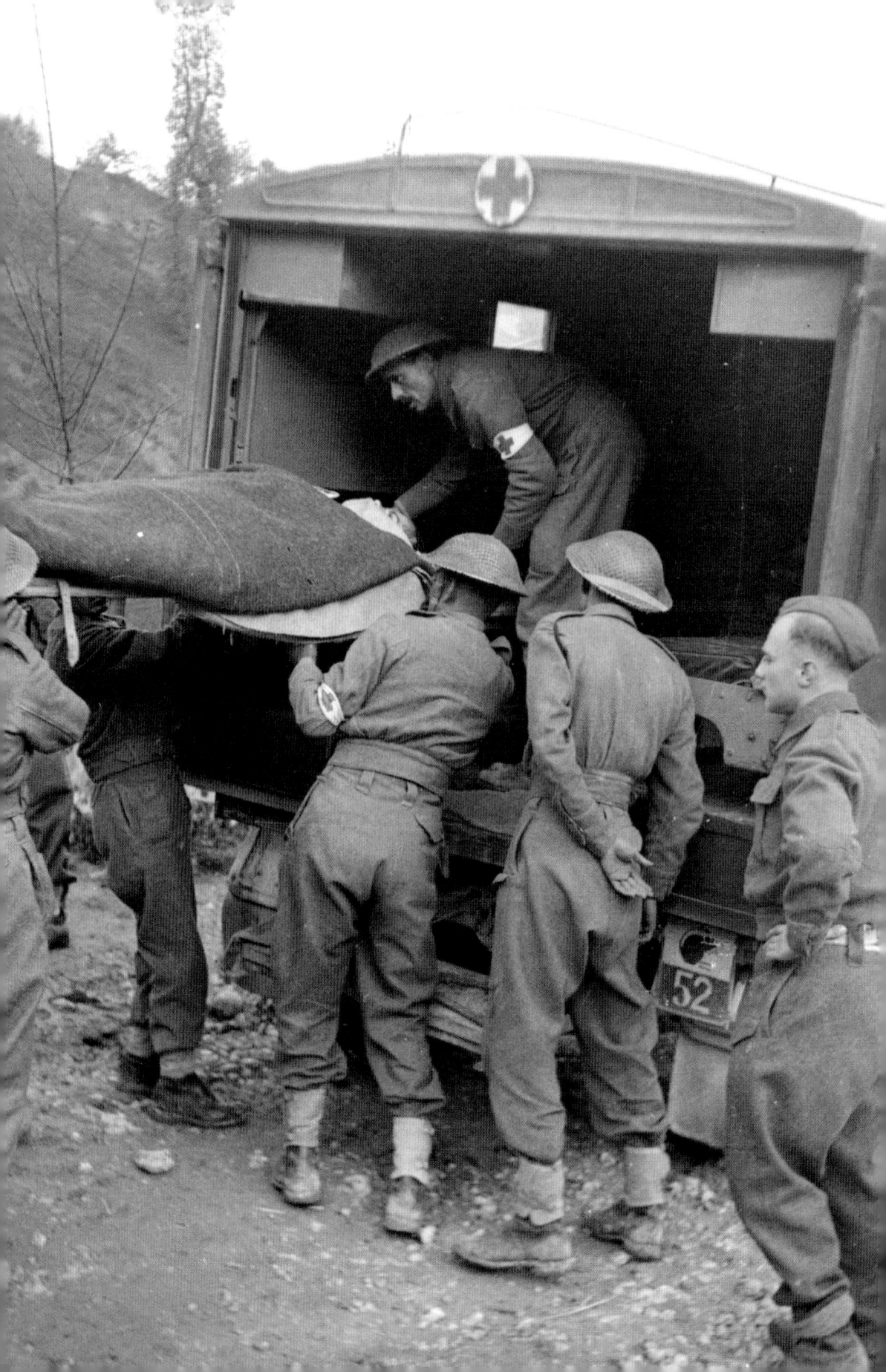

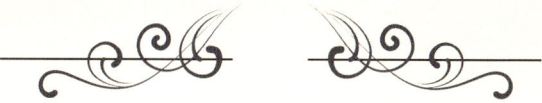

Chapter 1

TIMELINE FOR THE SECOND WORLD WAR

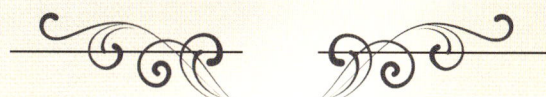

On 12 March 1938 Germany annexed Austria under what was termed the Anschluss or Union. This was done with the approval of the Austrian people. Adolf Hitler, the chancellor and Führer of Germany (1933–45), next turned his attention to the Sudetenland, where a German-speaking population of about three million resided.

Hitler annexed that region, and the annexation was sanctioned at the Munich Conference in September 1938 in the hope that it would satisfy Hitler's needs and that he would make no more territorial claims in Europe. However, on 14 March 1939 Hitler proclaimed the Protectorate of Bohemia and Moravia, thus swallowing up what remained of Czechoslovakia.

Six months later, in September 1939, Germany invaded Poland and war was once again to sweep across Europe, only twenty-one years since the end of the First World War.

Britain declared war on Germany on 3 September 1939, and, as in 1914, immediately dispatched a British Expeditionary Force (BEF) of 390,000 troops to France in an effort to thwart the German westward advance. The BEF and the French Army were posted along the Maginot Line of defence, which ran along the French border with Germany and neutral Belgium, to wait on Germany's next move.

Military operations on land were relatively quiet (a period known as the 'Phoney

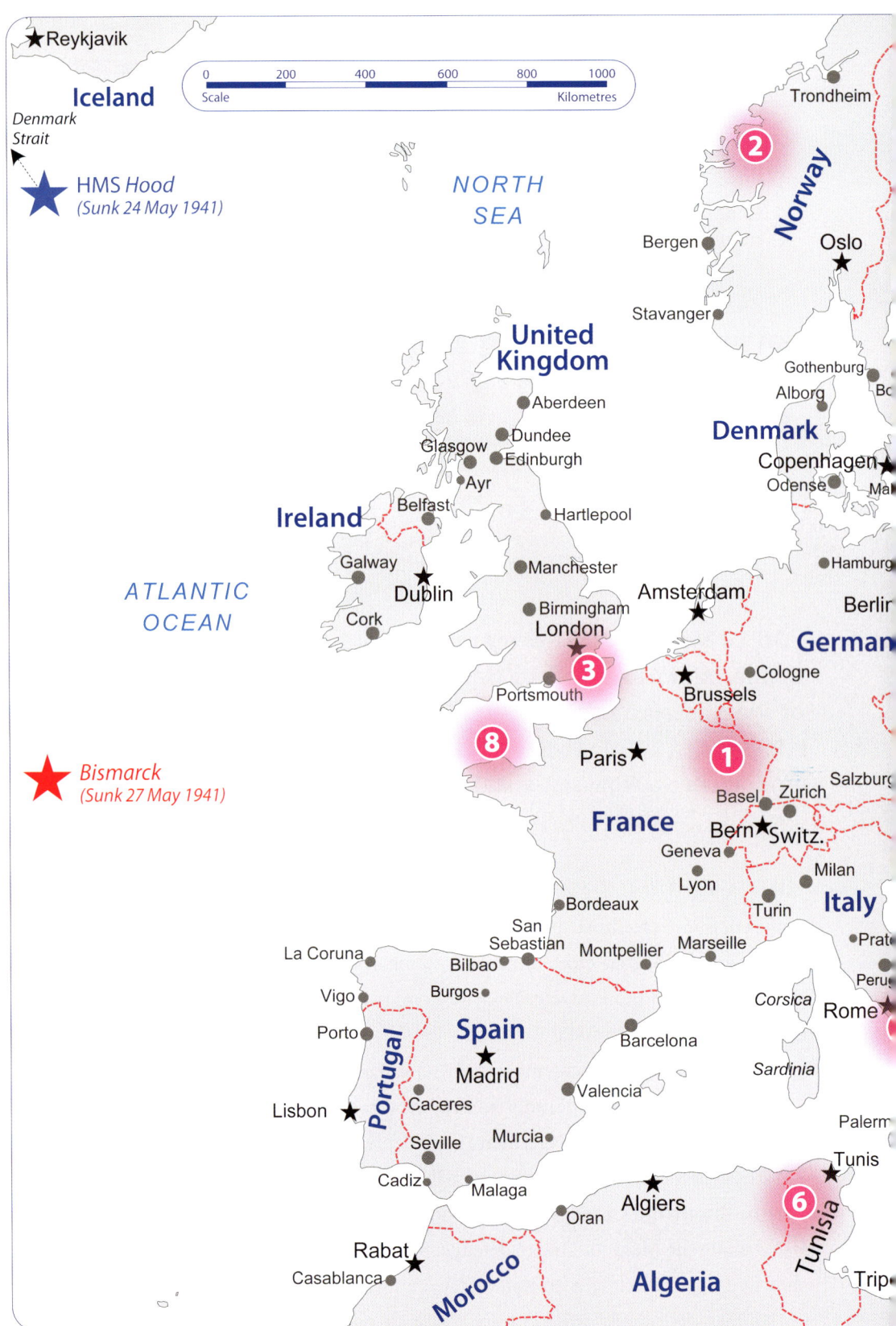

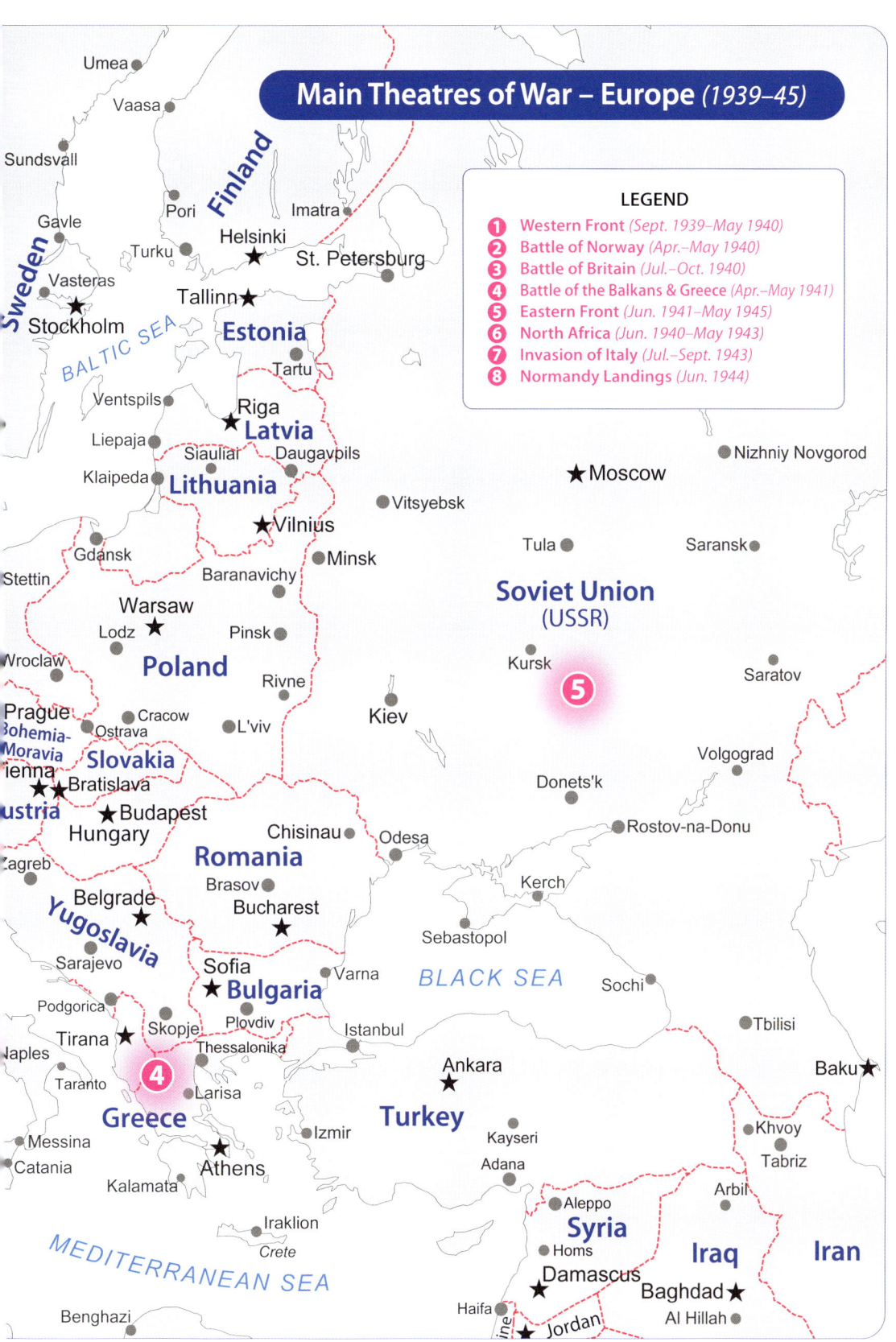

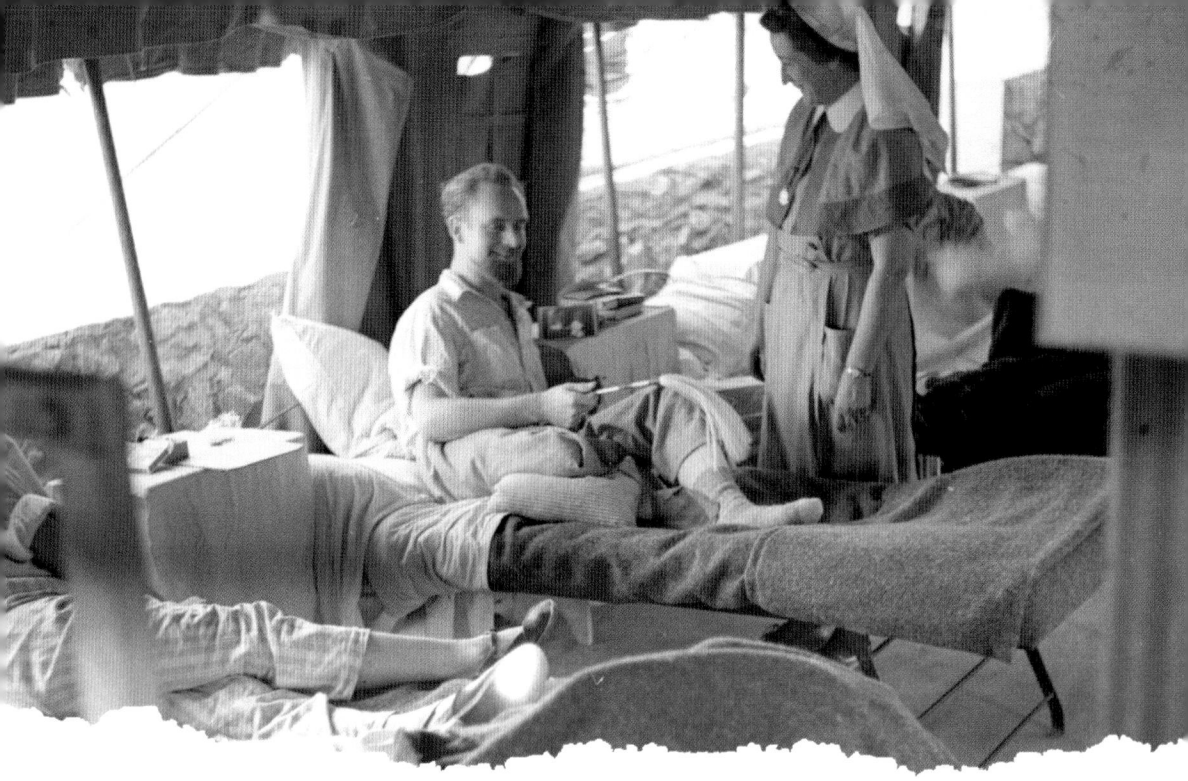

War') until in April 1940 when Germany invaded Norway and Denmark. Then, in May, Germany launched a major offensive against France, circumventing the Maginot Line on the Franco-German border by directing its attack at the neutral nations of Belgium, the Netherlands and Luxembourg.

This sudden German advance swept across the Low Countries and France and led to the evacuation of the BEF in May and June 1940, leaving Germany in control of most of Western Europe.

Benito Mussolini, the Italian fascist dictator, sided with Germany in May 1940 and declared war on Britain just days before the Germans occupied Paris unopposed on 14 June 1940. Mussolini then attacked south-east France and soon occupied a swath of French territory along the Franco-Italian border. Finally, in September 1940, Germany, Italy and Japan signed the Tripartite Pact, which became known as the Axis alliance.

Despite failing to subdue Britain in the Battle of Britain, which lasted between August and December 1940, the German military advance continued to spread across Europe, and the Allied forces were forced to retreat from Greece and Crete in May 1941. Shortly afterwards, Germany invaded Russia in June 1941. The conflict became a global affair after Japan launched offensives across south-east Asia and the Central Pacific in December 1941.

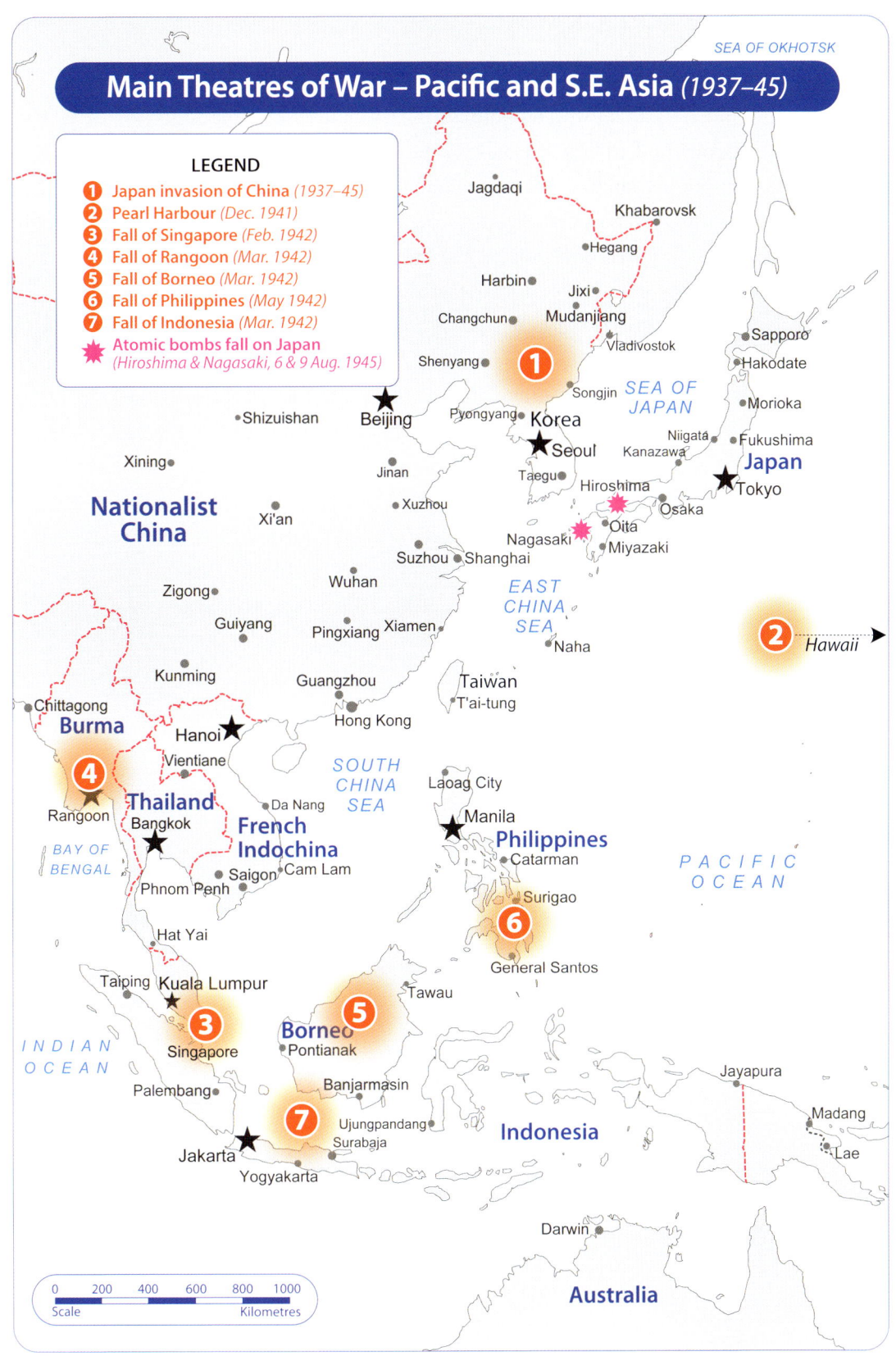

Initially the Axis forces won numerous military victories and the Allied forces were forced to regroup and re-arm on land, in the sky and at sea. Eventually, from 1943 onwards, the Allies began to get the upper hand, leading to their reinvasion of Western Europe in 1944 and the collapse of Nazi Germany in June 1945. The conflict in the Far East and the Pacific lasted until August 1945 and the Second World War finally ended when atomic bombs were dropped on the Japanese cities of Hiroshima and Nagasaki.

Just over 2,000 Irish doctors and medical students served with the British forces and saw action in all the British theatres of war, especially in Western Europe, North Africa, the Far East and at sea. Some ninety of them either died in service or were killed in action, while many of them served long periods in captivity and some suffered dreadful hardship, particularly under their Japanese captors.

Irish doctors and those medical students who gave up their studies to enlist accompanied the British armed forces into all the main theatres of war. Some remained where they were initially posted; others served in many other theatres of war as the conflict spread from Europe, Africa and the Far East to across the Atlantic and Pacific oceans.

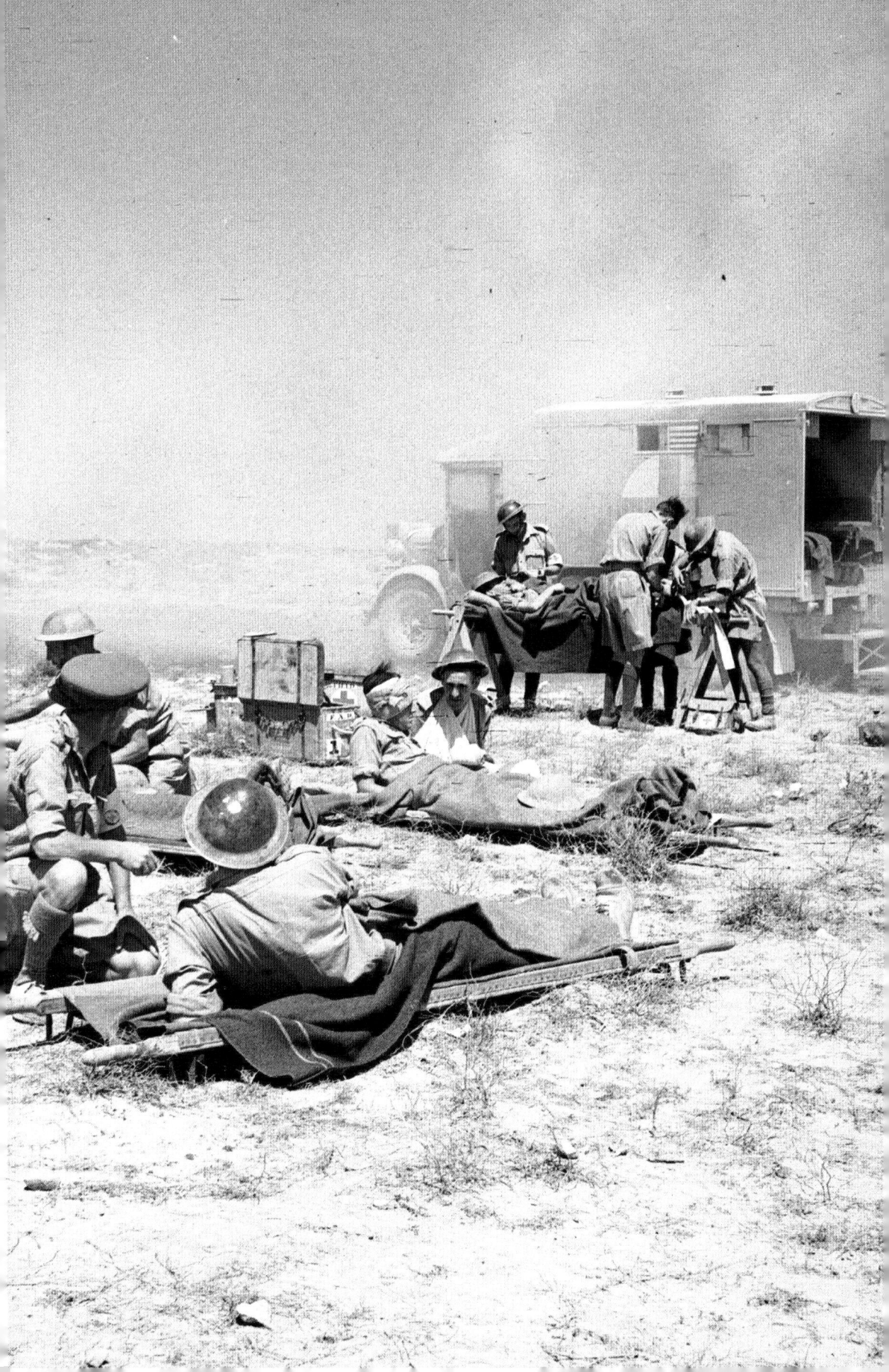

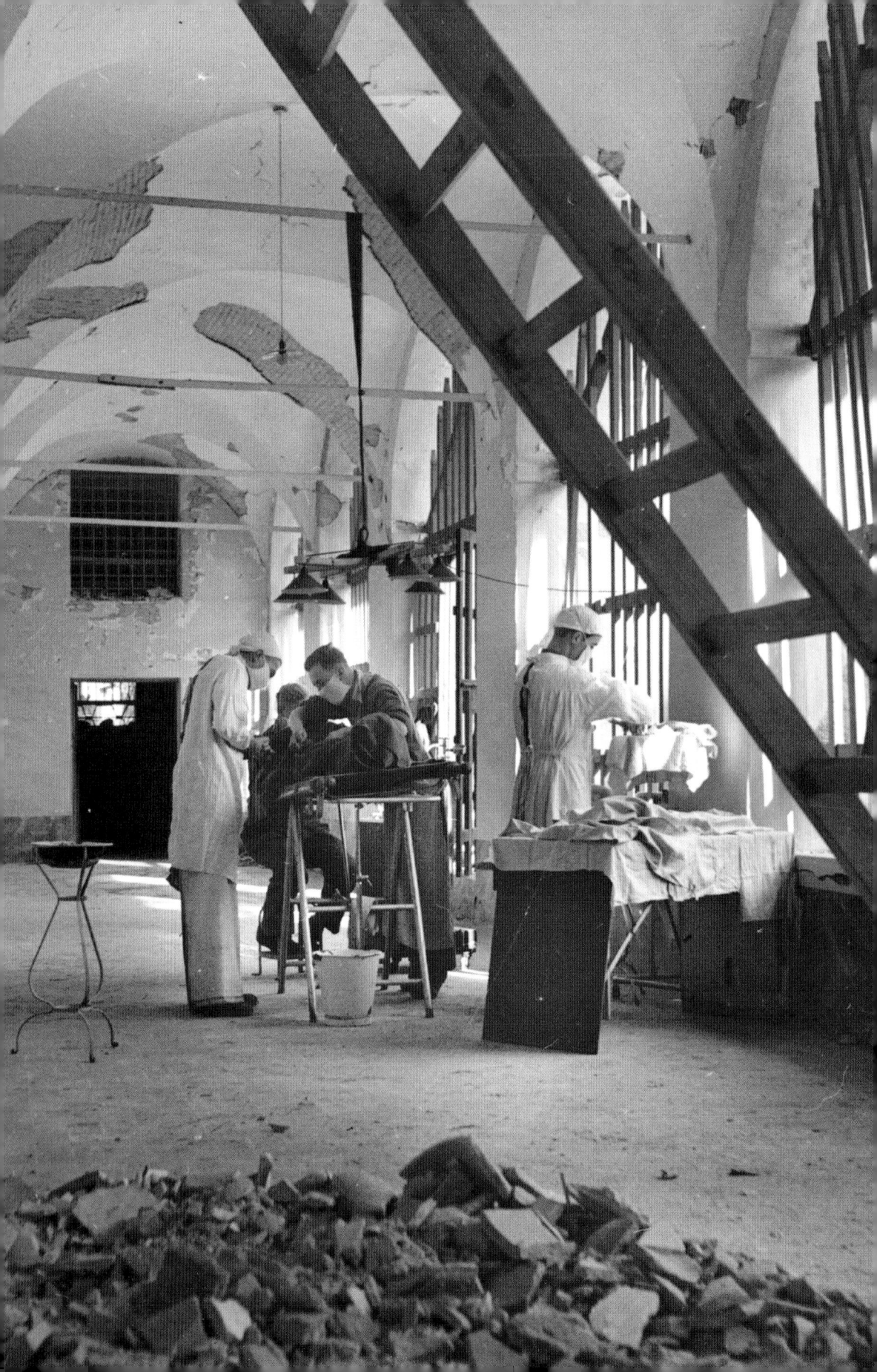

Chapter 2
MEDALS AND AWARDS

Many of the doctors who served with the British forces in the Second World War received medals either in recognition of their services or as acknowledgement of their participation in a particular campaign. The former type of medal can be divided into two categories, Medals for Gallantry in Action and Orders and Decorations. The following tables give an indication of the number of awards involved, but this information is far from complete.

Decoration	Total Awarded to Irish Doctors*	TCD	RCSI	QUB	NUI**	Other
Military Cross	43	15	5	17	4	2
Military Cross and Bar	1	–	–	–	–	1
DSO	11	3	1	6	1	–
OBE	58	26	4	15	12	1
CBE	10	8	2	–	–	–
Dispatches	150	53	4	85	5	3
Dispatches (>1)	17	5	–	12	–	–

Table 2: Military Decorations Awarded to Irish Doctors***
* Excluding awards from the First World War.
** UCD, UCC, UCG
*** From available information on Military Awards and Medals

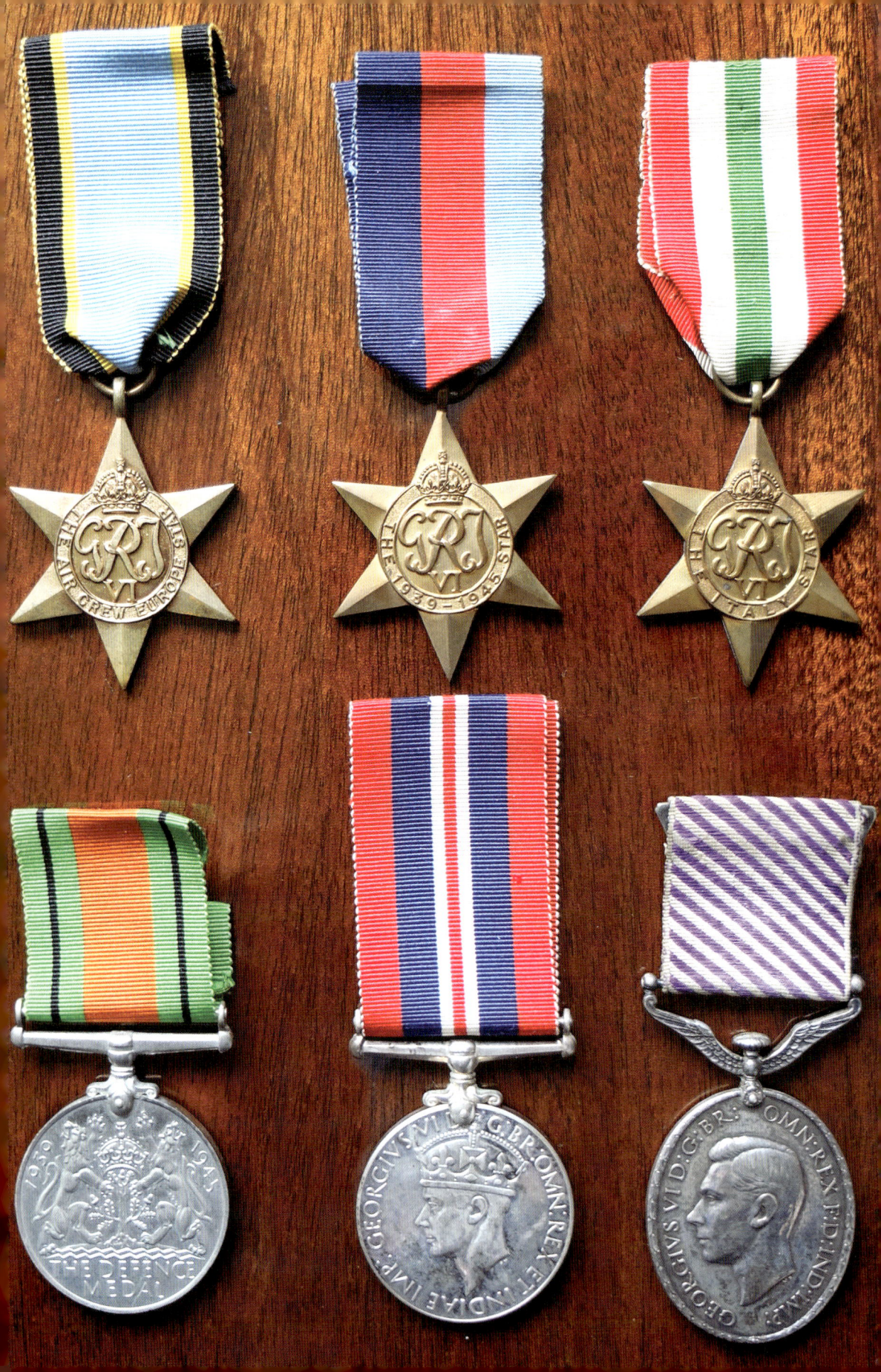

When the recipient of a certain medal received the award a second time, a bar was issued which was worn on the medal ribbon. This applied to the Victoria Cross (VC), the Distinguished Service Order (DSO) and the Military Cross (MC) amongst other Medals for Gallantry in Action.

MEDALS FOR GALLANTRY IN ACTION

Victoria Cross (VC)

The Victoria Cross was instituted in 1856 and is the highest award for bravery in the British Armed Forces.

Out of a total of 181 VCs awarded to officers of the British and Commonwealth Forces during the Second World War, one was awarded to a doctor serving with the RAMC. Of the 181 recipients, 85 (47 per cent) received their medals posthumously.

Distinguished Service Order (DSO)

The Distinguished Service Order is a military decoration of the United Kingdom awarded for meritorious or distinguished service by officers of the armed forces during wartime, typically in actual combat. The DSO was awarded to eleven Irish doctors in the Second World War.

Desmond Whyte received his award for his medical contribution to the Allied effort in Burma, while John Jordan merited the award for his assistance during the Dunkirk evacuation in 1940.

Ahern, Donal	Bradbury, William	Gilbert, Edward	Martin, Miles Patrick
Anderson, William	Doherty, Francis	Jordan, John	Whyte, Desmond
Barry, James	Fraser, Sir Ian	Kerr, Cecil	

Table 3: Distinguished Service Order Awards to Irish Doctors 1939–45

Military Cross (MC)

This was instituted by a Royal Warrant on 28 December 1914. The MC is granted in recognition of 'an act or acts of exemplary gallantry during active operations against the enemy on land' to all members of the British armed forces of any rank.

The MC was awarded to at least forty-seven Irish doctors during the course of the Second World War.

The MC and Bar were awarded to Edward Lewis Moore, from County Antrim, who had studied at Liverpool University, for acts of bravery in October 1943 and November 1945. The MC was also awarded to five medical students from Queen's University.

Officer of the British Empire (OBE)

Although initially intended to recognise meritorious service, the OBE was also awarded for gallantry. Member of the Most Excellent Order of the British Empire (MBE), Officer of the Most Excellent Order of the British Empire (OBE) and Commander of the Most Excellent Order of the British Empire (CBE) were awarded during the Second World War to the armed forces. Irish doctors and medical students serving with the armed forces were awarded fifty-eight OBEs and ten CBEs.

Ahern, Richard	Delap, Peter	McCollum, David	Parsons, Alfred
Aldwell, Basi	Dougan, Hampton	McCullough, William	Patton, George
Bannigan, Charles	Dougan, John	McWilliams, Lionel	Patton, Kevin
Boyd, Ringland	Ferris, Robert	Minford, Hugh	Robinson, George
Brittain, Herbert	Hayes, Gerard	Moore, Edward	Samuels, Leslie
Browne, Harold	Herbert, Leopold	Moore, John	Sheill, Gordon
Byrne, Aidan	Keatinge, Alan	Morrison, Eric	Smily, Thomas
Caraher, Edward	Leahy, James	Munn, Norman	Tully, Brian
Conway, Stephen	Lord, John	O'Neill, Desmond	White, Harry
Cowan, Jacob	Martin, John	Orr, James	Wright, Henry
Craig, Eric	McCartney, Ernest	Pantridge, James	

Table 4: Irish Doctors Awarded the Military Cross 1939–45

George Medal (GM)

The George Medal was instituted on 24 September 1940, and was intended primarily for civilians but could be awarded to members of the armed forces for actions of great bravery for which purely military honours are not normally granted.

Aidan MacCarthy from County Cork was awarded the George Medal for rescuing trapped airmen from a returning bomber that had crash-landed on a bomb dump at Honington airbase in 1941.

Mentioned in Dispatches (MID)

The names of personnel who contributed to outstanding or meritorious service were recorded in dispatches and an emblem in the form of an oak leaf records this fact. It is worn, in the case of the Second World War, on the ribbon of the War Medal. Individual Irish doctors and medical students were mentioned in dispatches at least 150 times with seventeen being mentioned more than once during the course of the war.

WAR CAMPAIGN MEDALS

Campaign Medals Awarded to Irish Doctors						
Medal	Awarded to Irish Doctors	TCD	RCSI	QUB	NUI**	Other
Atlantic Star	5	4	1	—	—	—
Africa Star	45	26	3	10	2	4
Pacific Star	13	5	1	3	4	—
Italy Star	28	12	1	7	3	5
Burma Star	20	12	3	2	2	1
France & Germany Star	24	14	2	5	2	1
1939–1945 Star	19	5	1	9	4	—
8th Army Star	17	9	2	3	1	2

Table 5: Service Medals Awarded to Irish Doctors during the Second World War
Clasps were granted for additional events of service in multiple theatres of war
** UCD, UCC, UCG

War Medal (WM)

This medal was awarded to full-time personnel of the armed forces, for twenty-eight days' service at home or abroad between 3 September 1939 and September 1945. This medal was also awarded to prisoners of war (POWs), many of whom spent most of the war as POWs in either German-occupied Europe or in the Far East when under Japanese control.

1939–1945 Star

This was awarded for six months operational service during the period but also for personal participation in commando raids such as Dieppe, St Nazaire and Sark, and those evacuated from Dunkirk or Norway.

Samuel Corry from County Down and Miles Martin from County Dublin were awarded the 1939–1945 Star for their medical support in the Dieppe raid in August 1942. The raid on Dieppe was an Allied amphibious attack on the German-occupied port in northern France. Miles Martin was also awarded the DSO for his involvement in the Dieppe raid.

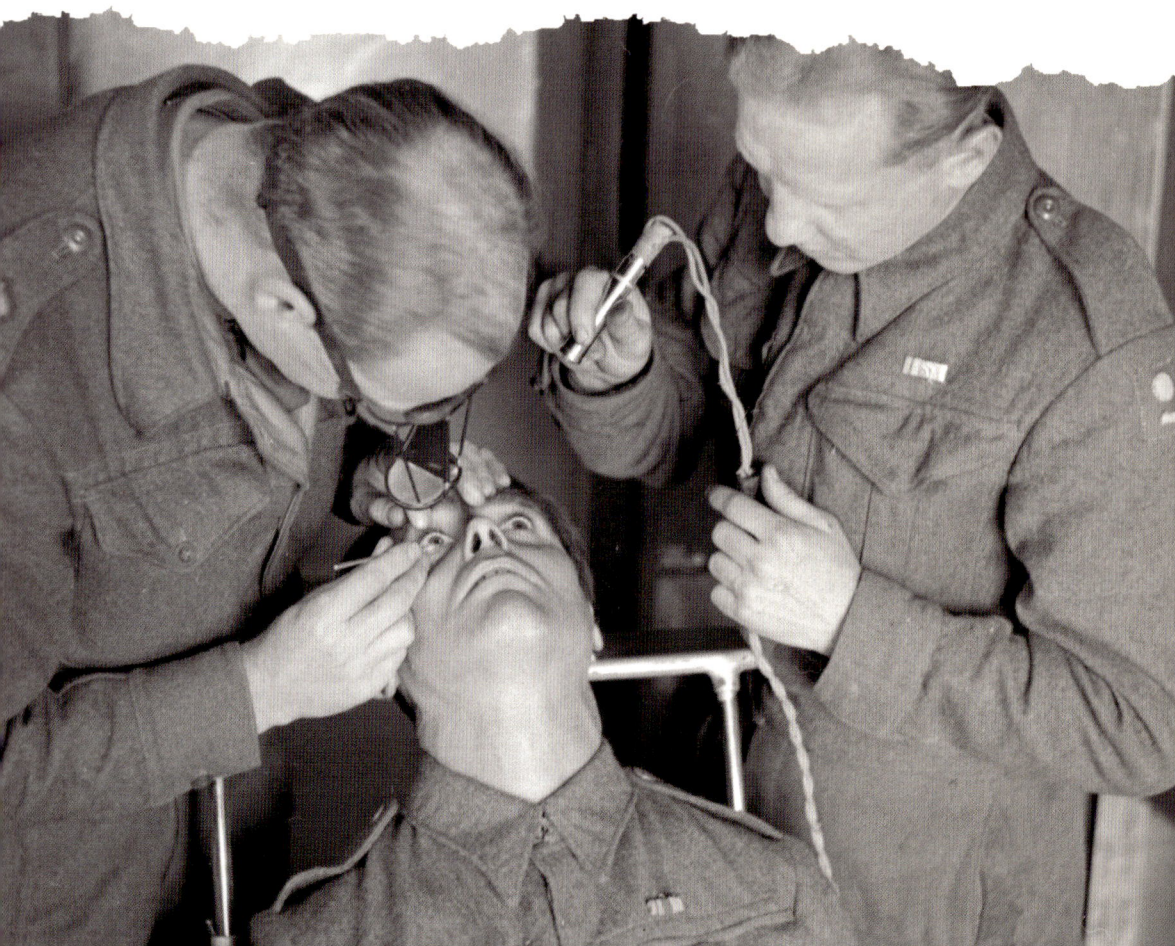

Atlantic Star

The Atlantic Star was intended to commemorate the Battle of the Atlantic, and was designed primarily for convoys, their escorts and anti-submarine forces, as well as for merchant ships that sailed alone. In addition to personnel of the RN and MN, air crew of the RAF were eligible through operations at sea, while army and RAF personnel serving on HM ships also qualified.

The Atlantic Star was awarded posthumously to Henry Hurst, Commander Surgeon on HMS *Hood* which was sunk in May 1941. It was also awarded to Dermot Walsh, one of the most decorated Irish doctors who served in the Second World War and who saw action in many of the principal theatres of war.

Africa Star

Eligibility was from 10 June 1940 to 12 May 1943, on entry into the operational area. Three bars were authorised: 8th Army and 1st Army, for those respective forces; North Africa 1942–1943 for the RN, MN and RAF.

Forty-six Irish doctors were awarded the Africa Star due to their posting to North Africa in 1941, following the retreat from Greece and Malta. Many of them went on to earn the 8th Army Bar or Clasp as the Allied Forces eventually gained control of North Africa under Field Marshal Montgomery.

Alley, George*	Field, Thomas*	McErvel, Thomas
Alison, George	Hamill, James	Moore, Edward
Allman-Smith, Edward	Hamilton, William*	Murphy, Richard
Atkins, Robert	Hughes, Brian	Odbert, Arthur*
Austin, Richard	Keatinge, Alan	Orr, James
Brennan, William	King, Francis*	Palmer, Philip
Bruce-Hamilton, William	King, Maurice	Plews, John
Carney, Philip	Lamkin, John	Robinson, William*
Clarke, William	Large, David	Sachs, Albert
Conwa, Stephen*	Martin, David	Trimble, Arthur*
Crean, Gerard*	Martin, John	Walmsley, George
Croker, William*	McCann, Henry*	Walsh, Dermot
Davidson, Thomas	McCloghry, Charles	Walsh, Ian
Devlin, Henry*	McConkey, George*	Whelton, Michael*
Dixon, Henry	McConvell, Dermot	Wilson, Dennis

Table 6: Irish Doctors Awarded the Africa Star
*8th Army Clasp

Italy Star

Many of the Irish doctors who supported the Allied forces in North Africa moved with the armed forces as the Allies reinvaded Europe in 1943, firstly through their occupation of Sicily and then with landings on mainland Italy. The Italy Star was awarded to those who contributed to the Italian Campaign, which lasted from June 1943 until the end of the war in May 1945.

This is the only star for which no bar was authorised.

Clarke, William	McCann, Henry	Sachs, Albert
Conway, Stephen	McErvel, Thomas	Sarsfield, Thomas
Crean, Gerard	Moore, Edward	Smyth, John
Davidson, Thomas	Odbert, Arthur	Tabuteau, Thomas
Eves, Thomas	Orr, James	Walmsley, George
Field, Thomas	Palmer, Philip	Walsh, Dermot
Hepple, Robert	Parkinson, George	Whelton, Michael
Hughes, Brian	Robinson, Johnson	Wilson, Denis
King, Francis	Robinson, William	
Magner, Jeremiah	Roddy, Francis	

Table 7: Irish Doctors Awarded the Italy Star

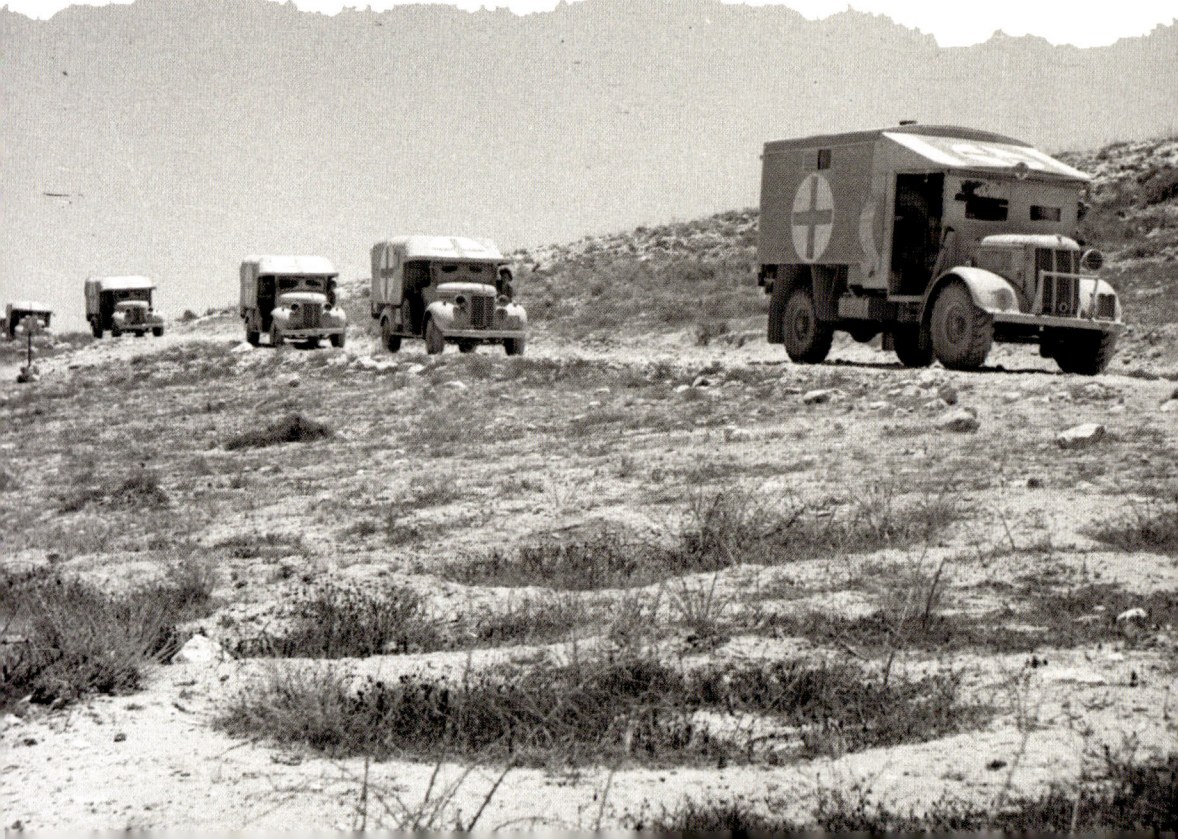

France and Germany Star

This star was granted for entry into operational service on land from 6 June 1944, in France, Belgium, Holland or Germany, until 8 May 1945, without prior time qualification. One bar was authorised, Atlantic, for those who qualified for the Atlantic Star after qualifying for the France and Germany Star.

At least twenty-four Irish doctors supported the Allied armies as they reinvaded Europe, firstly through Italy in 1943 and later on D-Day, 6 June 1944 until the surrender of the German Army in May 1945.

Burma Star

The Burma Star was a campaign medal awarded for service in the Second World War to the forces of the British Commonwealth, between 11 December 1941 and 2 September 1945. This campaign medal was also awarded for certain specified service in China, Hong Kong, Malaya and Sumatra. Twenty Irish doctors earned the Burma Star as the Allied forces firstly tried to halt the advance through the Far East of the Japanese Army in early 1942 and then as the Allies tried to recover the lost colonies.

Alexander, Hugh	Harris, Frederick	McGrath, John	Pennefather, Aubrey
Anderson, Robert	Holden, Ernest	Mitchell, Duncan	Steede, Francis
Austin, Frederick	King, Cecil	O'Dwyer, John	Walsh, Dermot
Barlas, Alexander	Lane, Wilfred	O'Neill, John	Whyte, Desmond
Chambers, Charles	McConnell, Dermot	O'Shea, Patrick	Woods, Thomas

Table 8: Irish Doctors Awarded the Burma Star

Pacific Star

The Pacific Star was awarded for entry into operational service in the Pacific theatre between December 1941 and 2 September 1945. Thirteen Irish doctors were awarded the Pacific Star, and John Joseph O'Dwyer and Dermot Francis Walsh were awarded the Burma Bar or Clasp.

Curra, Edward	MacCarthy, Aidan	O'Dwyer, John	Stringer, Charles
Hennessy, Edmond,	McQuillan, John	Smyth, Ernest	Walsh, Dermot
Huston, John	Murray, Francis	Stewart, William	
Kellet, John	Nolan, Colm		

Table 9: Irish Doctors Awarded the Pacific Star

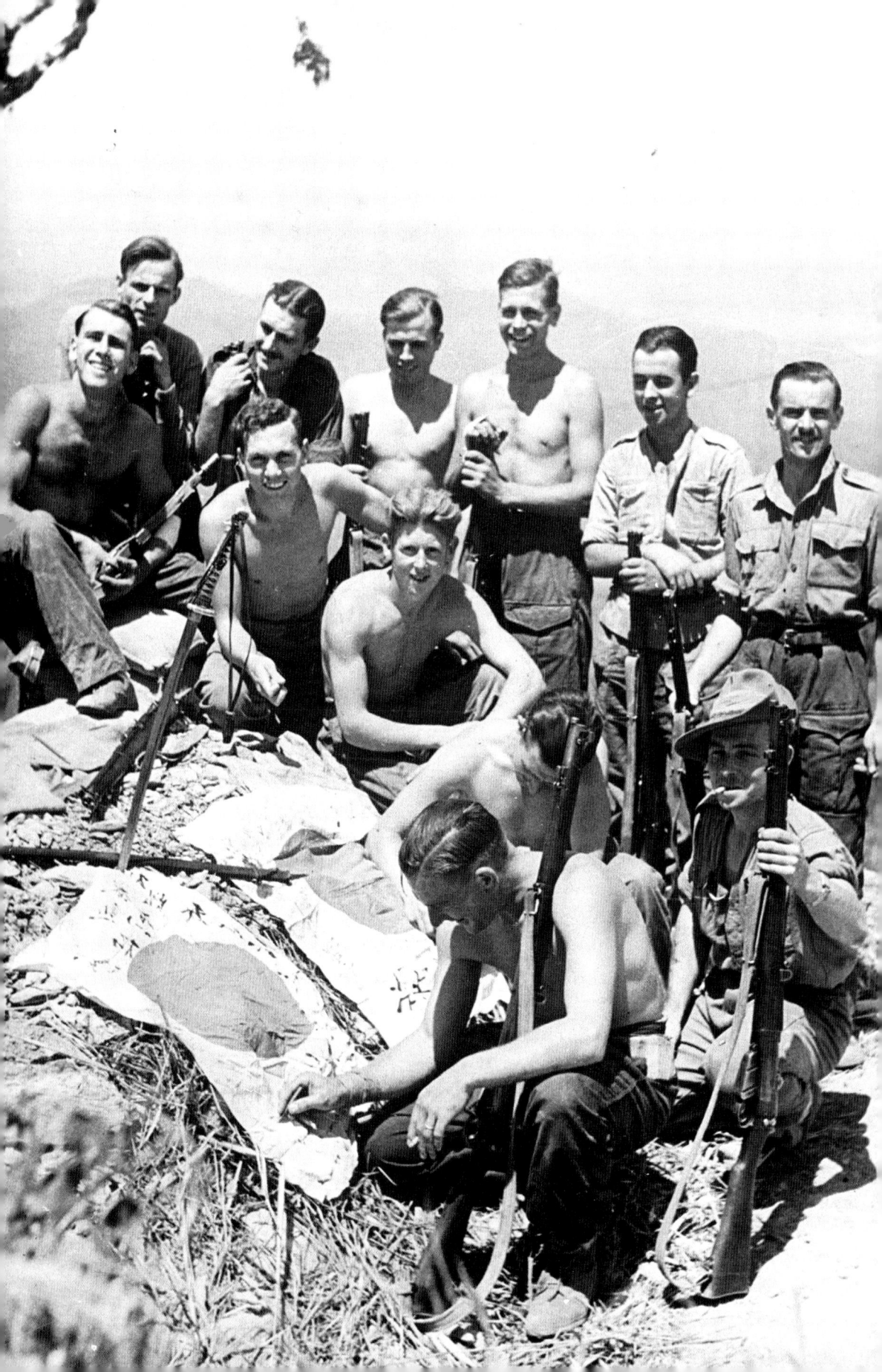

Chapter 3
IRISH DOCTORS IN EUROPE AND NORTH AFRICA 1939–45

The BEF had assembled along the Belgian–French border and by 27 September 1939 approximately 150,000 British soldiers had landed in France. Through the winter of 1939–40 the Dutch and Belgians strengthened their defences, the BEF expanded and the French Army received more equipment and training. By the end of April 1940 the strength of the BEF was nearly 400,000 men.

Accompanying the BEF were at least seventy-six Irish doctors supporting both the army and RAF forces. Amazingly, two of those doctors had travelled with the BEF in 1914 in the British response at that time to the invasion of Belgium by Germany.

William Brooke Purdon from Belfast travelled with the 1914 BEF and was later awarded the MC, the DSO and the OBE for his services and valour along with the Médaille d'honneur du Service de Sainte Militaire-Chevalier de la Legion d'Honneur. Joseph Andrew Wilson, a QUB graduate, was also a member of the 1914 BEF.

Allen, James	Dowse, John	King, Cecil	Parsons, Alfred
Allison, George	Draffin, David	King, Francis	Peacock, Pryce
Barlas, Alexander	Early, Edward	King, Maurice	Petit, Gerard
Bateson, William	Egan, Michael	Knight, William	Power, Michael
Beveridge, Arthur	Elliot, James	Large, Stanley	Purdon, William*
Blewett, Basil	Foot, William	Lord, John	Roddy, Francis
Browne, Harold	Gillespie, Frank	Lyburn, Rex	Russell, John
Carney, Philip	Graham, Roland	Magner, Jeremiah	Russell, Mortimer
Chesney, William	Gray, George	Maxwell, Peter	Ryan, Peter*
Clarke, William	Hayes, Patrick	MacCarthy, Aidan	Steede, Francis
Concannon, John**	Hepple, Robert	McVann, Henry	Stevenson, Alexander
Herbert, Conor	Herman, Myer	McConkey, George	Stevenson, Walter
Conway, Stephen	Hill, James	McGrath, John	Stuart, Charles
Coppinger, Francis	Houston, John	McQueen, Campbell	Summ, Julius
Creagh, Edward	Hughes, Brian	Mulholland, Henry	Todd, Andrew
Crean, Gerard	Hyde, Raymond,	Murphy, John	Tweedy, Ernest
Devlin, Henry	Keating, Victor	Napier, William	Whelton, Michael
Dixon, Kendal	Keatinge, Leslie	O'Meara, Francis	Wilson, Dennis
Douglas, Gerald	Kennedy, Alan	Orr, William	Wilson, Joseph*

Table 10: Irish Doctors Who Served with the British Expeditionary Force (BEF) September 1939–June 1940

* Irish doctors who served with BEF 1914–18
** Killed in action, June 1940

The Battle for Europe

The Western Front during the First World War was essentially a static line established in 1914 which separated the German and Allied armies and extended from the English Channel down through France to the Swiss border. The front moved a relatively short distance backwards and forwards over the four years of conflict until finally the Allies pushed the German Army eastwards to the French–German border, leading to the Armistice of November 1918. The increased mobility of the armies between the world wars and the availability of airborne firepower saw the European battlefront during the Second World War criss-cross the entire continent.

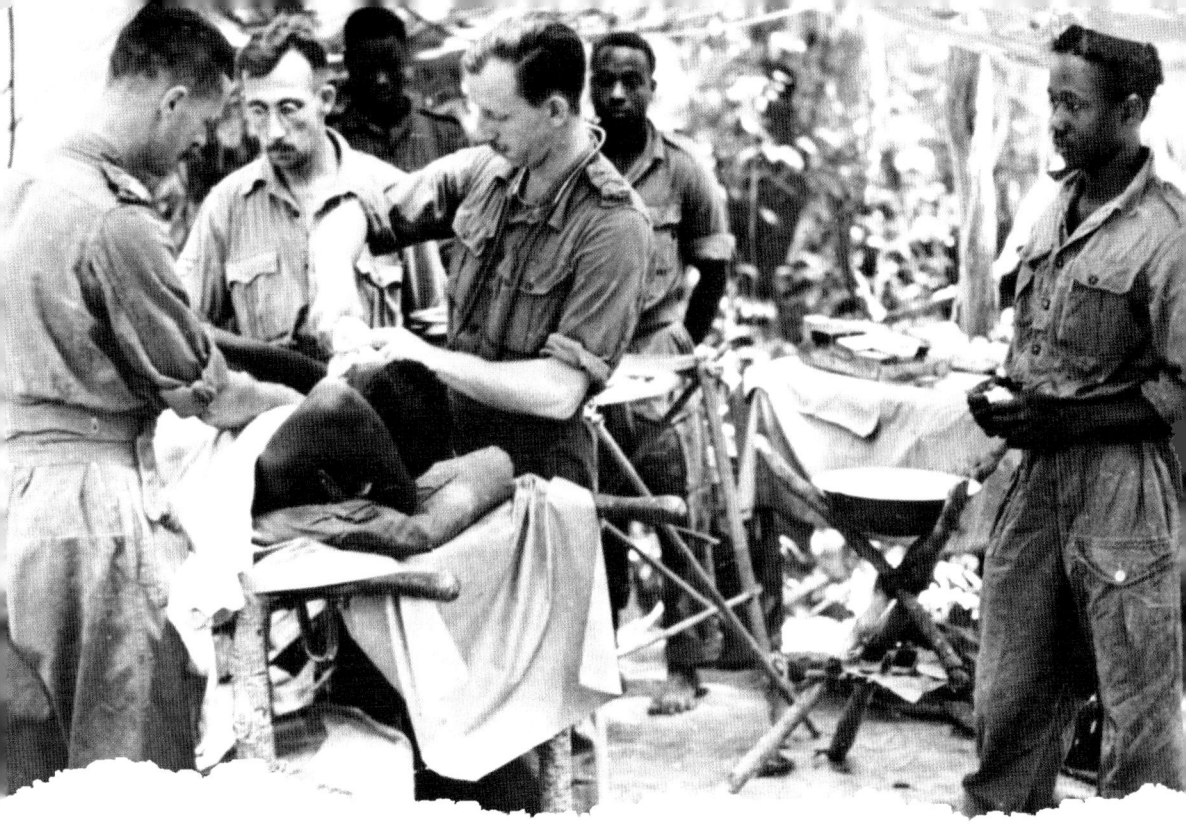

The period from September 1939 until May 1940 is referred to as the 'Phoney War', as the British Army in Europe saw no military action in the period. Aidan MacCarthy, a young graduate from UCC, had joined the RAF with two fellow graduates, Anthony O'Connor and Sydney Rosehill, shortly before the outbreak of the war. McCarthy was posted to France along with his RAF squadron in support of the BEF in December 1939. MacCarthy, in his book *A Doctor's War* describes the winter of 1939–40 during the Phoney War:

> *Each morning during the bad weather, we had to wait until a passage had been dug through the snow-drifts to allow us to go to the Mess for food. We spent endless days in the Mess, playing bridge, poker and back-gammon, reading books, writing letters, drinking, smoking, dozing – and bored to tears.*

The Phoney War came to an abrupt end when the German Army, supported by the Luftwaffe, invaded Norway and Denmark in early April 1940, as a prelude to the invasion of Belgium and France. Despite RN attempts to thwart the capture of the strategically important Norwegian Atlantic ports, the German forces quickly took control of the country, forcing the Norwegian king and his government to flee Norway to Britain. By occupying Norway Hitler had ensured the protection of Germany's supply of iron ore from Sweden and had obtained air and naval bases from which to attack Britain if required.

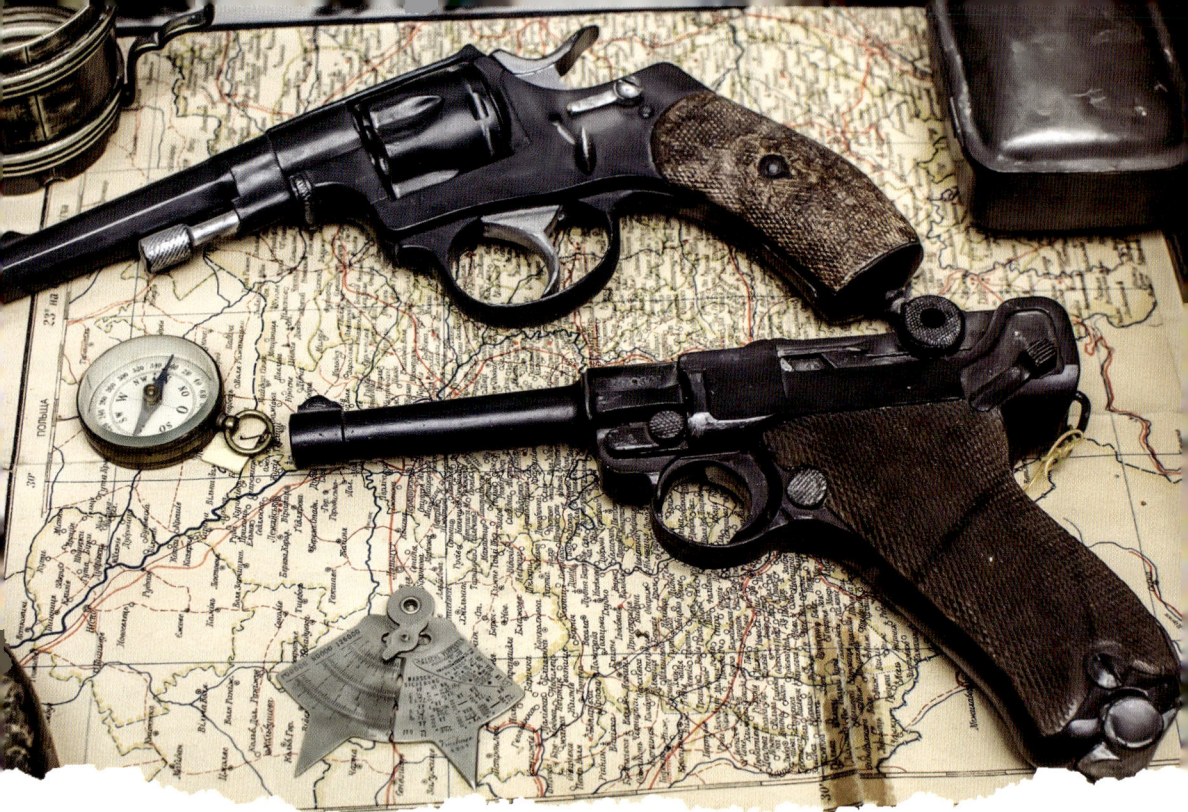

Arthur Joseph Beveridge, an NUI graduate from Rathgar in Dublin who had served with the RAMC, was awarded the Norwegian Military Cross 'for bravery and devotion to duty during the Norwegian Campaign'. He had also served with the RAMC during the First World War.

Beveridge, Arthur	Tyndall, William
Stewart, William Muir	Walmsley, George
Taylor, Robert	

Table 11: Irish Doctors who Served in the Norway Campaign, April 1940

Other Irish doctors who served in the Norwegian campaign included Robert Taylor, William Tyndall and George Walmsley, all of whom were TCD graduates, along with William Muir Stewart from QUB.

With Denmark and Norway invaded, Hitler ordered his army and air force to attack Belgium and France. On 10 May German troops swept through Belgium and the Netherlands, supported by their then familiar Luftwaffe blitzkrieg. With lightning speed, the German tank divisions rushed through the Ardennes and outflanked the Maginot Line, pushing deep into France despite a determined resistance by British and French forces who were unable to overcome the superiority of the Luftwaffe and the mobility of the German Army.

CHAPTER 3: IRISH DOCTORS IN EUROPE AND NORTH AFRICA 1939–45

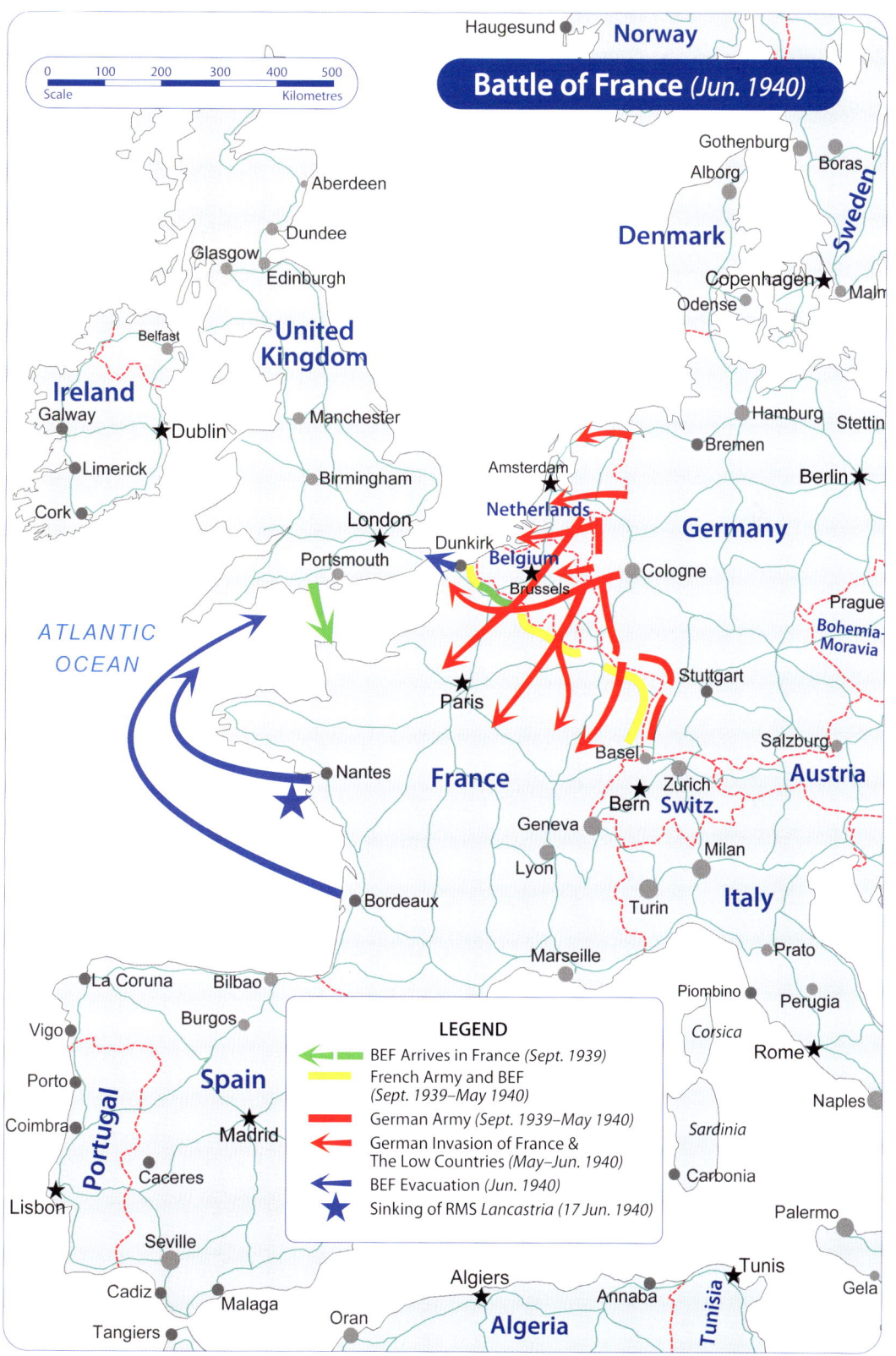

The success of the German rapid offensive deep into France placed the BEF in an impossible position, with the Atlantic to the west and the English Channel to the north. A general evacuation of all BEF and French forces was ordered, and between 26 May and 25 June 1940, some 560,000 military and civilian personnel returned to Britain, including 370,000 British troops. The initial evacuations took place at Dunkirk on the French north coast, starting on 26 May, and lasted ten days.

John Noel Concannon, from Dun Laoghaire, County Dublin and a TCD graduate, was killed in action on 1 June 1940 at the age of 29. He is buried in the De Panne Communal Cemetery, Belgium. De Panne village was the site of the final general headquarters of the BEF in June 1940, and there was a CCS on the beach, which was an embarkation point for the evacuation. From 27 May to 1 June 1940 the Germans strove to prevent the evacuation of the Allied troops by incessant bombing, machine-gunning and shelling. The first German troops reached the village on 31 May, and after heavy fighting, the commune was completely occupied on 1 June 1940.

The chaotic situation then facing Aidan MacCarthy, along with the RAMC and RAF personnel under his command as they retreated to the French coast for evacuation, is described by Bob Jackson in his book on MacCarthy's wartime experiences, *A Doctor's Sword*:

> *Complete chaos was unfolding across the front. The next order MacCarthy received was that his unit would be flown back to the UK from the city of Boulogne on the coast, 80 miles to the north west. He was instructed to take the ground staff of around 150 servicemen there. He assembled a convoy of about 15 vehicles including an ambulance, a water carrier, a fuel truck, troop carriers and five motorcycle outriders. As they headed west towards the town of Saint-Pol-sur-Ternoise they passed nervously through an ammunition park with stacks of bombs, shells, ammunition and petrol drums every 20 yards on either side of the road. He expected to be bombed at any moment by the enemy planes that seemed to be constantly overhead. The town was in pandemonium and the streets were choked with refugees … With the enemy already to the south and rapidly moving west, the trap laid for the British and French forces was closing.*

MacCarthy's convoy found no means of escape when they reached Boulogne and instead headed north to Calais in the hope of reaching Dunkirk, where they waited three days before being evacuated. Jackson describes how:

> *Due to the shallow nature of the beach, the group under MacCarthy's command filed along a long jetty that brought them to deeper waters where they waded out till the*

water was chest-high and got on small boats which took them to larger destroyers. The destroyers then transferred them to passenger ferries waiting further out at sea. They boarded a former Larne-to-Stranraer ferry, shattered but relieved. When they were about 2 miles off Dunkirk there was panic among the evacuees when they heard a load explosion below decks. They scrambled to the side where a gaping hole was visible on the waterline: the ship had been torpedoed by a German submarine. The quick-thinking ferry captain ordered everyone on the ship to move over to the opposite side, which tilted the ferry at an angle that kept the hole clear of the water. Luckily, the weather was calm as the ship limped its way back across the English Channel.

As the German Army took control of northern France, later evacuations were only possible at the French Atlantic ports of St Nazaire, Nantes and Bordeaux. The increased risk to later evacuations from air attacks became evident with the loss of the troopship RMS *Lancastria* just off the French west coast on 17 June 1940. About 2,500 passengers and crew were saved but 3,500 troops, RAF personnel and civilians died.

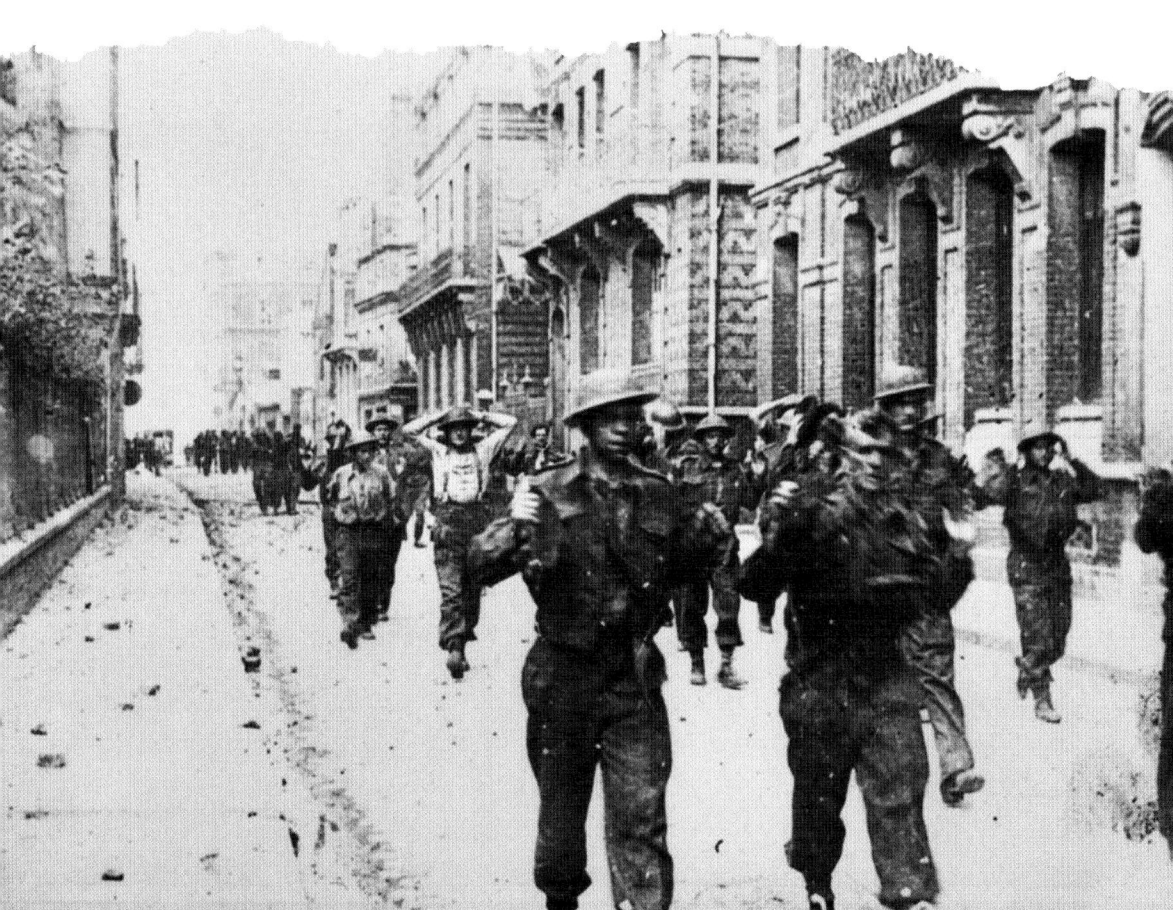

Thomas Bernard Kelly, a graduate of UCG, was to play an important role in the final days of the 1940 evacuation from France. He had served during the First World War and in 1918 was awarded the DSO 'in connection with military operations in Mesopotamia' (modern-day Iraq). After retiring from the IMS in 1926, Kelly served as a ship's surgeon with the Pacific Steam Navigation Company, which serviced British interests in South America. In September 1939, at the age of 69 and having been refused by the RN, he enlisted with the MN and acted as ship's surgeon on SS *Madura*. While on a return journey from East Africa, the *Madura* was diverted to Bordeaux to assist in the evacuation and successfully evacuated some 2,000 military personnel and families trying to flee the German onslaught. Kelly, along with some refugee nurses who were on board, looked after wounded British airmen and civilians who had been injured on their desperate journeys southwards.

The evacuation of the BEF ended on 25 June 1940. The BEF had suffered some 66,500 casualties, with 11,000 killed or dying of wounds and over 41,000 taken prisoner.

Many Irish doctors were captured during the German invasion of France when their positions were overrun or as they remained behind to look after the wounded who were too ill to be evacuated. Later the same fate would befall some Irish doctors as the Axis forces got the initial upper hand in the battle for control of North Africa.

Anderson, George	Ferguson, Ion	Martin, John	O'Meara, Francis
Barber, John	Gilbert, Edward	McCartney, Ernest	O'Neill, Stephen
Barrett, St Clair	Lewis, Joseph	McQueen, Campbell	Pollock, Robert
Brennan, William	Longmore, Louis	Mooney, Robert	
Caraher, Edward	Martin, John	Mulligan, James	

Table 12: Irish Doctors Who Were POWs in the European and African Theatres of War

Those prisoners captured in Western Europe were sent on forced marches into German towns, the march taking as long as twenty days. Others were moved on foot to the River Scheldt and were sent by barge to the Ruhr. The prisoners were then sent by rail to POW camps in Germany. Many spent all of the remainder of the war as POWs, while others were exchanged for their German counterparts after the Allied victory in North Africa in 1943. The German system of POW camps included the Camps Stalag Luft system, in which the Officers' POW Camps were titled Oflags and the other ranks' POW Camps were known as Stalags. Medical personnel, despite being of officer class, were required to attend to the health of the other ranks held in the Stalags and the associated work camps.

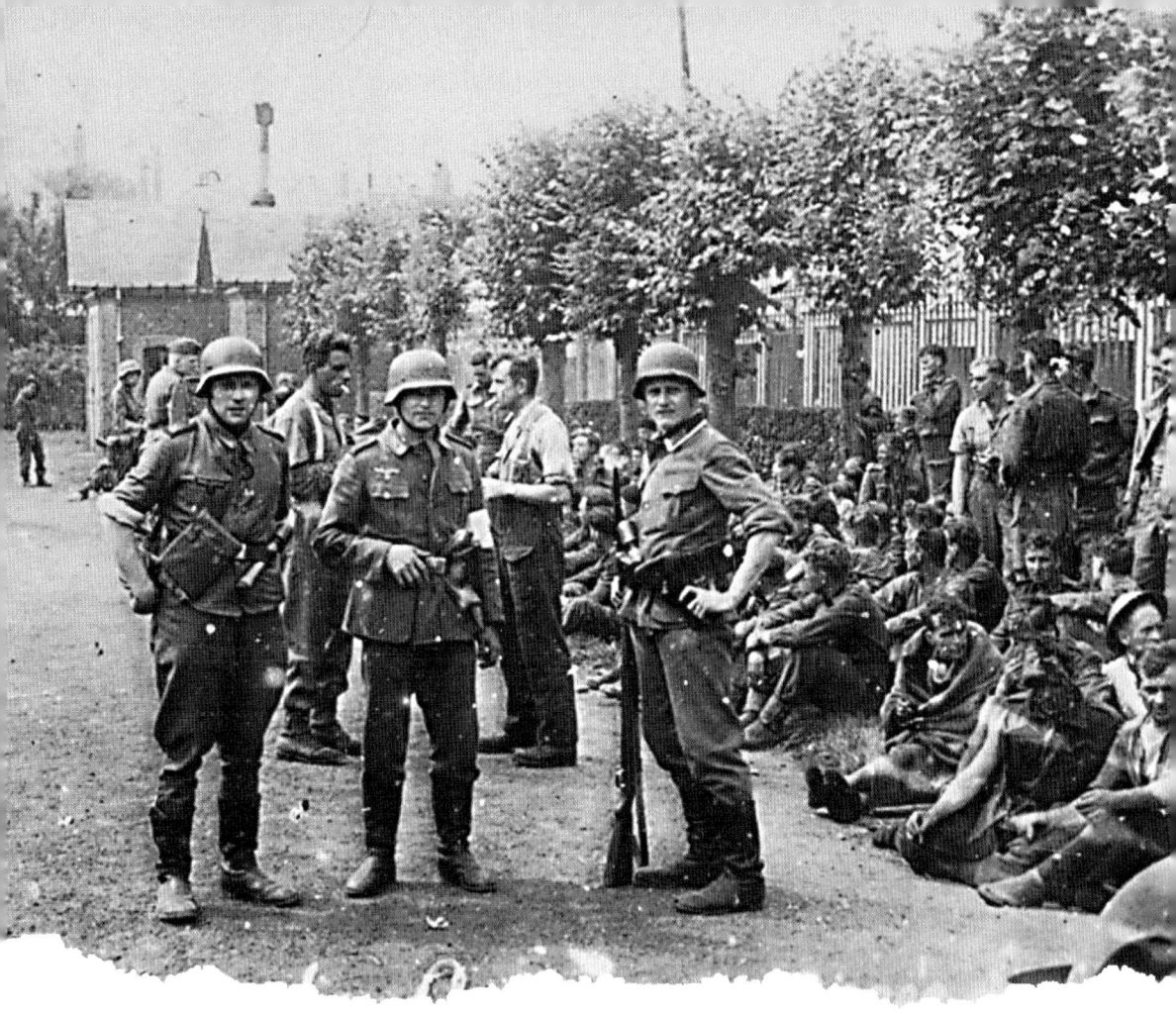

With much of continental Europe under German control, the German High Command set about a possible invasion of Great Britain by gaining air superiority, defeating the RAF and destroying Britain's armament production capability. Germany's attacks on RAF industrial installations and cities lasted from August to December 1940. The British victory in the Battle of Britain was achieved at a heavy cost in military and civilian casualties. Many thousands of airmen were killed on both sides, and it is estimated that some 23,000 civilians were killed and a further 32,000 wounded in the accompanying bombing of UK cities by the German Luftwaffe.

One casualty of the indiscriminate bombing of British cities was an Irish doctor, resident near Manchester, along with his wife and two children, on 22 December 1940. They were Dr Edward D'Arcy McCrea and Dr Edith Florence Wilcock, their son Patrick aged 13 and their daughter Biddy aged 10. Their house, The Cottage, located about 10 miles from Manchester, suffered a direct hit, and the entire family was killed instantly.

Edward D'Arcy McCrea was from Stillorgan in south County Dublin and had obtained his medical degree in TCD in 1917. On graduation he immediately joined the

RAMC, firstly as a lieutenant, being promoted to the rank of captain in July 1918. After the First World War he worked as a surgeon in St Patrick Dun's Hospital in Dublin, moving to Salford Royal Hospital in Manchester in 1922. Edward D'Arcy McCrea was also a talented tennis player who had represented Ireland in both the Davis Cup and the Olympic Games in 1924.

In 1925 Edward married Dr Edith Florence Wilcock, who, like her husband, was a Trinity graduate and a Fellow of the Royal College of Surgeons. Edward and Florence engaged in medical research and published several articles.

On the night of 2 December 1940 Edward and Edith were holding a dinner party at their home, unaware that a parachute bomb was drifting noiselessly towards them. When the bomb exploded it completely destroyed the house, killing everyone inside. That was the night of the heaviest raid on Manchester and its adjoining towns. There were 684 people killed and 2,364 injured when German bombers dropped 272 tons of high explosives and 1,027 incendiary bombs.

The Battle of Britain was an important turning point in the Second World War, as victory allowed Britain to rebuild its military forces and establish itself as an Allied stronghold, later serving as a base from which the liberation of Western Europe was launched in the summer of 1944.

Greece, the Balkans and Crete

As Hitler set about enforcing German control over occupied Europe and planned an invasion of Britain, Mussolini launched an attack on Greece.

The Italian invasion of Greece in October 1940 was one of Mussolini's greatest disasters. A totally inadequate Italian Army blundered into the mountains of north-west Greece where it was defeated and thrown back into Albania. War with Greece was far from inevitable. Although the king and sections of the political elite were Anglophiles, General Metaxas, the dictator who ran Greece, had far more in common with the Germans than with western democracies.

The Italian Army invaded Greece on 28 October. The 140,000 Italian troops faced a determined and tenacious enemy. They had to cope with a difficult mountain terrain where their superiority in tanks and artillery counted for little. By mid-November the Greeks had mounted a major counteroffensive and penetrated deep into Albania. This culminated in the capture of the Klisura Pass by the Greek Army in January 1941.

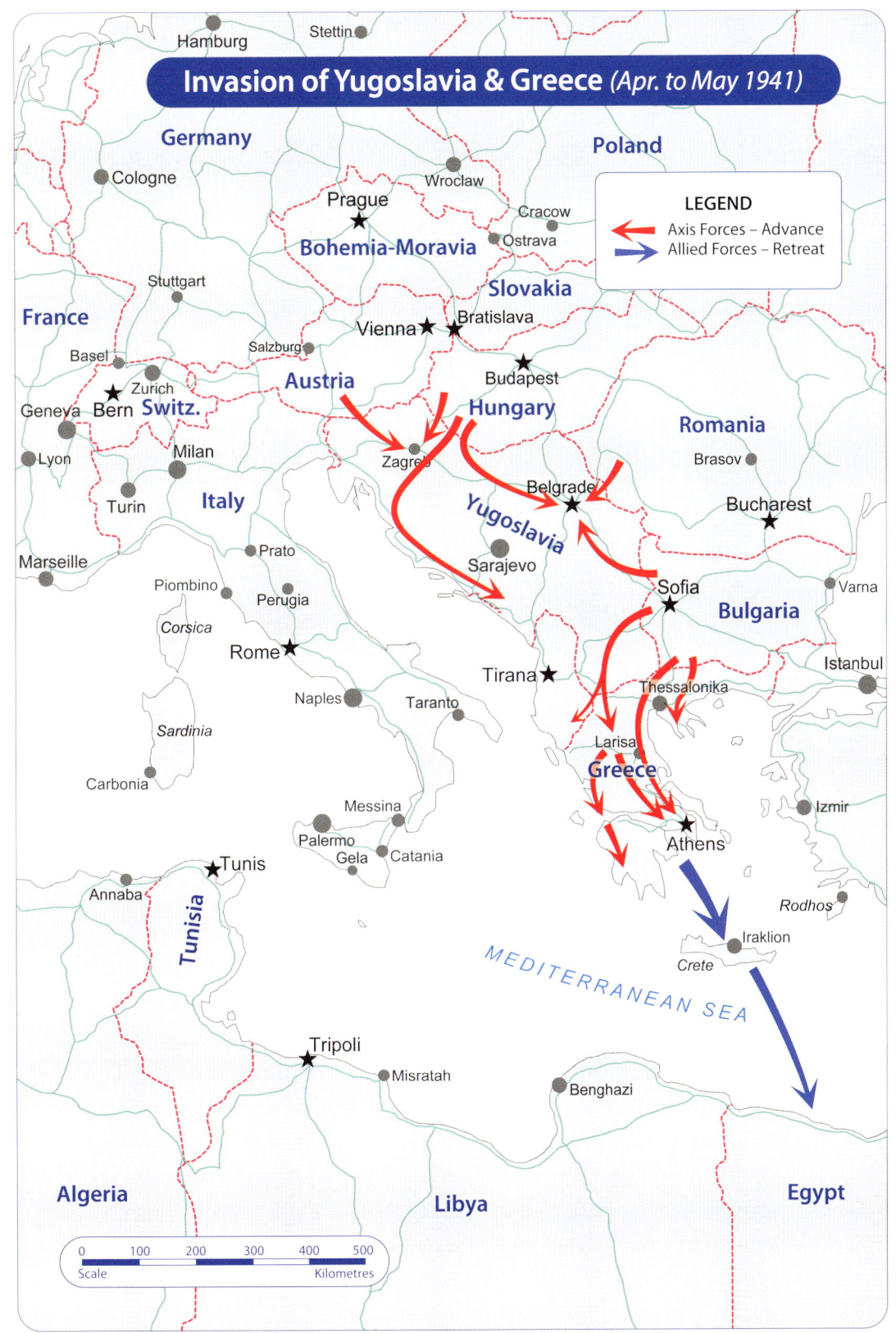

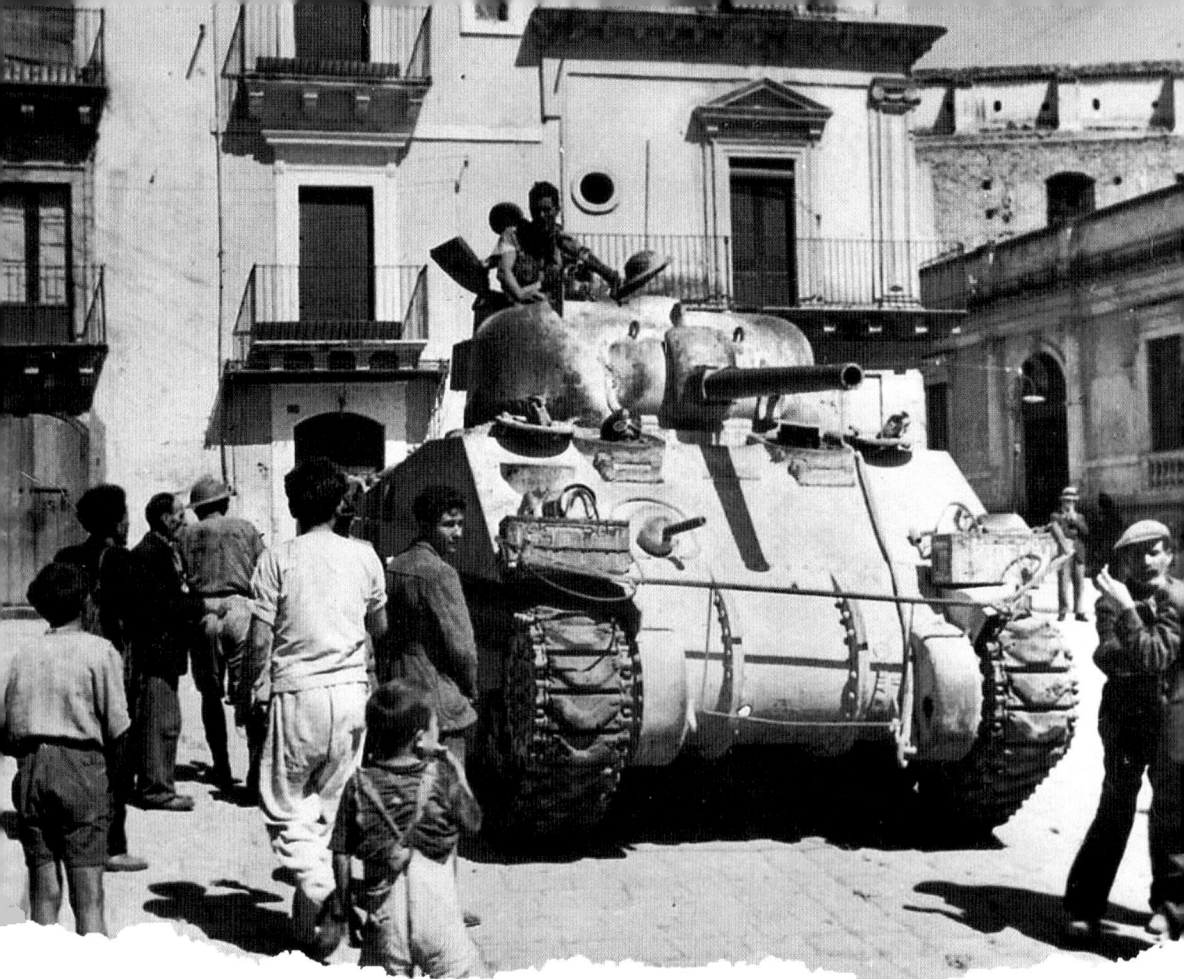

That location was 60km inside Albania and a highly strategic position. The front stabilised by February 1941, by which time both sides had serious losses. Despite Italian efforts to recover lost ground, their invasion of Greece failed and Italy finally withdrew its forces in March 1941.

The potential for Allied intervention forced Hitler to come to the aid of his Axis ally. German build-up in the Balkans increased after Bulgaria joined the Axis on 1 March 1941. Fearing another invasion but this time by Germany, the Allies agreed to send troops and air support to Greece. More than 62,000 Allied troops, mainly British, Australian and New Zealanders, were then deployed to help defend Greece.

When the German invasion began on 6 April 1941, the bulk of the Greek Army was on the Greek border with Albania, from which the Italian troops had attacked in October 1940. Germany launched its invasion from neighbouring Yugoslavia and Bulgaria and soon overran the Greek and Allied defences. By 20 April the Greek forces in Albania had surrendered. This allowed the German Army to advance southwards towards Athens. The British, Australian and New Zealand forces were also overwhelmed and forced to retreat, with the ultimate goal of evacuation.

The German Army reached the Greek capital, Athens, on 27 April and Greece's southern shore on 30 April, capturing 7,000 British, Australian, New Zealand and Yugoslav personnel, thus ending the German invasion of Greece with a decisive victory. Control of Greece was then divided up among Germany, Italy and Bulgaria.

The conquest of Greece was completed with the capture of Crete a month later in May 1941. With the fall of Greece, the Axis forces were now in control of much of Europe, allowing Hitler to turn his attention eastwards to an invasion of Russia.

As had happened when Germany invaded France and Belgium in May 1940, a similar dash by the Allied forces to the coast for evacuation was to happen as the Axis forces overran Greece in March and April 1941. And as had happened with the Dunkirk evacuation, some Irish doctors were left behind to care for wounded Allied soldiers and so became POWs.

Irish doctors who served in the 1941 Greece campaign included Hastings Fitzmaurice Deane, Charles Westland Greene from County Kildare, William Patrick Griffin, Louis Solomon from Dublin and Arthur Noel Odbert. Odbert went on to serve in the North Africa Campaign and was awarded the Africa Star with the 8th Army Clasp.

Among those captured was John Morgan Barber, from Bangor, County Down and a graduate of QUB, who was taken prisoner by the Germans on the Greek island of Leros. He was rescued after a month by the RN while being transported to the Greek mainland.

Ion Ferguson, from County Kildare and a graduate of RCSI, was not so lucky, as he was ordered to remain behind with the wounded at the No. 26 Hospital in Athens. Initially becoming a POW on 28 April 1941, he was sent to a POW camp at Corinth in late May before being transported to Stalag 18A at Wolfsberg in Germany at the end of June 1941. Ferguson was repatriated in January 1945 and his experience as a POW is described in Chapter 5.

North Africa and Italy

The initial engagement of the Allied and Axis forces in North Africa began with the failed attempt of the Italian Army to capture the Suez Canal by way of invading Egypt, then under British rule.

The Italian 10th Army crossed the Libyan–Egyptian border on 9 September 1940 and forced the British forces to retreat. The Italian Army set up a series of fortified camps just across the Egyptian border and awaited the development of a secure road along the Mediterranean coast. However, on 8 December the British launched a raid on Sidi Barrani, the main Italian encampment. The Italians were overrun and forced to retreat. The Italian 10th Army was destroyed and the few remaining units were forced to withdraw into the west of Libya.

Following this initial victory in North Africa in December 1940, the Allied forces were dispatched to Greece in anticipation of the German invasion, which began on the 1 March 1941. In the meantime, General Erwin Rommel landed in Tripoli with leading elements of the newly formed Africa Korps to reinforce the beleaguered Italian position.

By April 1941, under the command of Rommel, the Axis armies forced the Allies out of Libya back into Egypt. Benghazi had fallen once again and Tobruk was under siege. The Axis forces laid siege to Tobruk for 241 days until it was relieved by the British 8th Army in November 1941.

In January 1942 Rommel attacked again and this time took the surrender of Tobruk with the capture of 25,000 Allied prisoners. Among those captured at the fall of Tobruk was Stephen Gerald O'Neill. Douglas Bluett from County Wicklow was more fortunate, as he was evacuated from Tobruk the day before the city fell to the Axis forces.

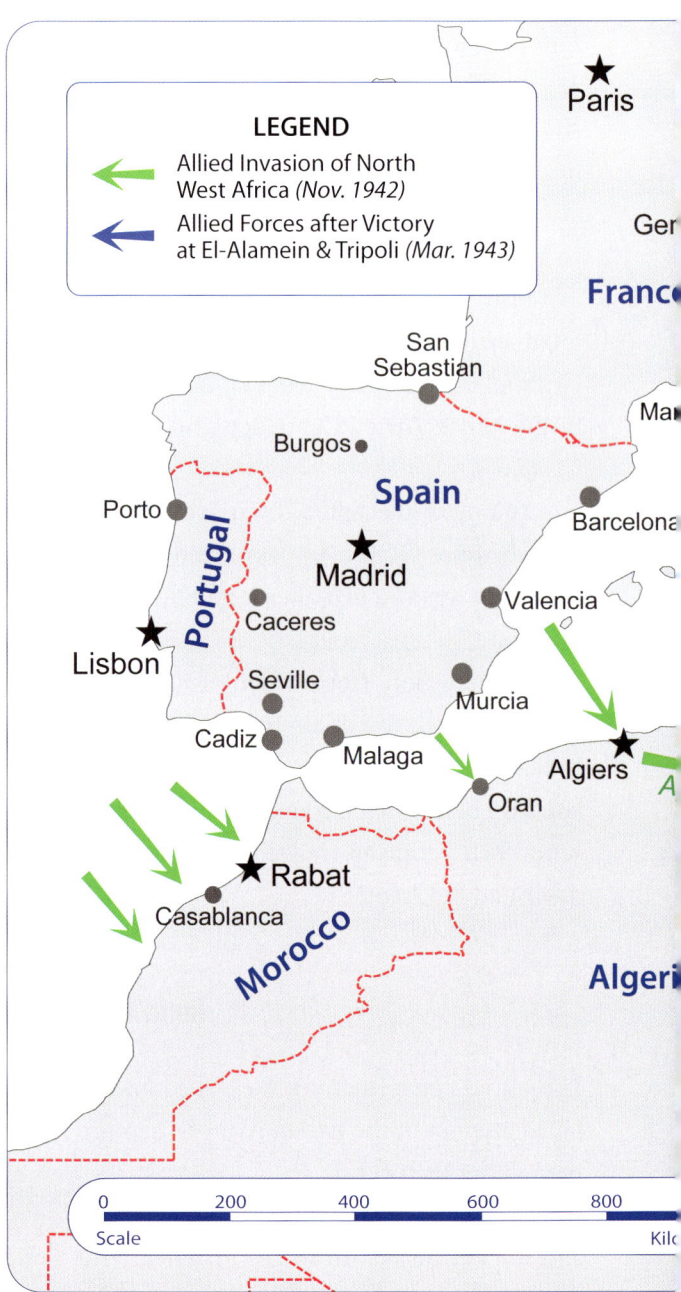

CHAPTER 3: IRISH DOCTORS IN EUROPE AND NORTH AFRICA 1939-45

The Axis forces continued their push eastwards but were eventually stopped in July 1942 at the 1st Battle of El Alamein, an important town on the Egyptian Mediterranean coast just east of Alexandria, the gateway to both Cairo and the Suez Canal.

Stalemate between the Allied forces and Axis forces continued on the Libyan–Egyptian border until the Allies, then under the command of Lieutenant General

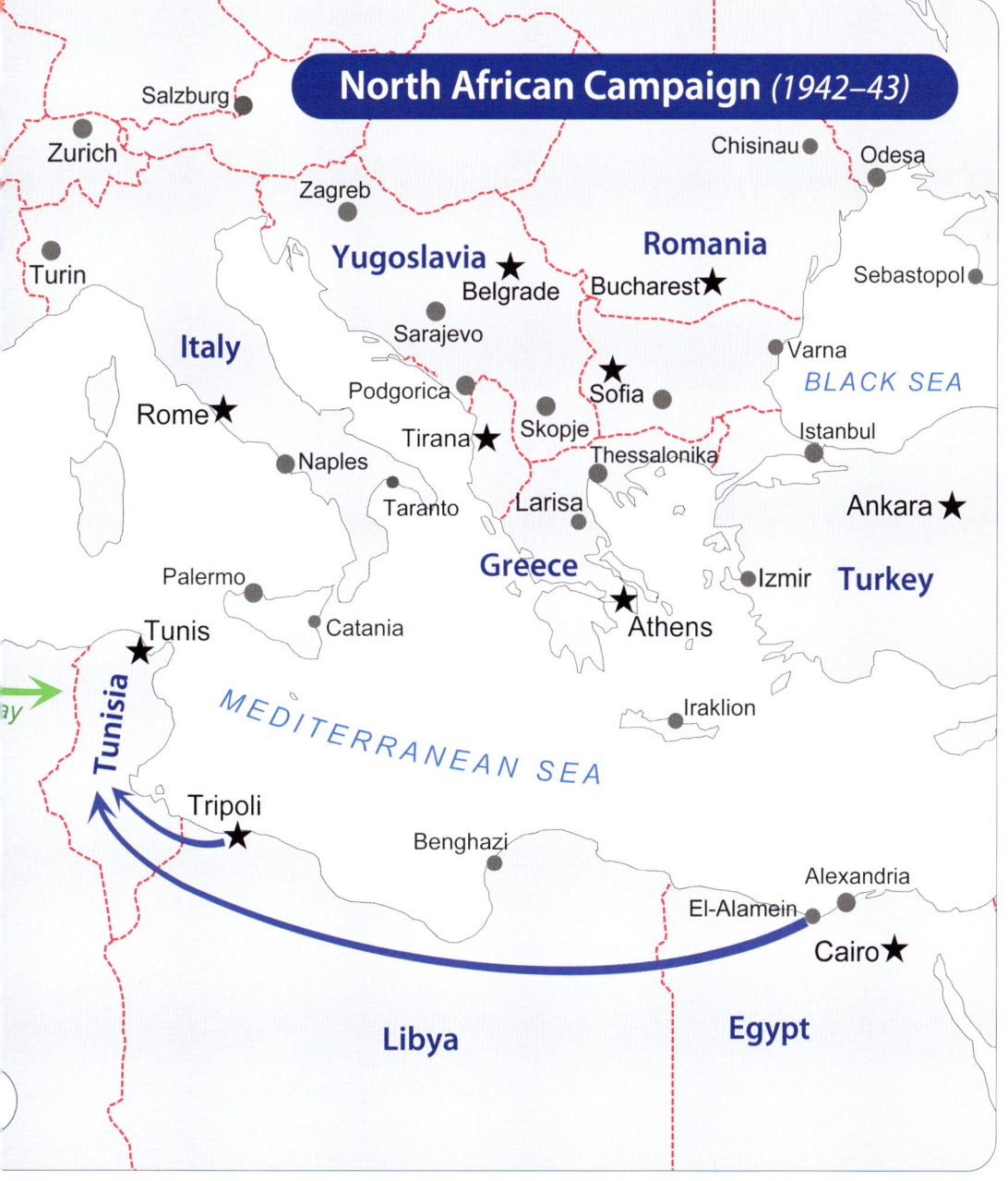

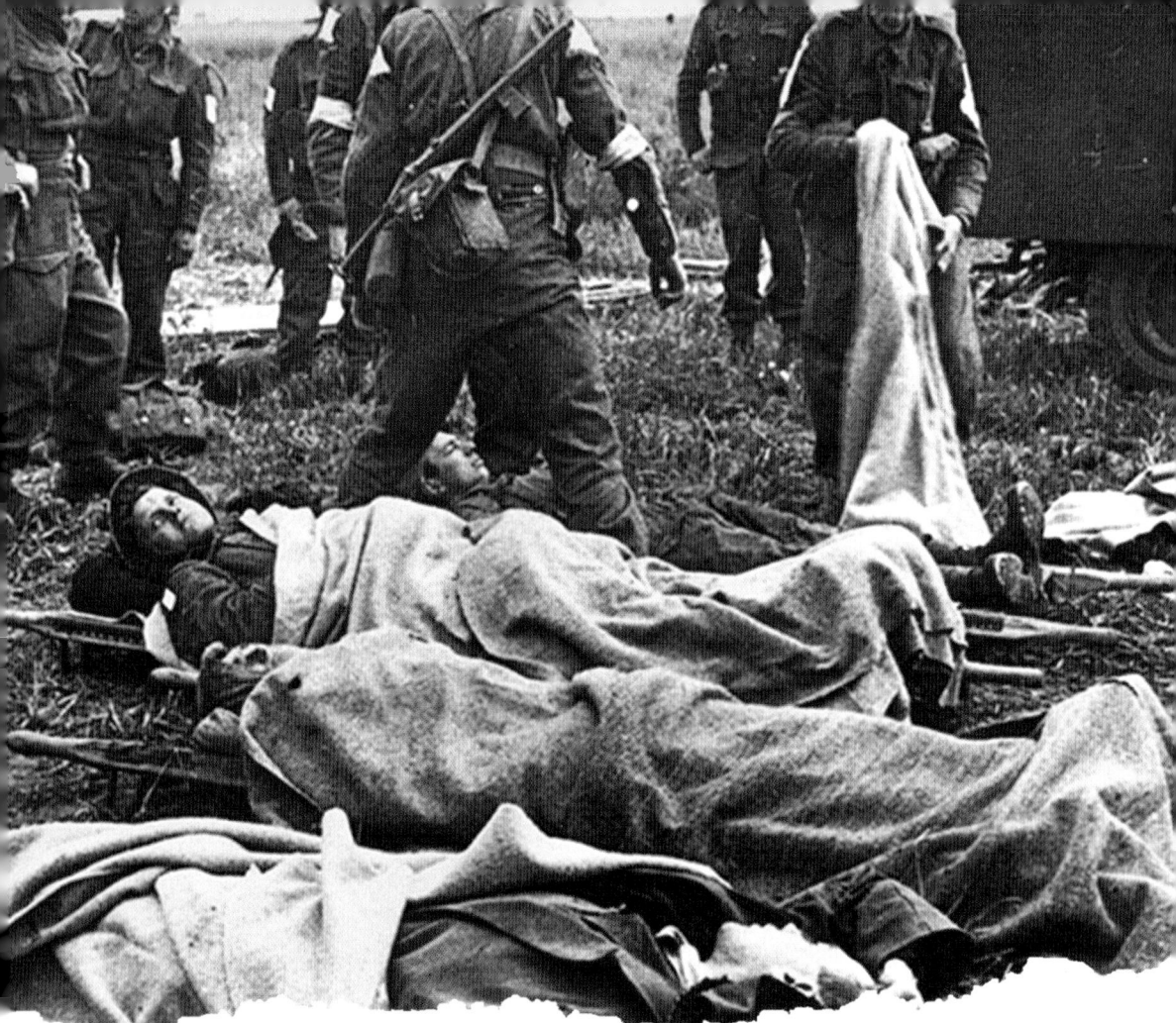

Bernard Montgomery of the British 8th Army, defeated the combined German and Italian forces in October 1942 at the Second Battle of El Alamein.

Among the Irish doctors who served in the African Campaign and the following invasion of Italy were Andy Parsons and Edward Caraher.

Edward Francis More Caraher MB was born in 1908 in Rathmines, Dublin. He graduated from UCD in 1932, enlisted with the RAMC in November 1940 with the rank of Lieutenant and served in the North Africa Campaign. He was taken prisoner in 1942 by the Axis forces and interned in an Italian POW camp from which he eventually escaped. Captain Caraher was awarded the MC on his repatriation in 1945 for his bravery during the attack in 1942 that ultimately led to his imprisonment in Italy.

His citation for the MC read:

Captain Caraher was in command of the advanced dressing station, 150 Field Ambulance, and under command of the late Officer Commanding 150 Brigade. During the period 29th May– 1st June, 1942, the Brigade Box was surrounded by the enemy and communication with M.D.S. some miles to the north-east was severed. This box was the left flank of the Gajala position, Western Desert. No evacuation of the wounded could take place. Throughout the above period enemy fire came from all quarters, and he continually attacked with armour, infantry and from the air, gradually whittling away the defences, shortening his range, improving his observation, and increasing the accuracy of his fire. Casualties were heavy, but although now only the more severe cases were sent to the A.D.S., it quickly became full to overflowing. Captain Caraher and his small staff worked day and night operating, bandaging, giving such blood transfusions as were possible, improvising beds and stretchers, and preparing hot drinks and food as best they could, while all the time the enemy fire continued and the wounded came streaming in. It was under these trying conditions that Captain Caraher set an example of courage, cheerfulness and devotion to duty which will rank high in the Annals of the Corps, and it is not too much to say that in his skill, ingenuity, and untiring care, many of the wounded owe their lives. In the early afternoon of the 1st June, the enemy finally overran the area and found Captain Caraher carrying on.

Captain Caraher died in 1984 and is buried in Balbriggan, County Dublin.

Alfred Denis (Andy) Parsons MB was born in 1914 in Athlone, County Westmeath. His family moved to Greystones, County Wicklow in 1920 and he attended Aravon school in Bray, County Wicklow and later Portora Royal School in Enniskillen, County Fermanagh. He graduated in 1936 from TCD.

He initially served with the MN before enlisting with the RAMC in 1939. After joining the BEF he saw action in May 1940 with the Inniskillings when Germany invaded France, and was eventually evacuated from Dunkirk.

In early 1941 Andy Parsons was sent to North Africa, initially to Egypt and Syria before joining the Royal East Kent Regiment (the Buffs) as that battalion trained alongside Montgomery's 8th Army for the offensive at El Alamein in October 1942. The battle of El Alamein ended on 4 November when Rommel ordered his Afrika Korps troops to withdraw. Over the following eight months the Allied forces harassed the German troops as they retreated into Libya, until the North Africa Campaign finally came to an end in May 1943.

He was involved in the landings at Anzio, but while in Italy he suffered a severe injury to his thigh which shattered his sciatic nerve. He was flown to Oxford to the neurosurgical unit there for reconstructive surgery, which was of limited success. Following the war he returned to Ireland but then emigrated to New Zealand. He disappeared in a boat with twenty-four other passengers in 1953.

For his medical support of the Allied troops in North Africa Andy Parsons was awarded the MC. The citation read:

Captain A.D. Parsons is a medical officer attached to the Buffs. Throughout a period of almost continuous action from early August 1942 to March 1943 the personal bravery and determined initiative of this officer have been responsible for the saving of a great many lives. On every occasion he was to be found at the spot where casualties were most likely to occur, and it is due to his complete disregard of danger, the calm skill and speed of his work, and his devotion to duty under fire that so many men owe their lives. The following are but a few examples of his consistent behaviour. On the morning of October 24th, 1943, he was with a company of Buffs behind the Miteiriya Ridge in a position which had just been captured by New Zealand battalions. A number of the New Zealanders had been lying for most of the night with severe wounds almost untreated.

Under continuous shell and mortar fire, Captain Parsons collected about a dozen severely wounded men from an area exposed to direct small arms fire in the middle of a mine field. He would not have failed in his duty had he devoted himself to casualties nearer at hand and less exposed to fire. Throughout the twelve days of the Alamein battle he repeatedly recovered wounded men from forward slopes under fire, who must otherwise have lost their lives. On January 19th south of Tarhuna under heavy shellfire, a General was severely wounded. Captain Parsons at the time was characteristically returning in his jeep with a badly wounded man from the most shelled area, but on being informed he put the man in an ambulance and under continued fire went to the General, and there is little doubt that his calmed skill saved a valuable life. Again on the morning of January 22nd, in the Tarhuna pass at a time when four men had just been killed by close-range heavy mortar fire, after dressing several wounds Captain Parsons crawled out onto a forward slope under direct fire to rescue a man believed to be alive. West of Zavia on January 25th, 1943, his work under very heavy shelling while others were taking cover, again saved several lives. It is in fact not possible to speak too highly of the sustained and unselfish courage of this officer in saving life throughout eight months of nearly continuous periods of action.

The Allied victory in the Egyptian Western Desert was followed by Operation Torch, which saw American troops invade the Vichy French colonies in Northwest Africa. The American troops, including airborne divisions, had been based in Northern Ireland where they had been gathering since January 1942. With Allied forces both to the east and west of the retreating Axis forces, the North African campaign ended in May 1943 with the capture of several hundred thousand German and Italian POWs.

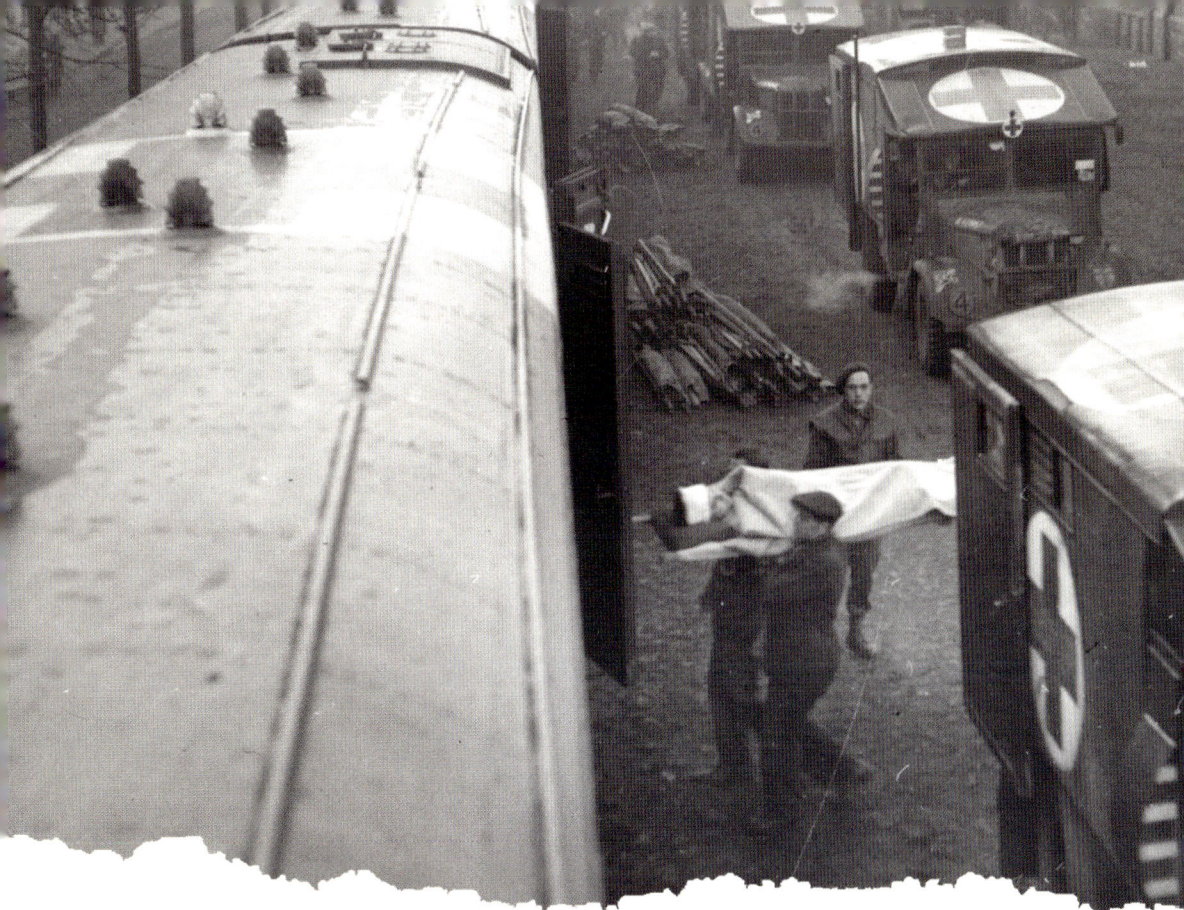

Reinvasion of Europe

Victory in North Africa allowed the Allied forces to invade Italy and so open another European front, a long-sought demand of the beleaguered Russian army on the Eastern Front. Firstly, the Allies invaded and captured the island of Sicily in July and August 1943 before attacking the Italian mainland. Then, in September, the Allies launched a major offensive by landing troops at Salerno, Taranto and the toe of Italy. The invasion of Italy followed the overthrow of the Italian fascist leader Mussolini on 25 July and the official withdrawal of Italy from the war on 8 September 1943.

Despite the success of the invasion, the Allied advance north to Rome and the borders with Germany was slow, due to the dogged defence of the German forces, coupled with the mountainous character of the Italian peninsula. In January 1944 the Allies landed at Anzio, 50km south of Rome, with the objective of bypassing the German forces in central Italy and then taking Rome. It was also hoped that the landing at Anzio would draw German forces away from Monte Cassino and facilitate an Allied breakthrough there. Unfortunately, the invasion force at Anzio failed to move inland as speedily as expected, and while the liberation of Rome did eventually come in June 1944, German forces had relocated to the north of the city.

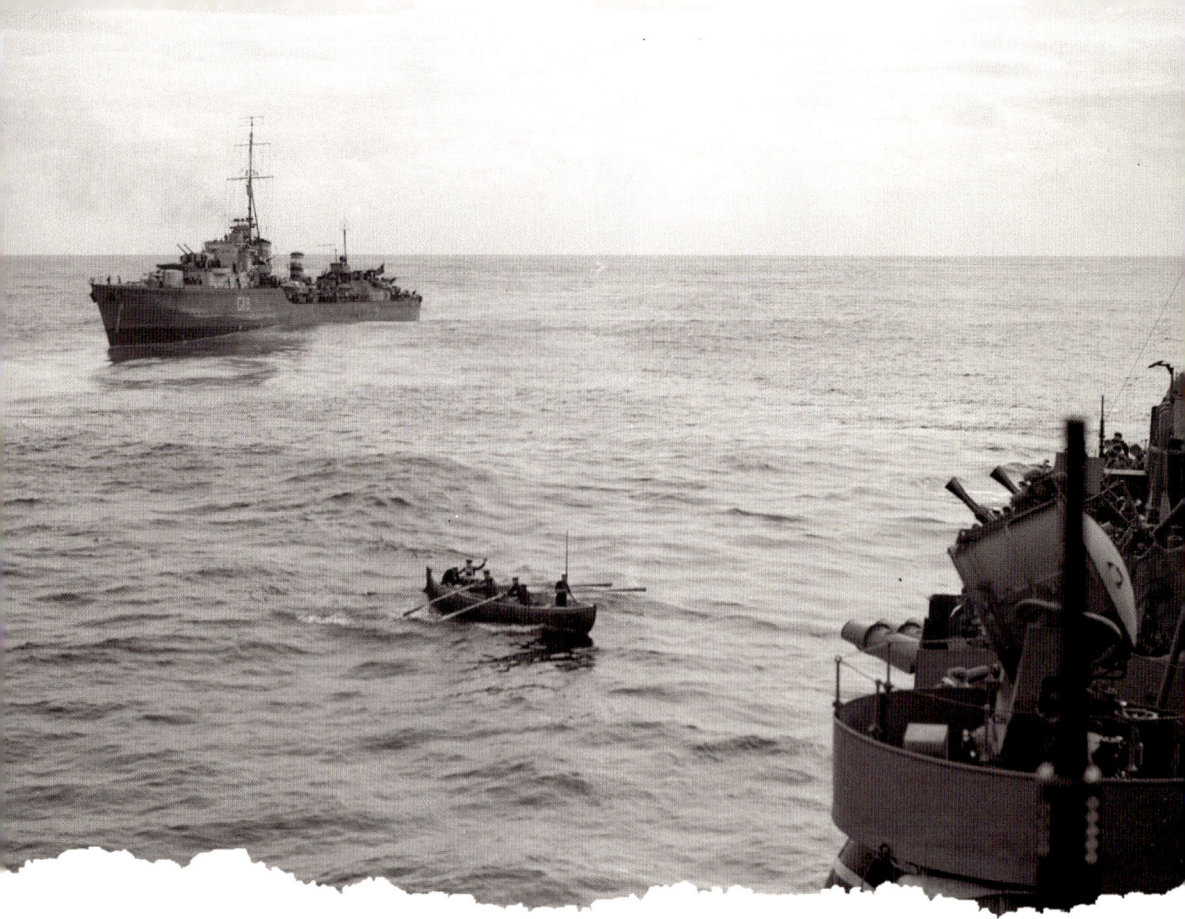

The final victory over the Axis forces in Italy did not come until the spring offensive of 1945, leading to the surrender of German forces there on 2 May 1945, shortly before Germany finally surrendered, ending the Second World War in Europe on 8 May 1945.

The War at Sea

As in the First World War, the war at sea in the 1939–45 conflict was dominated by the German U-boats' capability to attack both Allied navies and merchant shipping, especially the relieving convoys coming from America and to a lesser degree from Canada. The Allies gradually gained the upper hand by firstly overcoming the German surface fleet by the end of 1942 and then defeating the U-boats by mid-1943, although losses due to U-boats continued until the end of the war.

Unlike the situation on land where there was a stand-off between the Allies and German forces along the Maginot Line, the outbreak of the war saw British and French navies immediately establish a blockade of German ports and engage with the German Navy. The summer of 1939 then saw a flurry of activity as the German U-boats attempted to minimise the British and French navies' control of its access to Atlantic waters. On

14 September, Britain's most modern aircraft carrier HMS *Ark Royal* was damaged by torpedoes and another carrier, HMS *Courageous*, was sunk three days later by a U-boat. Further German successes followed with the sinking of numerous merchant ships and the sinking of HMS *Royal Oak* at anchor at the British naval base at Scapa Flow in the Orkney Islands with the loss of 833 lives in October 1939.

The British Navy also had some early successes, notably the trapping of the German battle cruiser *Admiral Graf Spee* in Montevideo harbour, leading to it being scuttled by its captain on 17 December 1939.

The German occupation of Norway, the Low Countries and France in May 1940, coupled with the Italian entry into the war on the Axis side, transformed the war at sea, particularly in the Mediterranean, where the Axis forces barred the direct route through the Mediterranean Sea to the Suez Canal, forcing British shipping to use the long alternative route around the Cape of Good Hope.

A further blow to the Allied naval forces was foreseen should the large French naval fleet fall to enemy control with the fall of France in June 1940. Initially Britain used diplomacy to request that the Vichy government, which had signed armistices with Germany and Italy, disable their ships to avoid them falling into German hands. With no diplomatic success, the French warships located in southern British ports were taken over by armed boarding parties with few casualties. In other ports in Allied control – as in the Egyptian port of Alexandria – French naval ships were blockaded in the harbours. A tragic outcome took place on 3 July 1940 in the French North African port of Mers-el-Kebir, in French Algeria. The British Navy mined the entrance to the port and tried to persuade the French Navy to scuttle their ships. After a day of diplomacy failed, they fired on them and badly damaged the four battleships present. Altogether 1,297 French sailors were killed and 350 wounded.

On 8 July 1940 the Vichy government officially severed all diplomatic ties with Britain, allowing the U-boat fleet direct access to the Atlantic with friendly ports on the French coast. The British Navy also had to protect the British mainland from a German invasion.

The spring and early summer of 1941 saw the large battle cruisers of both the British and German Navy fight it out in the Atlantic. Firstly, the mighty German battleship *Bismarck* sank the British battle cruiser HMS *Hood* on 14 May 1941 with the loss of over 1,400 lives, while only three crew survived. The *Bismarck* was damaged in the firefight and headed for a friendly port in France. However, it was spotted on a routine patrol by a Catalina flying boat out of Castle Archdale on Lough Erne, County Fermanagh, and was sunk by the British Navy on 27 May. With the loss of the *Bismarck*, the remainder of the war in the Atlantic was dominated by the German U-boat fleet. In response the Allies developed systems to protect convoys, coming mainly from America and Canada, from submarine harassment. They also deployed locate-and-destroy tactics to essentially neutralise such threats. The port of Derry in Northern Ireland, along with the Catalina flying boats stationed on Lough Erne, played a key role in the protection of Allied convoys coming from North America.

Ultimately, the threat from the German U-boat fleet was reduced, allowing for the flow of strategic supplies to Britain and the build-up of troops and supplies needed for the Allied invasion of Europe in June 1944. During the Battle of the Atlantic, the Allies lost 3,500 merchant ships and 175 warships and about 72,000 sailors lost their lives. German casualties numbered 783 U-boats and about 30,000 sailors.

A number of Irish doctors became casualties while fulfilling their duties, either as part of a medical team on board one of the ships of the RN or in the course of being transferred to or from a scene of conflict.

The controversial sinking of the aircraft carrier HMS *Gloucester* took place on 8 June 1940. The ship was on its way back to the United Kingdom, escorted by two destroyers, HMS *Ardent* and HMS *Acasta*, having been used to evacuate aircraft from Narvic in Norway. They encountered two German battle cruisers, one of which was the *Scharnhorst*. No aircraft were in the area to protect the *Gloucester* and no aircraft were launched, though the weather conditions were perfect. The *Scharnhorst* opened fire and HMS *Gloucester* was hit in the forward upper hangar and the bridge, leaving a gaping hole in the flight deck and starting a serious fire. Another shell hit the aft of the carrier and five minutes later the order to abandon ship was given. Twenty minutes later HMS *Gloucester* rolled over and sank, taking with her 76 officers, 2,086 other ranks and 41 RAF personnel. The dead included 37-year-old George Passmore Pearse from Glenageary, County Dublin. There were forty-three survivors, who were picked up by Norwegian vessels during the next few days. Questions that remain unanswered are why a valuable aircraft carrier was sent to Norway to evacuate seventeen worthless aeroplanes, ten of which were biplanes, and why did the commanding officer, Captain Greg Doyly Hughes, not keep aircraft in the air to protect his ship?

In the same engagement that saw the loss of HMS *Gloucester*, the two destroyers HMS *Ardent* and HMS *Acasta* were sunk by German gunfire. They were hopelessly outranged and outgunned. HMS *Ardent* was hit and sank with a loss of 10 officers and 142 ratings. Among the officers killed was 27-year-old surgeon Lieutenant Dermot Harry Tuthill Duggan from Foxrock, County Dublin.

One of the most iconic battleships of the Second World War was the battle cruiser

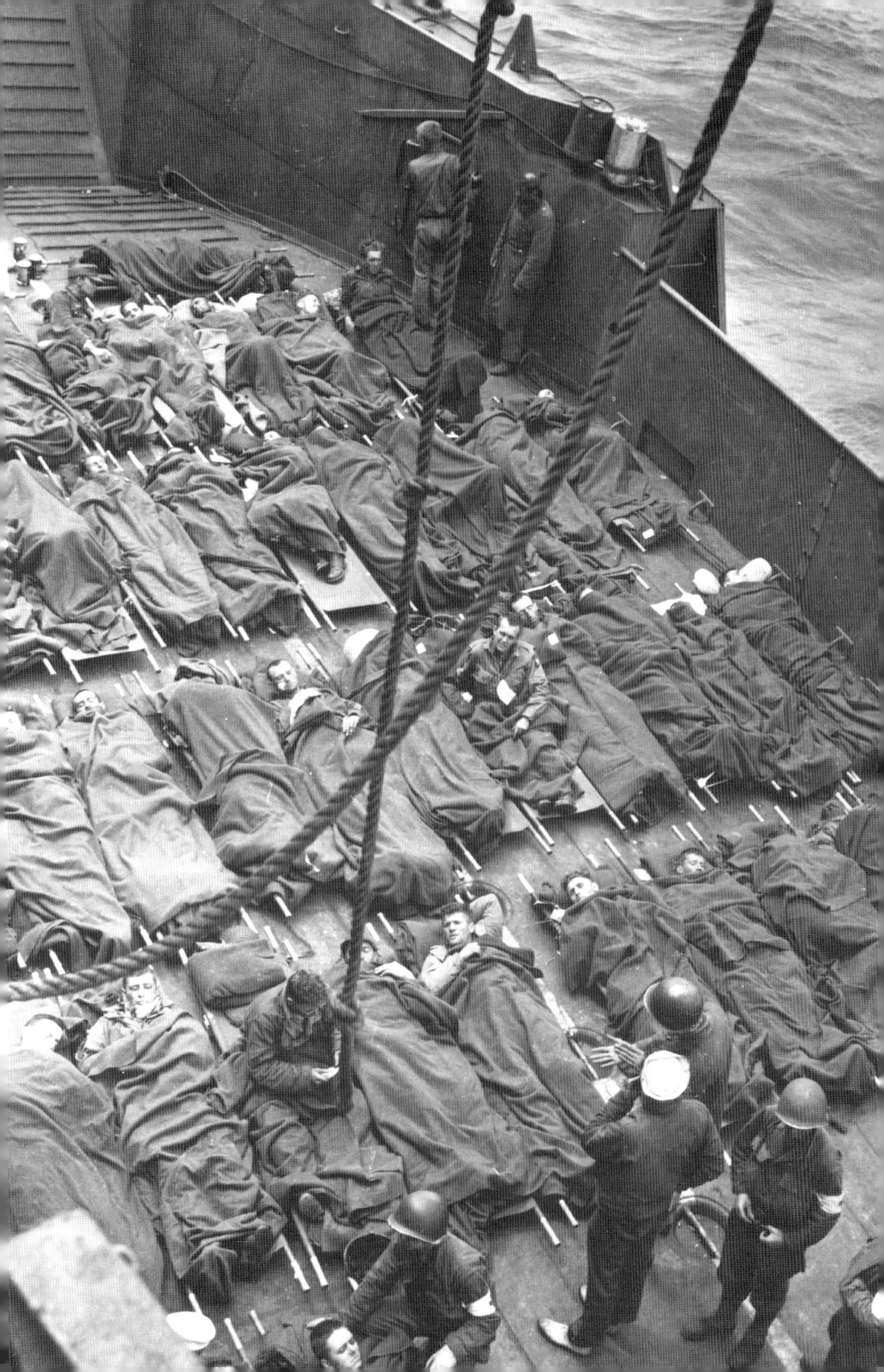

HMS *Hood*, which was launched on 2 August 1918 and sunk by shellfire on 24 May 1941. On hearing that the German battleships *Bismarck* and *Prinz Eugen* were on their way to the Atlantic, the *Hood*, under the command of Captain Ralph Kerr and accompanied by six destroyers, left Scapa Flow on 22 May 1941, and steering north-west on 24 May met with and engaged the German flotilla steering south-west. The fifth salvo from the *Bismarck* struck HMS *Hood*'s starboard quarter, and the explosion that followed sent the forward section of the ship into a vertical position before it sank. There were only three survivors, and among the 1,418 casualties was surgeon Commander Henry Hurst from Bantry, County Cork, an RCSI graduate who had joined HMS *Hood* on 16 August 1940.

The aircraft carrier HMS *Hermes* was launched on 11 September 1919 and on 9 April 1942 it was intercepted by the Japanese, having left Trincomalee in former Ceylon. The ship requested fighter cover, but due to communication difficulties this never arrived. After being ordered back to Trincomalee as fast as possible, the ship was attacked by Japanese aircraft from every direction and suffered over forty hits. Just after Captain Onslow ordered to abandon ship, she rolled over and sank. Amongst the 307 casualties was surgeon Commander James Michael McNamara from Coleraine, County Londonderry.

Surgeon Lieutenant Hugh Marks RNVR, from Randalstown, County Antrim, was posted to a RN ship in the east and travelled from England on a passenger ship in a convoy, in order to take up his position. The convoy was attacked by an armed raider on 25 March 1941 and the boat on which he was a passenger was sunk. Surgeon Lieutenant Marks died of exposure after two days on a raft.

Hospital ships did not avoid attack in spite of their markings and clear medical status. The hospital ship St David was attacked and sunk by German aircraft on 24 January 1944 off Anzio and Lieutenant Colonel Thomas Preston Eaves (RAMC) from Donnybrook in south Dublin was reported missing at sea. He had been awarded the DSO and Bar for services during the First World War.

The Eastern Front

With most of Europe secure, Germany turned its attention eastwards and in June 1941 invaded Russia. Under the code name 'Operation Barbarossa' Germany allocated almost 150 army divisions totalling some three million men supported by 3,000 tanks and 2,500 aircraft. This formidable force was further strengthened by thirty divisions of Finnish

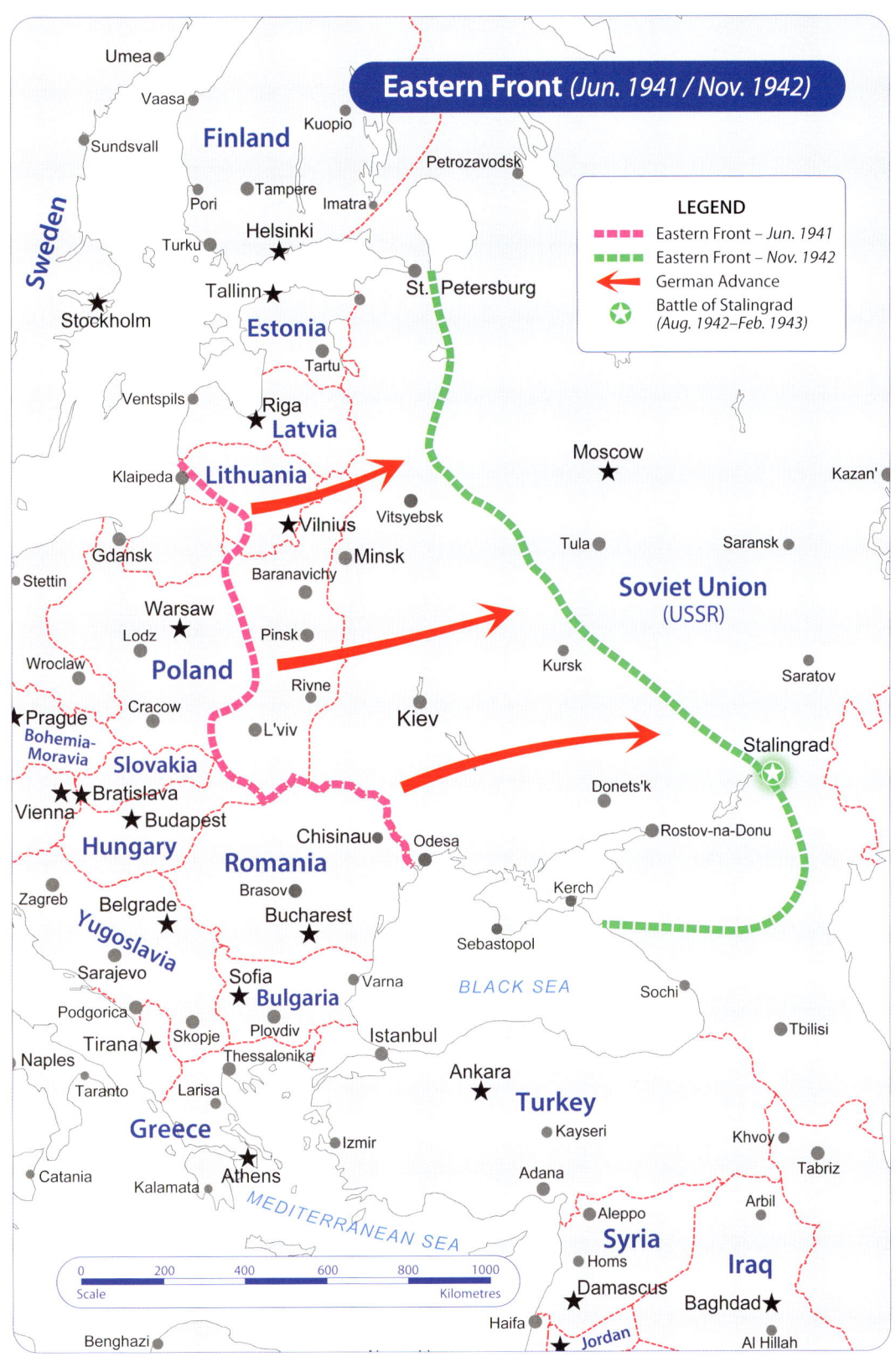

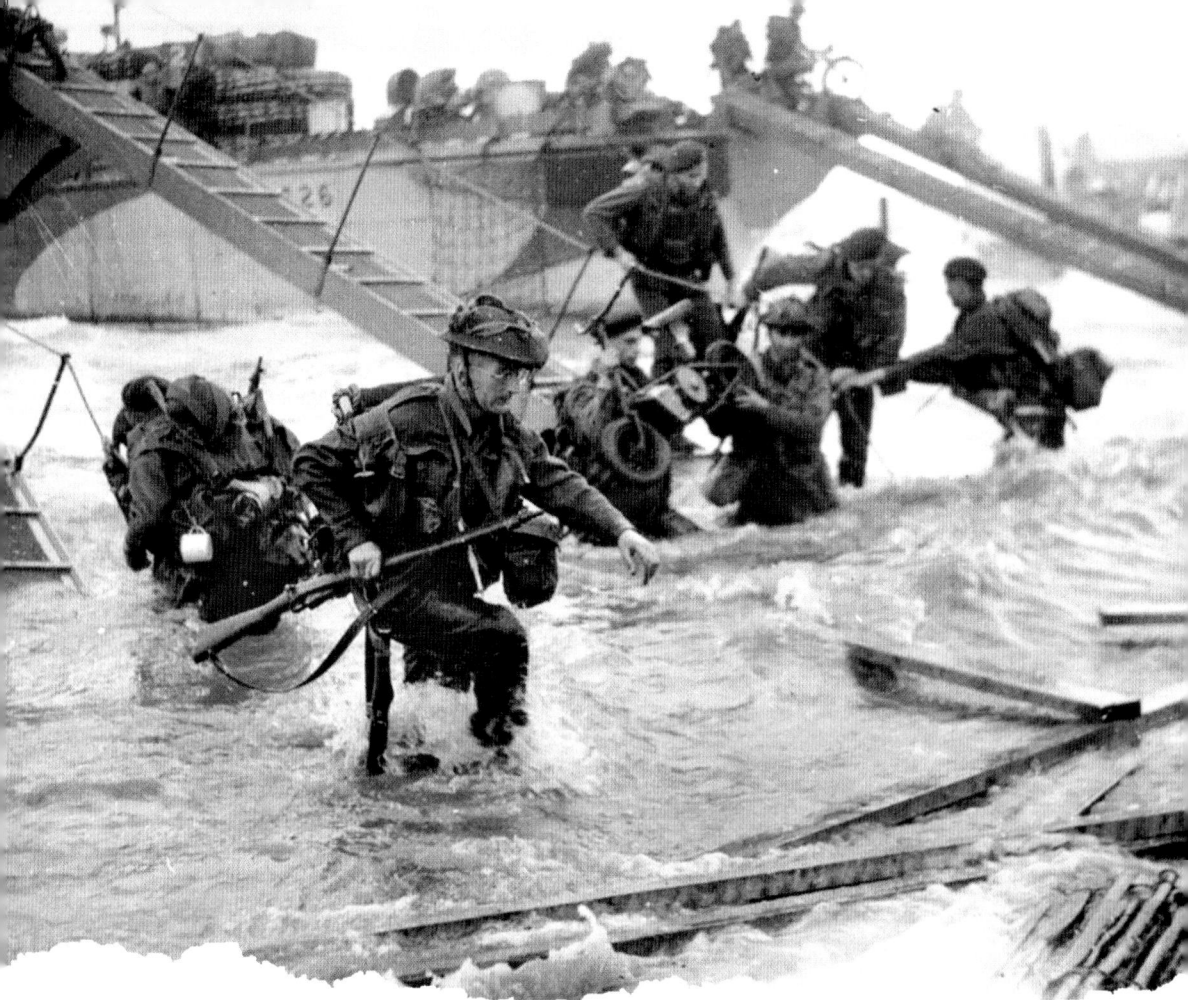

and Romanian troops. Despite stubborn Russian resistance, the German advance was rapid and by mid-July the German Army had advanced more than 650km and was less than 300km from Moscow.

However, despite this early progress the German advance was eventually stopped at Moscow. With the onset of a winter – the most severe in decades – and Russian counteroffensives, the German Army fell back and suffered enormous casualties. The war in Russia continued throughout 1942, eventually culminating in the battle for Stalingrad, considered by some to be the greatest battle of the Second World War.

In October 1942, with the Volga river at their backs, the Russian troops stopped the German advance on Stalingrad which had begun in August. Finally, following a massive counteroffensive by the Soviet troops in November 1942, the German forces, numbering some 91,000 frozen and starving men, surrendered in January 1943.

The Battle of Kursk in July and August 1943 was the greatest tank battle of the Second World War, involving 6,000 tanks, 4,000 aircraft and one million men. The defeat of the Nazi Army at the Battle of Kursk halted the German invasion of Russia and heralded the start of the end of this global conflict.

The End of the Second World War in Europe

The Western Front had remained static until the Allied forces launched their decisive invasion of Europe in June 1944 in the Battle of Normandy, code-named 'Operation Overlord'. Landing 150,000 American, British and Canadian forces using 5,000 ships and 11,000 aircraft, the Allies established a secure beachhead on France's Normandy coast.

A number of TCD graduates took part in Operation Overlord. William Anderson was wounded while accompanying the Allied Airborne Army ahead of the landings on the Normandy beaches. James Hearn and Robert Taylor were killed in action in June and July 1944 respectively.

The German Army put up stiff resistance, but by August the Allies had managed to break out from the Normandy coast landing area and liberate Paris, and by the end of 1944 they were at the German border. Gordon Sheill, a TCD graduate, had survived the Normandy invasion but was later killed in action in March 1945 during the Rhine crossing.

Victory over Germany soon followed with the fall of Berlin and the German unconditional surrender of 7 May 1945.

On 15 May 1945 the following article appeared in *The Irish Times*, quoting from a letter sent home by an Irish doctor with the RAMC to his family in Ireland:

> *Yesterday I spent about an hour-and-a-half in one of the German concentration camps (at a place called Belsen). There has been much publicity of it in the papers in the last week, but the reality is, at least, 20 times as bad as the photographs. Apart from beatings, hangings and shootings, the real keynote of the Nazi methods of getting rid of dangerous persons, or people they dislike, is by a process of slow starvation.*
>
> *In the camp there were about 60,000 people (about two-thirds of them women and children of all ages). Some had been there only a week or two, some for many months. For at least two months before the British army captured the place the daily ration was, morning and evening, rather less than a pint of turnip soup. In addition, once a week they received one-twelfth of a loaf of bread. The result is that the inmates present a picture of all the gradual stages of starvation – some of them literally skin and bone – diseases of every kind are rampant.*
>
> *When the troops arrived there were thousands of corpses lying about on the ground, and even now there are about 300 deaths a day. The Nazi guards have been put to the burial work. They comprise both men and women members of the S.S.*

The wretched prisoners were not criminals – just individuals whom the Nazis did not like – and for no crime they were allowed to die in the coldest and most callous manner that the human mind could devise. The place made a deep impression on me, and I came away very embittered against Germany and Germans.

Just before I left the officer who took me round – a little Scotchman with an apt turn of speech said – 'And we have got to remember that for the grace of God and the man who invented the Spitfire we would have this sort of thing in England.' That was the message which I brought away from Belsen. (Perhaps he might have included Ireland also.)

In the same article another Irish officer, an army chaplain with the RAF, is quoted as reporting to his family back in Ireland:

I visited one of Germany's concentration camps the other day, and the things I saw are incredible. When the camp was overrun by the army they found it infested with every disease known to man; typhus especially was rampant. The camp was a graveyard filled with thousands of dead bodies unburied. For the most part those that were alive were in no condition to bury the dead. They were mainly animals, living like animals and acting like them; their minds were gone and their bodies emaciated to such an extent that it would be possible for your finger and thumb to meet around their thighs.

In all there were 50,000 men and women of every European nationality. During the last month (March) it had been discovered that 17,000 men and women have been cremated in this camp. Such a figure may be difficult to believe, but you can take it as correct.

During the last four days the army has buried 3,000, and they are still dying like flies. Nothing can save them. They are too far gone.

You have been reading in the newspapers about the atrocities perpetrated in those camps. Well, if you multiply what you read by 100% you will arrive at something like the truth. The absolute horror of it is incredible.

If the Nazis had conquered England then the best thing we could have done would have been to shoot ourselves. Those who were killed immediately on entering these prison camps were lucky.

All these facts that I have given you are absolutely true. Folks in Ireland have been slow to believe such things. They need to be shaken badly.

They don't understand the horror of this war because it has not been brought home to them. They have spun their own little cocoon and have been indifferent to a great extent to the sufferings of humanity.

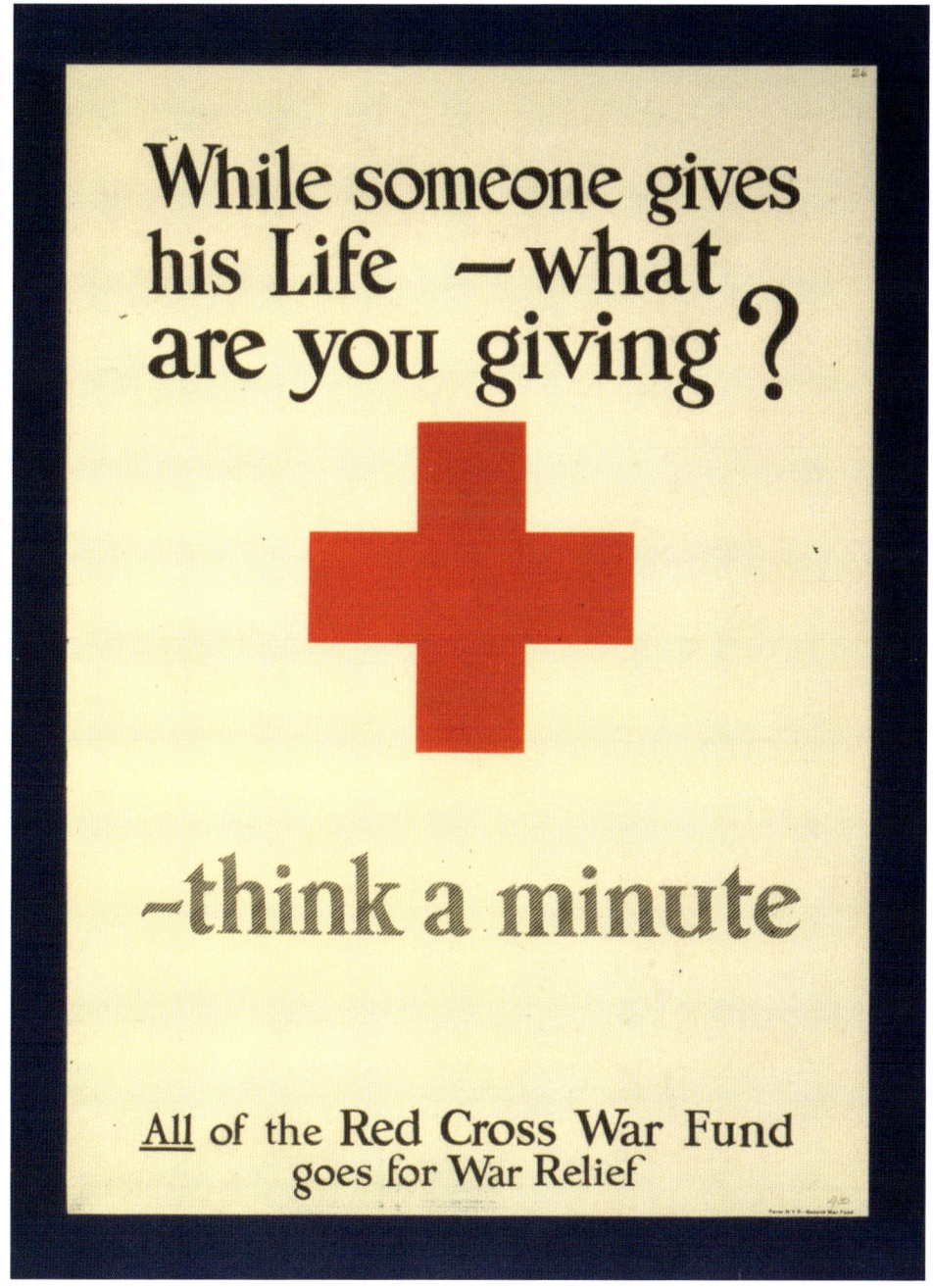

A number of Irish doctors are known to have attended at the Belsen concentration camp, including Nigel Kinnear and Francis Waldron of the RAMC and Martin Clancy of the RAF, along with Robert Collis of the Red Cross. William Hughes was the senior medical officer at the Belsen camp for a period in 1945.

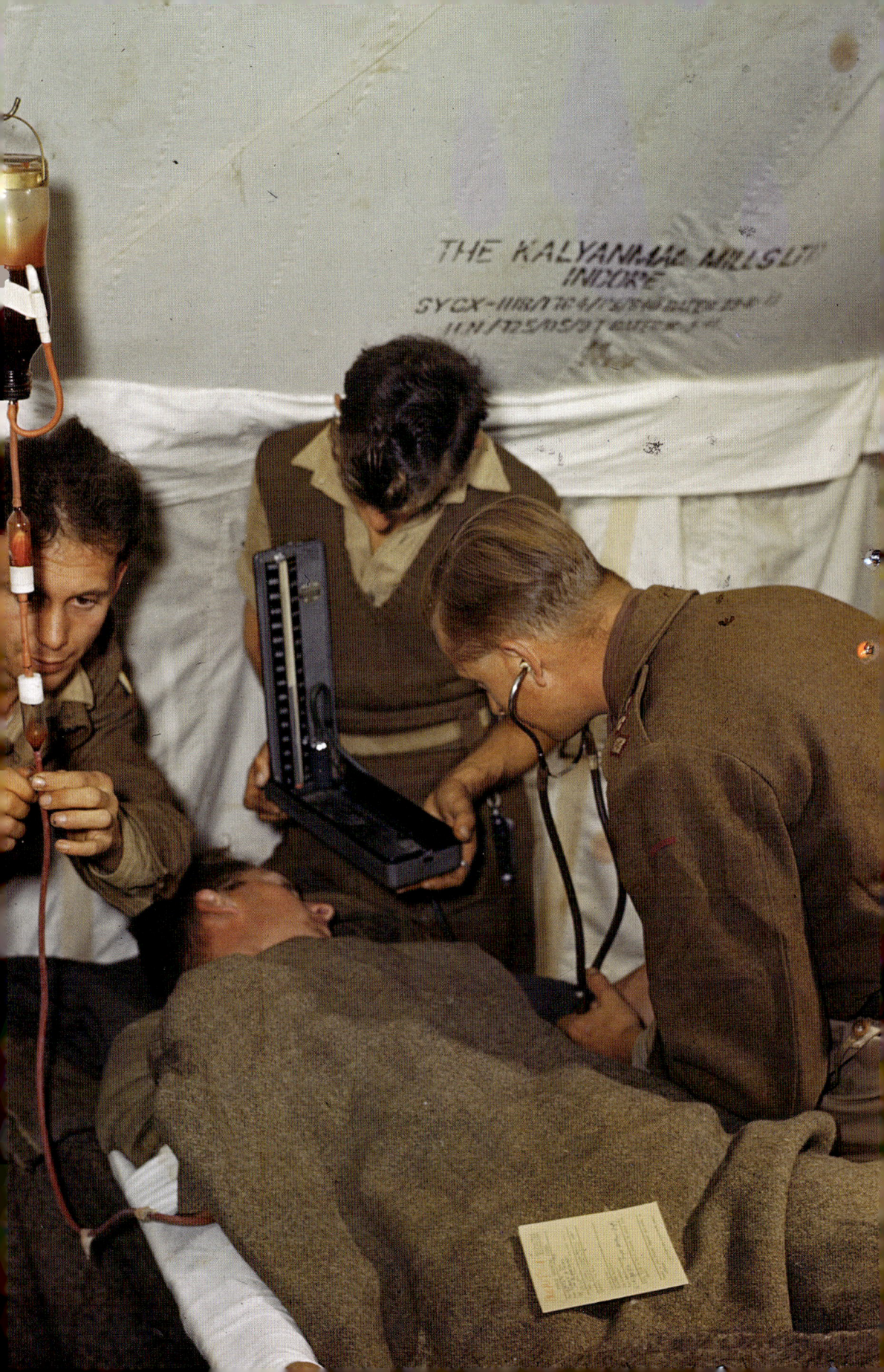

Chapter 4
IRISH DOCTORS IN THE FAR EAST

As had been the case in Europe, the Second World War in the Far East had its origins in the early 1930s. In 1931–32 the Japanese had invaded Manchuria in north-east China and created the Japanese-controlled puppet state of Manchukuo.
In July 1937 Japan captured the former Chinese imperial capital of Peking and in 1938 occupied Guangzhou (Canton) and several other coastal cities in south China. When war broke out in Europe in 1939 it opened up new horizons for Imperial Japan in south-east Asia and the Pacific Rim.

The Dutch East Indies (now Indonesia) along with French Indochina and British-held Malaya contained raw materials including tin, rubber and petroleum products. Control over these natural products would make the Japanese Empire self-sufficient and a dominant power in the Pacific. The German victories over France and the Netherlands in 1940 encouraged the Japanese strategists to look at the Far East colonies controlled by the British, French and Dutch, along with the Philippine islands.

Japan, then ruled by Emperor Hirohito, entered the Second World War when it sided with Germany and Italy in September 1941 and invaded French Indo-China. An attack on the United States' Atlantic fleet stationed at Pearl Harbour in Hawaii on

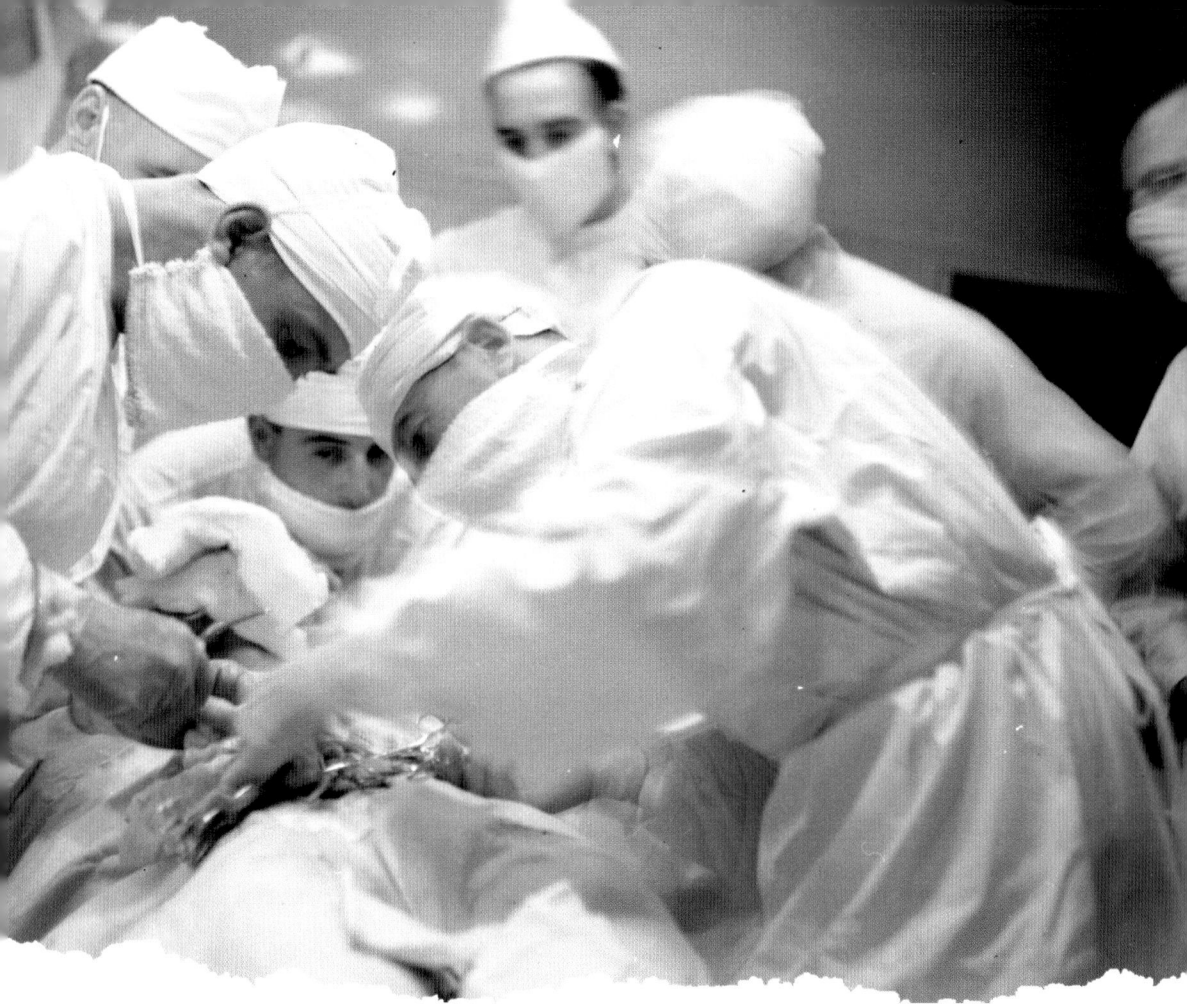

7 December 1941 heralded the Japanese expansionist policy. Following the Japanese attack on Pearl Harbour, the then American President Franklin D. Roosevelt obtained a congressional declaration of war against Japan. On 11 December 1941 Japan's allies, Nazi Germany and Fascist Italy, declared war on the United States. In response the United States formally joined the Allies and entered the European theatre of war.

Coinciding with the attack on Pearl Harbour, Japan launched an offensive against the British Crown colony of Hong Kong, which surrendered on Christmas Day 1941. With the sinking of the British battleship HMS *Prince of Wales* and battle cruiser HMS *Repulse* in the South China Sea off Malaya, the Japanese took control of the seas.

An Irish doctor casualty of the Japanese advance down the Malayan peninsula was William Anthony Cavanagh from Greencastle in County Donegal. A recent graduate of RCSI, he was a Surgeon Lieutenant on HMS *Repulse* when it was sunk by the Japanese Air Force off Malaya on 10 December 1941, having decided to remain with the injured.

The battle cruiser HMS *Repulse* sailed from Singapore on 8 December 1941, accompanied by HMS *Prince of Wales* and four destroyers, with the intention of thwarting a Japanese attack on the east coast of Malaya. Hearing that reports of this attack were untrue and having been spotted by the Japanese, the flotilla headed back towards Singapore. The *Repulse* received one hit from the first wave of high-level Japanese bombers, which caused a small fire that was quickly extinguished. The ship survived a second high-level and torpedo bomber attack an hour later, but during the third attack the *Repulse* was hit by five torpedoes and began to list heavily. Shortly after the crew were ordered to abandon ship it rolled over and sank.

Following the capture of Hong Kong, the Japanese forces invaded the Malayan Peninsula and speedily advanced south towards Singapore. As the Japanese forces advanced down the Malayan Peninsula, Allied outposts were overrun with the capture and imprisonment of Irish doctors who had been serving with the MMS. These doctors included John Ernest McMahon, Colman Nairnsey, Ernest Albert Smyth from County Laois and Charles Herbert Stringer from Armagh.

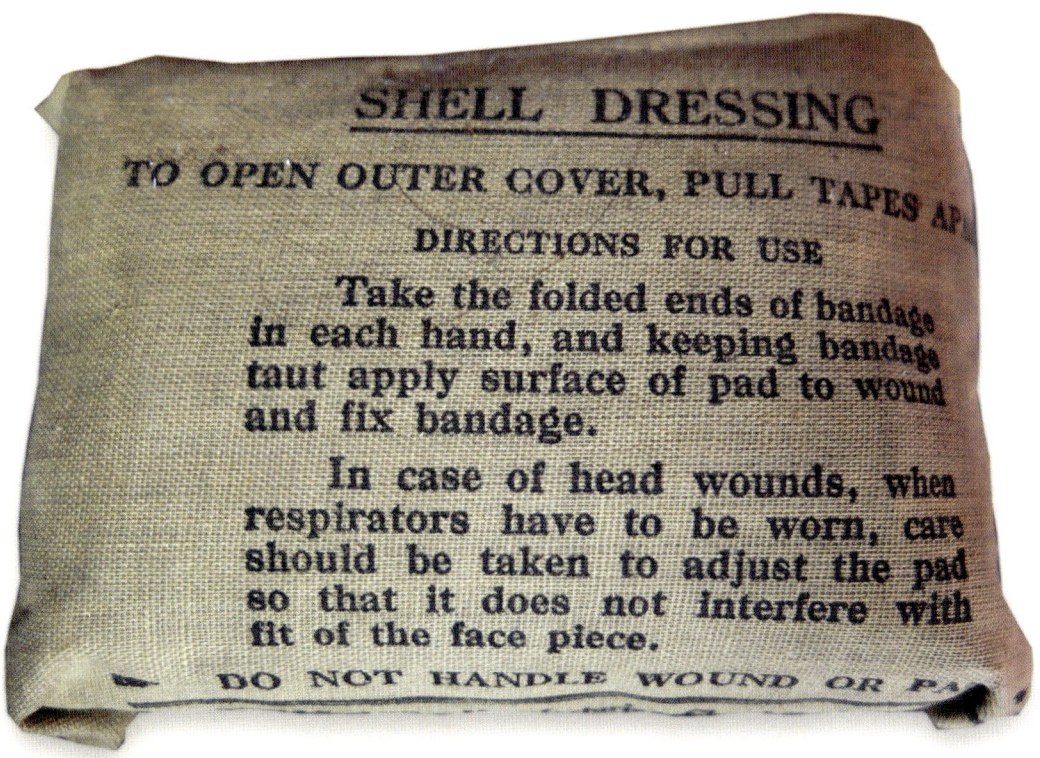

Within weeks of the attack on Pearl Harbour, Japanese forces had captured Manila in the Philippines and Kuala Lumpur on the Malaysian Peninsula and had invaded the Dutch East Indies (Indonesia) and Burma (Myanmar). The Japanese continued their advance through the region with the surrender of the Philippines in January 1942 and the capture of 70,000 American and Filipino POWs.

The harsh and often deadly treatment that those who surrendered to the Japanese forces were going to receive throughout the Second World War was announced on Christmas Day 1941, when the British colony of Hong Kong was captured by the Japanese Army. St Stephen's College at Stanley in the south of the colony had been a school for boys but was being used as a hospital for wounded soldiers. On entering St Stephen's, the Japanese soldiers set about bayoneting wounded soldiers while they lay in their beds. This was followed by the indiscriminate slaughter of other soldiers, doctors and nurses. There were 150 people killed and their bodies cremated. The Irish doctors who escaped the slaughter but remained as Japanese POWs for the following three years and eight months included John Allison Page from Glenageary, Dublin, Edward Joseph Curran from Glanmire, County Cork, Edward William Hackett and Sterling Tomlinson.

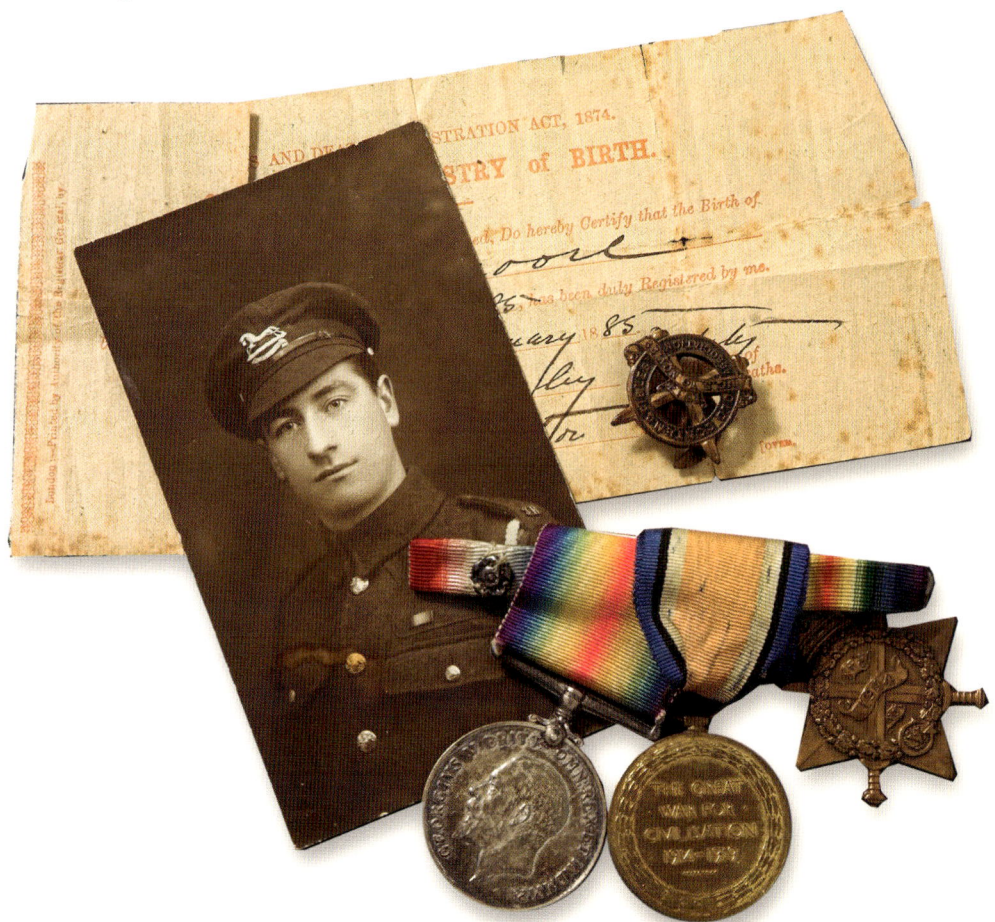

By February 1942 Japan had subdued much of the Malaysian Peninsula and was advancing on Singapore, the key British outpost in the Far East. Fighting started in the outskirts of Singapore on 8 February and lasted until the colony surrendered on 5 February, making it the largest British surrender in history. Humphrey Barron Thomson from Belfast, a recent graduate of QUB, was killed in action earlier in a Japanese attack on Singapore on 14 December and is commemorated on the Singapore War Memorial.

The fall of Singapore to the Japanese took place in February 1942, along with the capture of an estimated 80,000 Australian, Indian and British troops who joined the 50,000 of their compatriots who were taken during the Japanese invasion of Malaysia. The capture of the British colonies in the Far East, especially Singapore, included the capture of many Irish doctors who were serving there with the British forces.

The same dreadful treatment was experienced at the fall of Singapore as the surrendering forces had experienced at Hong Kong. When the Japanese captured Singapore their troops went through the first floor of the Alexandra Military Hospital and bayoneted every person there. They then entered the operating room, where a soldier was undergoing an operation. They bayoneted him, the anaesthetist and the surgeon. Afterwards they went to the second floor, and to other parts of the building, removed the patients and nurses and massacred them all.

Ransome McNamara Allardyce from Rathmines in Dublin, a 1926 medical graduate from TCD, was bayoneted to death when the Japanese overran Alexandra Military Hospital, Singapore, on 15 February 1942, and is buried in Kranji War Cemetery, Singapore. That cemetery is the final resting place for Allied soldiers who perished during the Battle of Singapore and the subsequent Japanese occupation of the island from 1942 to 1945 and in other parts of south-east Asia during the Second World War.

Allen, George	Hennessy, Edmond	MacFarlane, Gordon	O'Driscoll, Gerard
Anderson, Henry	Holmes, William	McNeilly, James	Pantridge, James
Egan, Eugene	Huston, John	McQuillan, John	Stewart, William
Grove-White, Robert	Hutchinson, William	Murray, Francis	Wilson, Robert

Table 13: Irish Doctors Who Were Captured at the Fall of Singapore on 15 February 1942

The surrender of Singapore in February 1941 was followed by the invasion of Bali in the Dutch East Indies later that month and the fall of the Philippines in May 1942. The capture of such colonial territories led to the incarceration of tens of thousands of Allied personnel, including Irish doctors in POW camps in the Far East and on mainland Japan.

When the Indonesian island of Java was captured, two more Irish doctors were taken prisoner – Flight Lieutenant Joseph Aidan MacCarthy from Castletownbere in west Cork and Flying Officer Frederick William Parke from Dalkey, County Dublin. RAF reinforcements had been originally directed to support the defence of Singapore, but unfortunately arrived too late and were instead redirected in Java where they would eventually surrender, along with their Dutch allies, to the Japanese in March 1942.

The Japanese victories in 1942 were the beginning of three-and-a-half years of harsh treatment for the Allied prisoners, including atrocities like the Bataan Death March and the misery of Japanese prison camps, along with the 'hell ships' on which Allied men were sent to Japan to be used as slave labour in mines and factories. Thousands were crowded into the holds of Japanese ships without water, food or sufficient ventilation. The Japanese did not mark 'POW' on the decks of these vessels, and some were attacked and sunk by Allied aircraft and submarines, leading to the death of thousands of Allied prisoners.

Allen, George	Huston, John	McQuillan, John	Smiley, Thomas
Anderson, Henry	Hutchinson, William	Moss, John	Stewart, William
Canton, Nathaniel	MacCarthy, Aidan	Murray, Francis	Stringer, Charles
Curran, Edward	MacFarlane, Gordon	Nairnsey, Colman	Tomlinson, Sterling
Egan, Eugene	MacFarlane, Lennox	O'Donnell, Thomas	Wallace, Hugh
Egan, John	Mayne, Brian	O'Driscoll, Gerard	West, George
Grove-White, Robert	McCarthy, Charles	Page, John	Wilson, Robert
Hackett, Edward	McCartney, Ernest	Pantridge, James	Wilson, Thomas
Hennessy, Edmond	McMahon, John	Parke, Frederick	
Holmes, William	McNeilly, James	Smyth, Ernest	

Table 14: Irish Doctors Who Were POWs in the Far East Theatres of War

The Allied naval victories over Japan in the sea battles of Coral Sea and Midway in May and June 1942, along with the land offensive on Guadalcanal in the Solomon Islands from August 1942 to February 1943, marked a transition by the Allies from defensive operations to offensive ones and allowed them to take the strategic initiative in the Pacific theatre of war from the Japanese.

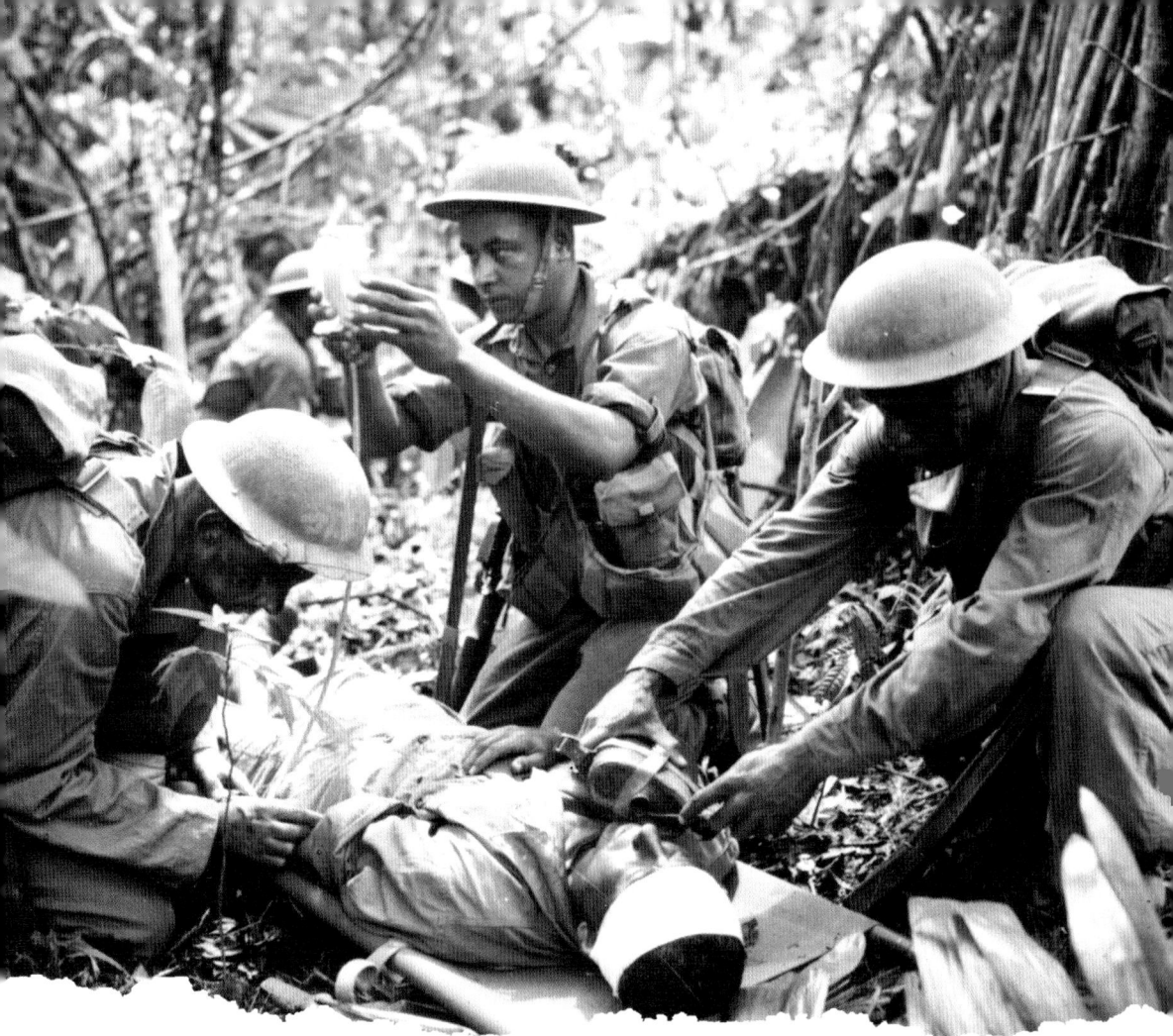

    The Allied success in the Solomon Islands was soon followed by a further defeat of the occupying Japanese forces on Kwajalein in the Marshall Islands in January 1944 and on Saipan in the Marianas, and the capture of Guam island in August 1944. The Allied push into the Philippines was followed by the taking of islands closer to the Japanese mainland: Iwo Jima in March 1945 and Okinawa in June 1945. Along with their advances in the Pacific islands, the Allies were also having success on land, with the capture of the Burmese city of Mandalay in March 1945 and of Rangoon (Yangon) in May 1945.

    The refusal of Japan to surrender to the Allied forces in July 1945 was followed by the dropping of the world's first atomic bomb on Hiroshima on 6 August, followed by a second dropped on 9 August on Nagasaki. The surrender of Imperial Japan was announced by Japanese Emperor Hirohito on 15 August and formally signed on 2 September 1945, bringing the hostilities of the Second World War to a close and the release of many thousands of Allied POWs from their years of harsh incarceration.

One of the first doctors to enter Yokohama Harbour on the east coast of mainland Japan to tend to the thousands of sick POWs was George Frederick Hunt, an NUI graduate from Coolaney in County Sligo. He was then commanding a hospital ship that was operating with the Pacific Fleet strike force.

The experiences of QUB graduate Francis Joseph Murray and UCC graduate Joseph Aidan MacCarthy as POWs, both of whom ended their years of incarceration as commanding officers of POW camps on the Japanese mainland, are recounted in Chapter 5.

The Second World War ended with the unconditional surrender of Japan on 2 September 1945. The war had caused devastation all over the world. Over nineteen million human beings, both military and civilian, had died in the conflict, and vast swaths of cities in both Europe and Asia had been levelled. The Irish doctors in the accompanying Roll of Honour took part in this global conflict and in doing so brought great honour both to themselves and to their country.

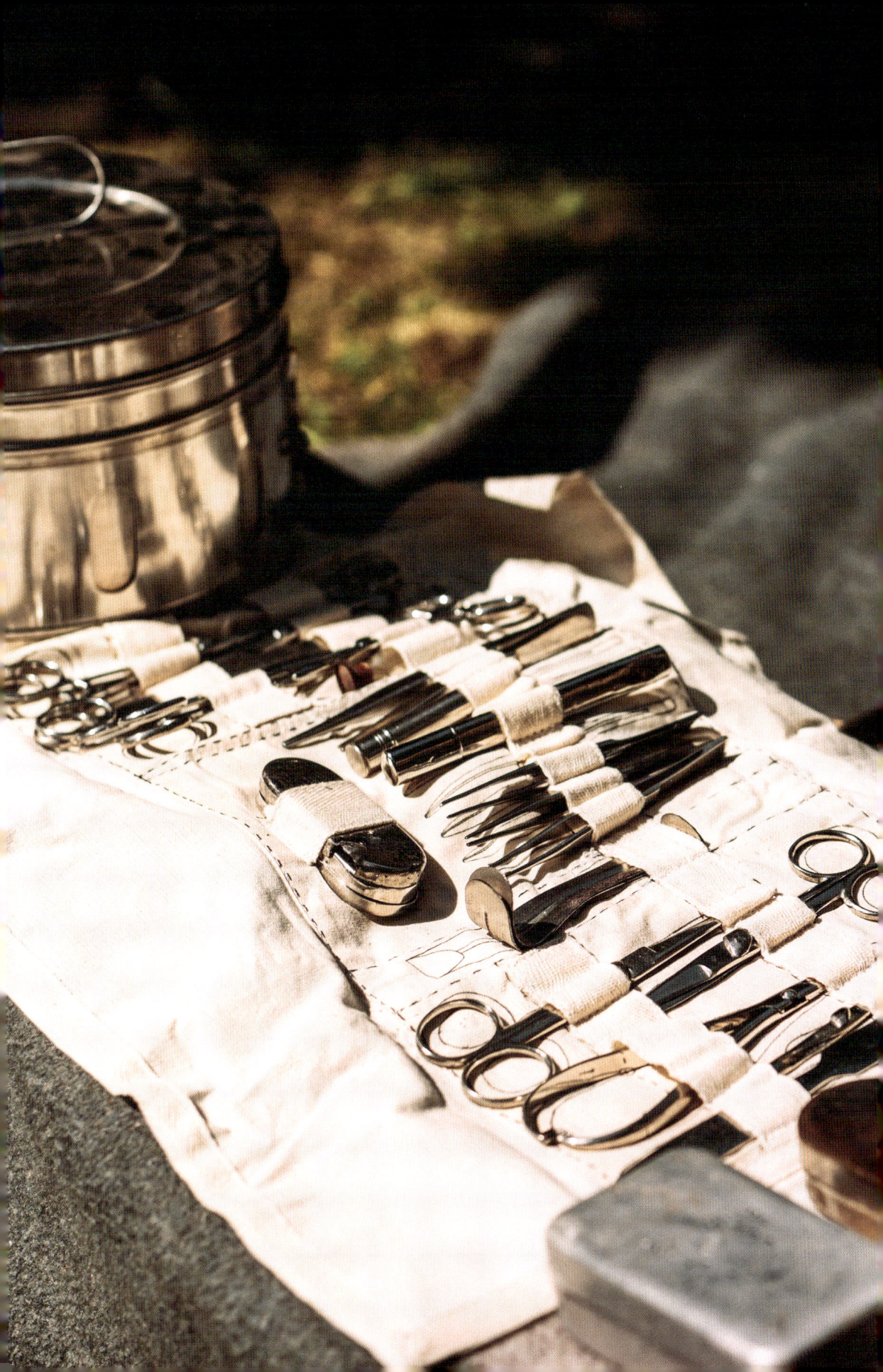

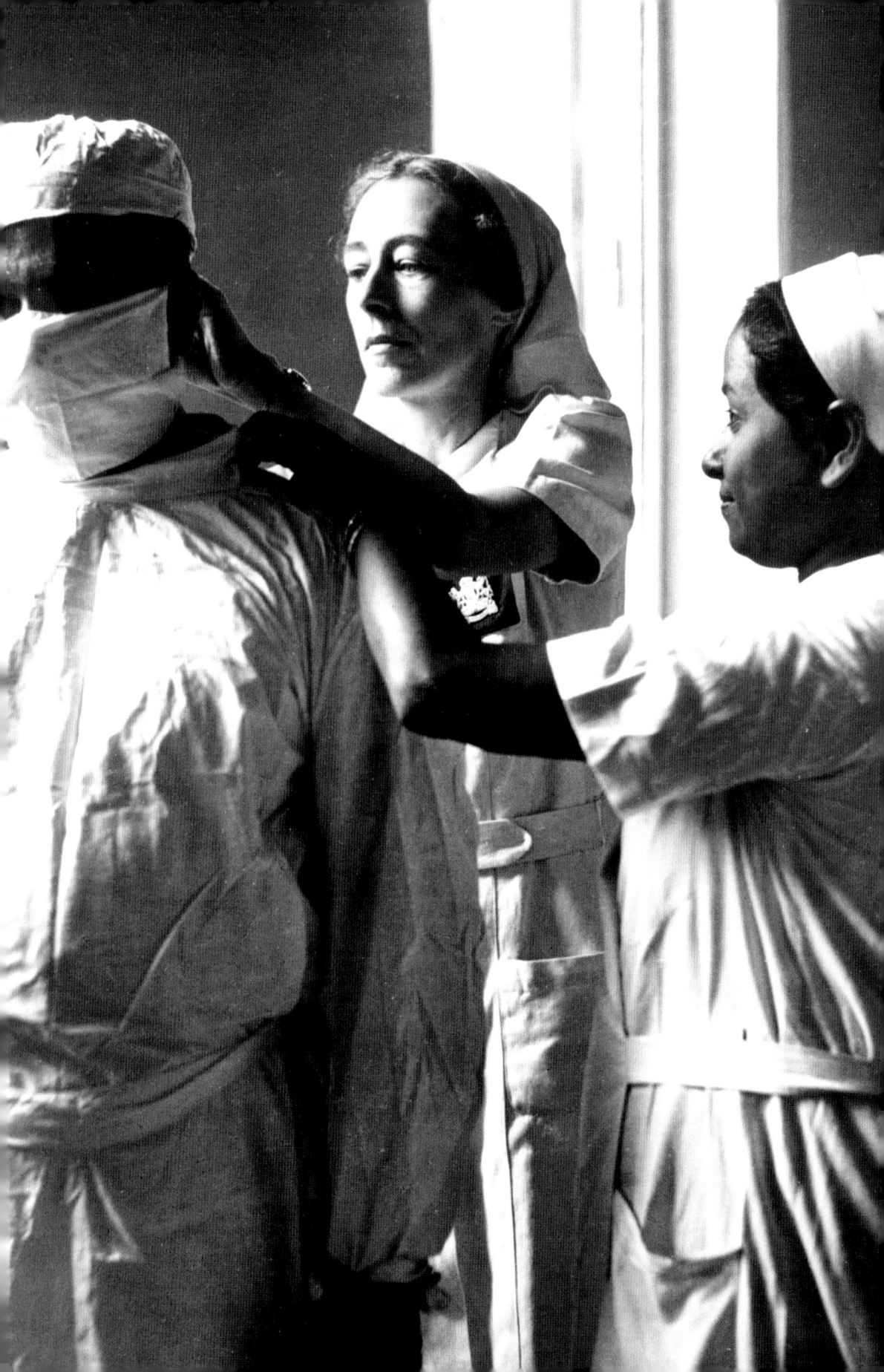

Chapter 5
IRISH DOCTORS AS PRISONERS OF WAR

A prisoner of war is someone who is held captive by a belligerent power during an armed conflict. They are held in custody for a variety of legitimate and illegitimate reasons. These include isolating them from enemy combatants still in the field, demonstrating military victory, punishing them, prosecuting them for war crimes, exploiting them for their labour, recruiting them, collecting intelligence from them or even indoctrinating them.

The Geneva Convention on the Treatment of Prisoners of War was signed in Geneva on 27 July 1929 and came into force in 1931. It is this version of the Geneva Convention which covered the treatment of POWs during the 1939–45 war. The Allied armies were ordered to treat Axis prisoners of war strictly in accordance with the 1929 Geneva Convention. Germany and Italy also generally treated Allied prisoners in the same way. Japan had not signed the Geneva Convention by 1941 and so did not feel bound to conform to the protections it afforded to POWs. Cultural differences between Western and Far Eastern nations were also to play a major role in the contrasting treatment between POWs held by the Allied and Axis forces in Europe and those captured by Japan.

Article 12 of the 1929 Geneva Convention states that medical personnel may not be retained after they have fallen into the hands of the enemy and that they should be returned to their parent country as soon as possible. Sadly, this did not happen.

Under the 1929 Geneva Convention, doctors, being commissioned officers, were not required to work, although many were put to work and did so willingly as medical officers in their camp. In general, they were treated well, the main complaint being the lack of food. It was the same for the German and Italian troops, especially in the latter years of the war. They were very grateful for the food parcels which arrived regularly via the International Red Cross. In some camps the officers were allowed out of the camp into the surrounding towns on condition they did not try to escape. For most officers the camps were an opportunity for learning something different from their regular work and for entertainment, since they put on musical shows on a regular basis.

Also under the 1929 Geneva Convention, POW camps should be open to inspection by authorised representatives from a neutral power. Article 10 required that POWs should be housed in buildings with adequate heat and lighting, where conditions were the same as for their own troops. Articles 27–32 detailed the conditions of labour. Enlisted men were required to perform whatever labour they were asked and able to do, so long as it was not dangerous and did not support the captor's war effort. Senior non-commissioned officers (sergeants and above) were required to work only in a supervisory role. Commissioned officers were not required to work, although they could volunteer. The work performed was mainly agricultural or industrial, including coal or potash mining, stone quarrying, or work in sawmills, breweries, factories, railway yards and forests. The workers were also supposed to get one day of rest per week.

During the early years of the war in Europe, especially during the retreat to Dunkirk in June 1940 and the fall of Tobruk in June 1942, many male members of the medical services were captured and spent the rest of the war in captivity. Overall, they were treated in compliance with international laws, but some experienced harsh conditions when held in camps in Eastern Europe.

In the Far East both male and female members of the medical services were captured and suffered appalling deprivations, often in jungle and remote camps. A large number of those taken prisoner in the Far East were captured when Singapore surrendered on 15 February 1942, while others were captured when Burma and the Dutch East Indies were overrun.

These members of the medical services, suffering as a result of deprivation and disease, carried on and provided medical care to their fellow prisoners, often with little or no medical supplies. Where there was a shortage of supplies their ingenuity prevailed and they improvised their equipment and medicine.

The treatment of POWs by Japanese forces was particularly harsh and brutal but fitted in with their belief that those who had surrendered to them were guilty of dishonouring their country and family and, as such, deserved to be treated in no other way. Japanese POWs were subject to murder, beatings, summary punishment, brutality, forced labour, medical experimentation, starvation rations and poor medical treatment.

More than 170,000 British and 120,000 American prisoners were taken by German and Italian troops during the war and were held in 1,000 POW camps stretching from Nazi-controlled Poland to Italy. These POW camps were separate from the concentration camps, which had an entirely different purpose.

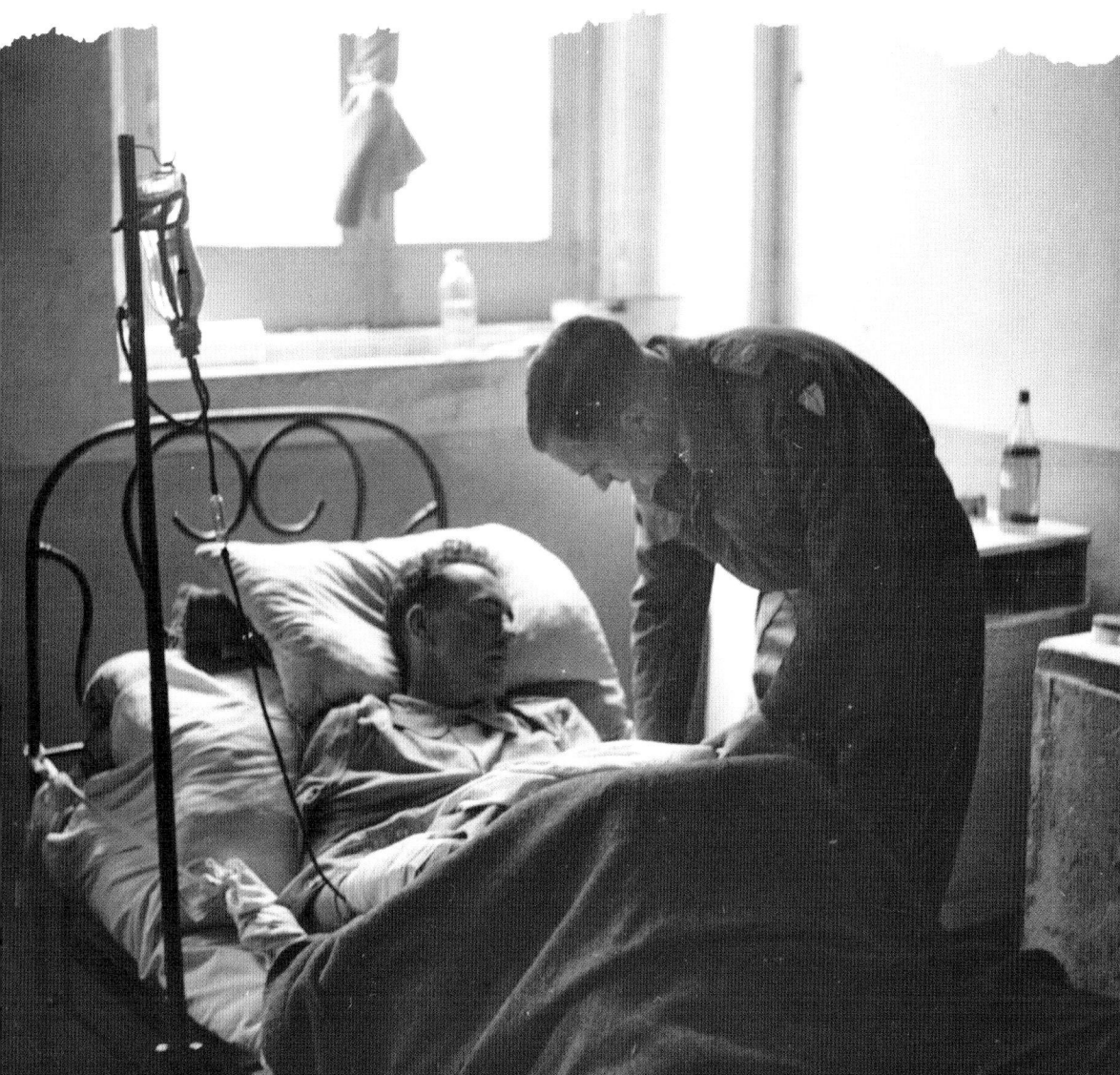

Japanese armed forces captured nearly 140,000 Allied military personnel in the south-east Asia and Pacific areas. About 36,000 were transported to the Japanese mainland to supplement shortages in the workforce, and compelled to work at coal and other mines, shipyards and munitions factories. By the time the war was over a total of more than 30,000 POWs had died from starvation, diseases, and mistreatment, and some 11,000 POWs tragically had lost their lives when Allied air and submarine forces attacked ships transporting POWs to Japan.

Fifty-two Irish doctors became POWs between 1940 and August 1945 before the war in the Pacific ended. The Axis forces held eighteen in Europe and North Africa, while at least fifty Irish doctors were taken prisoner by Japanese forces as they swept through the South China Sea, including some who were members of the MMS, who had been serving the civilian population on the Malayan Peninsula.

A number of Irish doctors have described their treatment and experiences as POWs. Francis O'Meara and Ion Ferguson were German POWs between 1940 and 1945. Aidan MacCarthy and Frank Murray were captured in different parts of the Far East, but both ended up as POWs on the Japanese mainland by the time the war finally ended in 1945. The contrast between being a POW in Europe and in the Far East is clearly highlighted by the following testimonies.

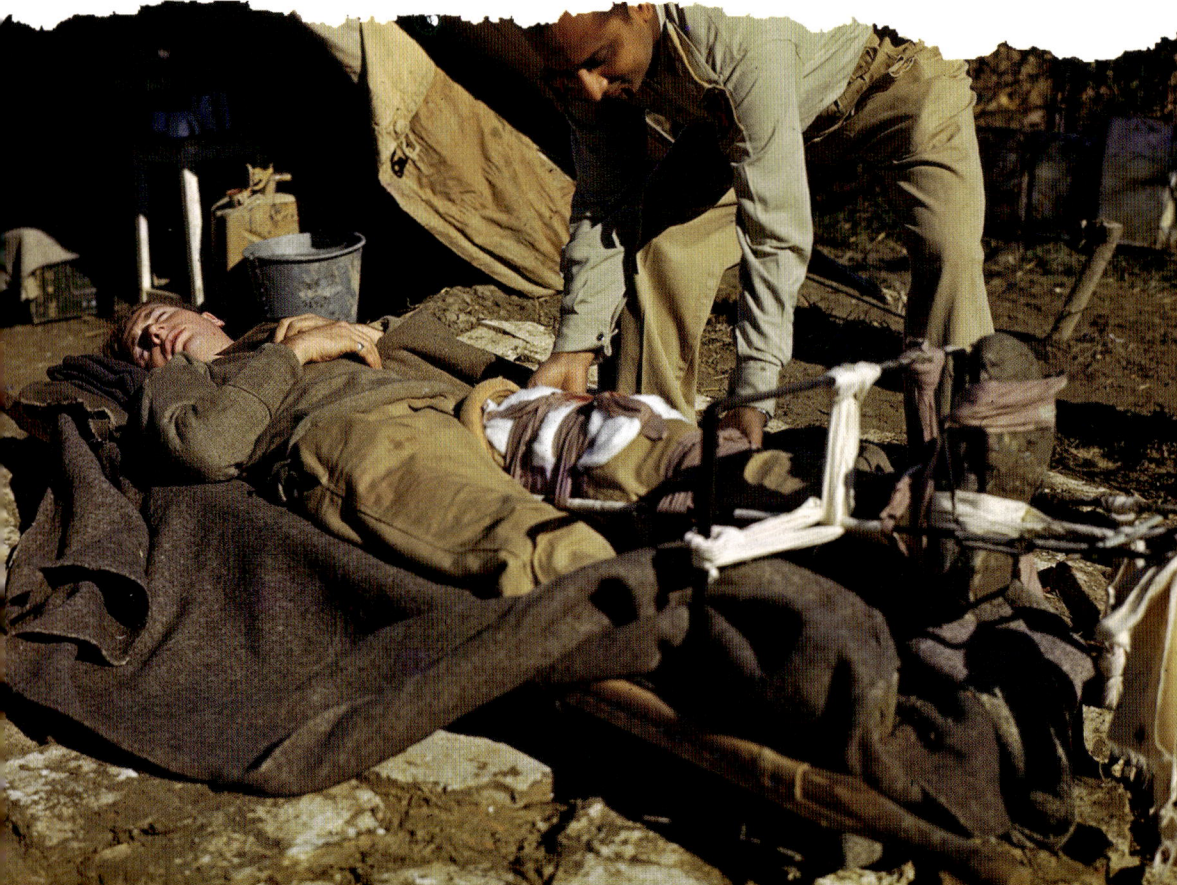

Major Francis O'Meara

Francis O'Meara, from Skibbereen in County Cork, qualified from TCD (1923) and RCPI (1926). After serving in the college's Officers' Training Corps (OTC), he became a captain in the RAMC in 1927 and was promoted to major in 1934. He was posted to France as part of the BEF and was captured at Fontaine la Bourg, north of Rouen, on 9 June 1940, and was taken by lorry with five others to a POW camp in a field 32kms to the rear. Each succeeding day they marched 20kms towards Germany.

On 29 January 1941 he was escorted into Germany from Cambrai via Brussels to Cologne. The destination was Spangenberg in Hesse-Kassel in the middle of Germany. There the officer's camp had been organised in a forestry school and was divided into two camps with a headquarters in the town. The *ober* or upper camp was in a fortified castle on top of a hill dominating the town. It was surrounded by a moat containing a wild boar and two sows. Major O'Meara was consigned to the *unter* or lower camp in the nearby village of Elbersdorf. This was a wired enclosure in the centre of the village around the buildings of the forestry school.

The organised life of the village and its animals and fowl, particularly the geese, was a source of constant interest. When he arrived it was mid-winter, the ground was frozen and there was snow everywhere. The British Red Cross Society had been active during the stalemate of 1939–40 and had supplied a library of 5,000 books to the camp. The officers had organised themselves and there was an active education programme in place, a weekly magazine and a dramatic society which organised a concert or play every Saturday night. And so the winter passed.

In August 1941 O'Meara was sent to Bad Sulza, Thuringia, to a men's camp of between 30,000 and 40,000 prisoners, where he worked as the British Medical Officer. His job was to examine the British patients as they arrived in camp and present their history to the German doctor when he visited the next day. During the time he was there, there was an outbreak of typhus in the camp which required Major O'Meara and the medical orderlies to quarantine for forty days. Even so, the German doctor and a number of the orderlies died of the infection.

The long, weary winter of 1941–42 came to a close and in April 1942 Major O'Meara was sent to another camp, this time in Hildburghausen in the state of Thuringia. This was an unspoilt baroque town in a very beautiful setting of wooded hills and was a pleasant time in his life as a POW, made better since he was brought shopping by a German interpreter.

Early in 1943 he was moved to a camp in Stadtroda, where he became an internist without pay. That involved a good deal of X-ray screening of patients with respiratory symptoms to pick out the POWs with tuberculosis, which was quite common. He worked there until May 1944, when he was repatriated. He insisted that all the British medical personnel be repatriated together.

They went by train to Metz and then down the Rhone valley to Marseilles. There they boarded a hospital ship which took them to Barcelona, where they were exchanged for German POWs. They were then transferred to a Swedish liner staffed by the American Red Cross, being lavishly entertained and treated very kindly. They sailed to England by a complicated route via Algiers, the Azores, the mid-Atlantic and up to Belfast. There, after a civic reception, they were transferred to a West Indian ship for the journey to Liverpool, where they were given a second civil reception.

Major Francis O'Meara was promoted to the rank of major general in 1955 and ultimately retired to Hertfordshire.

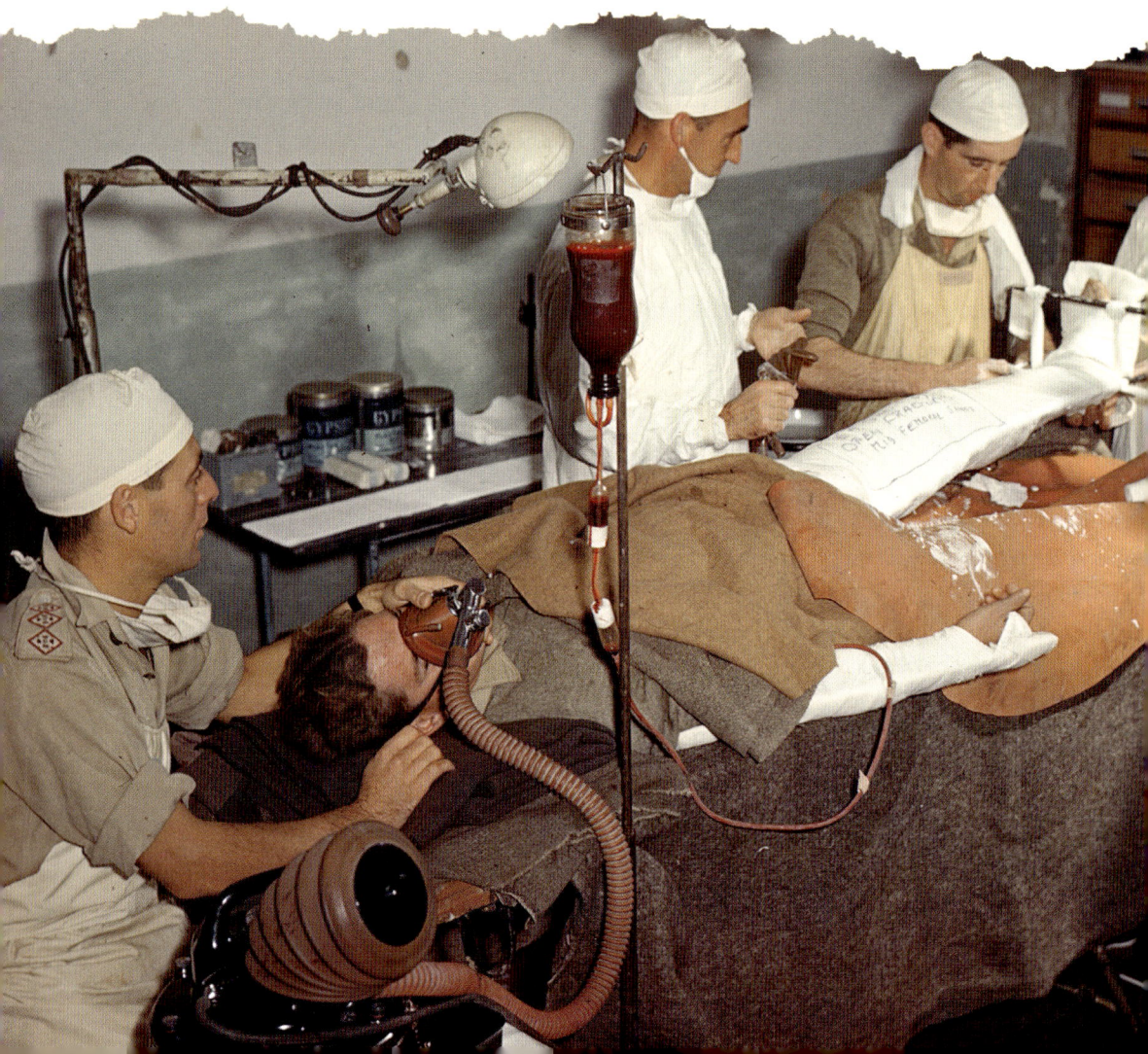

Ion Thomas Ferguson

Ion Thomas Ferguson from County Kildare qualified from RCSI in 1939 and enlisted in the RN. After a period of duty serving with HMS *Mackay* on convoy protection duty in the Atlantic, Ferguson was invalided out of the RN due to his debilitating seasickness. After a period in civilian life, he enlisted in the RAMC in May 1940 and was posted to a military veterinary hospital in Palestine. In spring 1941 he was transferred initially to the 30th RAF Squadron at Eleusis in Greece and shortly afterwards to the 26th General Hospital in Athens.

Following the German invasion of Greece and the evacuation of the Allied forces, Ferguson became a POW on 28 April 1941 and was incarcerated in a POW camp in Corinth. At the end of June 1941 he was transferred to Stalag 18A at Wolfsberg in Austria, and then to an *arbeitskommando* camp (i.e. a work detachment or subcamp for POWs to be used as labour camp) close to the Austrian–Yugoslavian border.

Ferguson, in his book *Doctor at War*, describes how the POWs were sleeping 100 to a hut in very overcrowded conditions, but nonetheless the quarters at the *arbeitskommando* were better than those he had endured in Corinth or Wolfsberg. Ferguson's task as medical officer was to ensure that sufficient men out of the 400 under his care turned out to work every morning at the nearby dam. He was continually a difficult officer for the camp commander to deal with, as he would not certify sufficient numbers of men as fit for work as deemed appropriate by the German High Command. His continued obstructiveness eventually led to him being transferred to Oflag IVc, Colditz, in August 1942. Most of the men in Colditz Castle had been confined there for their constant attempts to escape from other camps.

Ferguson describes that while the physical health amongst officers was very good, in many cases their mental health bordered on the psychotic side of normal behaviour. This was primarily due to the boredom that followed from their inability to carry out any meaningful tasks or work. Every day followed a set pattern, starting at 7 a.m. with the morning *Appell*, when all ranks of every nationality lined up in separate groups in the courtyard. When the numbers turning out tallied, the German officer would dismiss the parade, but the prisoners made it a point of honour never to move, unless and until they received a command to do so from a senior officer of their own nationality.

After morning *Appell*, the prisoners returned to their quarters to wash and have breakfast. Then the dishes had to be cleaned and the dining room brushed out. By about 10 a.m. most of the tables were reoccupied by men who were using their enforced leisure to learn a foreign language. Ferguson describes how the chronic escapers among the POWs 'could be seen making ropes from bed covers and Red Cross string or anything else that would serve their purpose. The passport forgers, the map copyists and the compass manufacturers were to be found busy in corners, each closely guarded by a look-out.'

After lunch, 'which usually consisted of watery and lukewarm sauerkraut soup which congealed on the plates as soon as it was placed there, the bell would sound for the afternoon *Appell*'. After the roll call the prisoners made their own recreation. The table-stooges served some tea at 4 p.m. and then until 6 p.m. 'most of the chaps walked around the *hof* (central courtyard) in the eternal circle'.

The evening meal was at 6 p.m. and was the most substantial of the day. 'We often got bully beef or spam then, from the Red Cross parcels, with hot potatoes, and tea and bread and cheese followed.'

The time of the evening *Appell* varied, but it was usually around 7 p.m.:

> *The soul-destroying part of it all was that we had nothing constructive to do. The psychological effect on men being doomed to undertake no constructive task during those years of their lives when they would normally have been most energetic, created a feeling of deep frustration … Lights out at 9.30 pm came as a blessed relief for it meant the end of another wasted and useless day.*

In early 1943 Ferguson decided on a ruse to get himself released from Colditz. On St Patrick's Day he wrote a letter to Éamon de Valera, the son of the then Irish prime minister, who had been a student colleague but not personally known to Ferguson.

> *I decided to write to him in Dublin and to give the impression that he was a close personal friend of mine and that I was a frequent visitor to the de Valera household before the war. I slipped this letter into the prisoners' post box in the hof, knowing full well that the Germans would never let it through, but realising that it would probably be sent to the OKW for their observations.*

A fortnight later, after *Appell* one afternoon, Ferguson was sought out and was told: 'Herr Doctor, the Kommandant has received instructions from the OKW that you are to be released and sent to work at a Stalag.'

At the beginning of April 1943 Ferguson walked through the great stone archway of the castle 'with an overwhelming sense of gratitude that I was out of Colditz, alive and sane'.

Ferguson was transferred to Stalag IVd at Torau: 'My new prison was Res Lazarett Schmorkau situated about 20 miles from Dresden.' The Stalag 'housed many nationalities, Yugoslavs, Russians, Poles, French, Dutch, British and Dominion troops'. Ferguson was the senior British officer and in addition to his responsibility for the physical health of the prisoners he also cared for the mental department, 'which was full to capacity'.

In late 1944 Ferguson decided that he would convince a visiting Swiss Repatriation Commission that he was insane, suffering from *Haft Neurosis* (detention neurosis) and so was suitable for repatriation. He managed to get himself certified as a lunatic and on 23 January 1945 he started his journey back to England via Constance in Switzerland and Marseilles to Liverpool after three years and ten months as a POW. Ion Ferguson returned to civilian life and practised medicine in Whitworth, England.

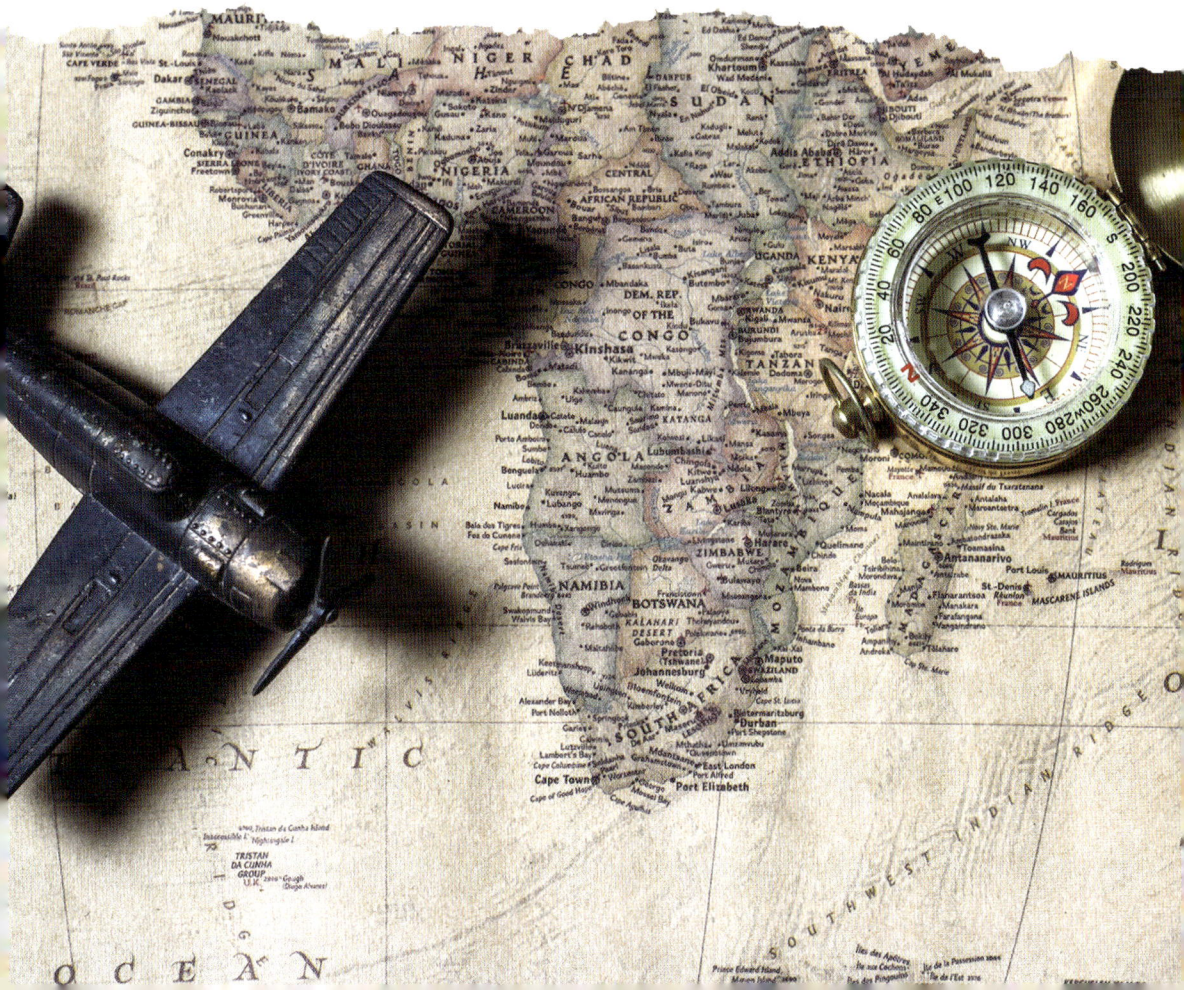

Alexander Draffin

Alexander Draffin from Ballybay, County Monaghan, qualified from QUB in 1939. At the outbreak of the war, he volunteered for the RAMC and became the medical officer to the 2nd Battalion of the Royal Norfolk Regiment. The Royal Norfolks travelled with the BEF to France and Belgium, with Draffin becoming the youngest person to serve as a regimental medical officer with the BEF.

Draffin was captured when the German Army overran France in May and June 1940, and remained under German imprisonment for most of the war. However, he was troublesome to his captors, even as a prisoner. He was notorious for multiple escape attempts and acts of rebellion. Due to this behaviour, he was transferred to many different camps. At one camp he managed to save ninety of his fellow prisoners during one of his escape plans. Unfortunately, he was wounded and captured before he escaped. His constant efforts to escape resulted in multiple terms of solitary confinement and camp transfers, but when these measures failed to faze him, he was transferred to Colditz Castle. He remained there from August 1943 until September 1944.

Draffin continued his escape attempts even while in Colditz Castle, but he never succeeded in escaping from the Germans. He finally managed to escape captivity only after the Russians had taken over from the Germans. His last escape was as eventful as the rest of his imprisonment. Before he escaped, he saved six German nurses with a smart move. He asked them to hide in the cellar and he wrote on the door 'Typhus Ward – Keep Out' in German, Russian and English. Because of his distrust of the Russian Army, he swam across the River Elbe to the American Second Army to ensure his liberation.

He married Margaret R. Lyle in July 1948 in Newcastle-upon-Tyne. That year he obtained the Diploma of Laryngology and Otology and started working as an otolaryngologist. He worked in various hospitals, including the Hospital of St Cross in Winchester, the Manor Hospital and George Eliot Hospital in Nuneaton and South-East Kent Hospital Group. He was also active academically and published several medical articles with international citations. He published about his eponymous invention, the 'Draffin Bipod', in 1951 in the *British Medical Journal*. This was a device to hold a gag mouthpiece in place during ear, nose, throat and dental procedures. The device was a complete success and became popular around the world.

Despite his active career in clinical practice and research, he never passed the examinations for the Fellowship of the Royal College of Surgeons and therefore he was never officially a consultant. He was also a very successful businessman and was involved in real estate dealings.

On 30 March 1967 he was found dead in his flat in West Kensington, London.

Frank Murray

Frank Murray from Belfast qualified at QUB in 1937 and moved to Birmingham to practise as a doctor. In December 1939 he was commissioned into the RAMC and was posted initially to India but was soon transferred to Malaya as second in command of a field ambulance based at Ipoh, Kroh (Keroh) and finally at Kuantan, on the east coast of the Malaya Peninsula. Soon after Japanese forces invaded Malaya in December 1941, he was appointed commanding officer in charge of a motor ambulance convoy and was ordered to move to Singapore in January 1942, where he eventually became a POW following the surrender of the British colony on 15 February 1942.

As a POW, Major Frank Murray was firstly interned at Changi camp on the eastern coast of the Singapore island. Changi camp was one of the more notorious Japanese POW camps and was used to imprison Malayan civilians and Allied soldiers.

In the summer of 1943 Murray was transported to Hokkaido, the northernmost of Japan's main islands. There he moved between the Hakodate camp, Yakumo camp, Muroran camp, Raijo camp, which is near Nisi Ashibetsu, Utashinai camp and finally Akabira camp, where he was liberated in early September 1945, following the surrender of Japan on 15 August.

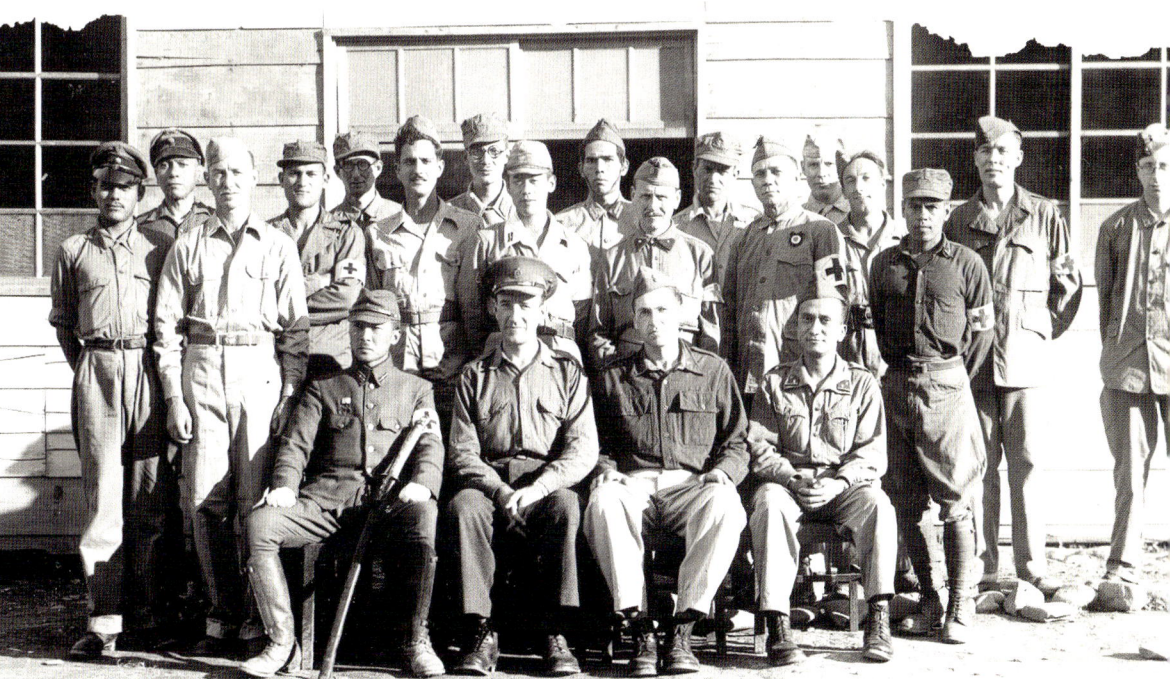

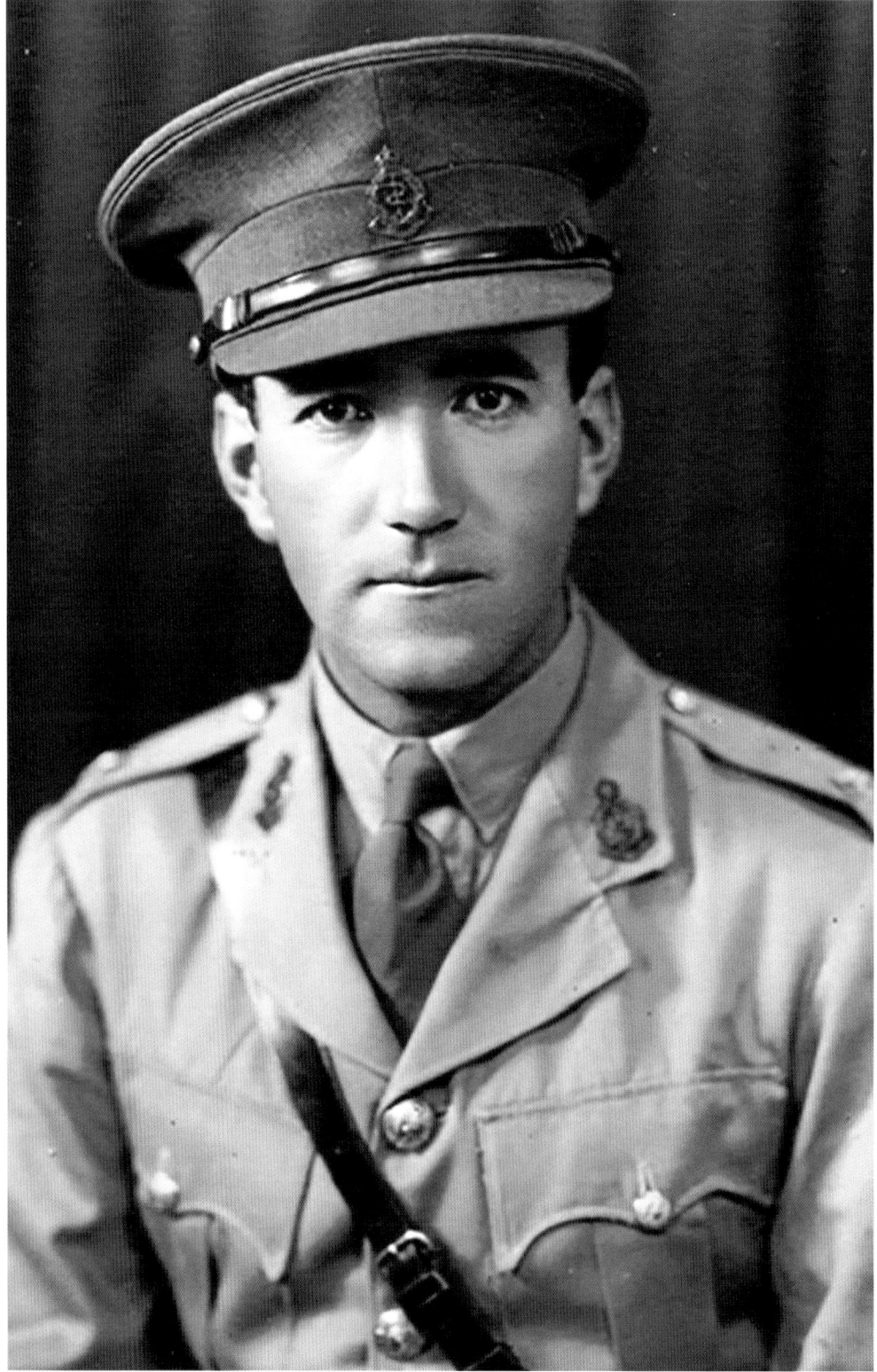

In February 1944 Major Frank Murray became the officer commanding the troops in the Muroran POW camp when more senior officers were moved to other camps. The exemplary manner in which Murray carried out his duties both as a commanding officer and as a doctor while a POW is best summarised by the moving testimonial (see below) presented to him and signed by 348 former fellow POWs on 6 September 1945, shortly after the surrender of Japan.

Frank Murray returned to Belfast in November 1945, married his fiancée Eileen O'Kane in February 1946 and was awarded an MBE in the same year. He settled down and ran a family medical practice in Belfast until he retired in 1974.

Major F. J. Murray
Royal Army Medical Corps

Dear Major Murray,

In this moment of our release from the purgatory of Japanese incarceration, we feel your absence and wish you were here to share our happiness as you shared our want and humiliation till seven weeks ago, when you were removed from this camp. The great majority of us have known you for over three years – since the 'Mucky' Maru of May 1943. You were our only Medical Officer at the Prisoner of War Camps at Hakodate, at Yakumo and during the worst period at Muroran. Since early last year you have been Officer Commanding British and American Prisoners of War and Senior Medical Officer at Muroran and here. During these two years – the blackest period of our lives – you were at all times and in all places a genuine friend to each and all of us.

Your quiet and indomitable struggle for our health and welfare in the face of obstructive and often vicious Japanese inhumanity; your tenacity in carrying on though it fell to you at times to watch, helpless, men suffering and dying for want of food and simple but essential medicines and surgical instruments; your dignity in dealing with the Japanese and patience with their interfering swashbuckling medical orderlies; the tonic of your dry humour which exorcised any tendency for self-pity; your extraordinary memory and intimate knowledge of every one of sometimes more than four hundred men; your ability to maintain discipline, without force to back you, in very trying living conditions; your understanding of and forbearance with the occasional aberrations of some of us, which we now sincerely regret; the reforms you introduced and vigilantly enforced to ensure honest distribution of the little food and Red Cross supplies available; the utilization of your private funds for the benefit of the sick; your unwavering patience with each of us according to his needs; all this, and much else, we shall never forget.

Many of us would not be alive at this happy moment but for your care; from the point of view of health all of us owe you more than we can express. You have been an inspiration to everyone and to very many of us a source of spiritual refreshment and courage.

Whatever wider recognition you may, as we hope, ultimately receive, we all, the men of the British Navy, Army, Air Force and Mercantile Marine and the American Army now in this camp want you to know that [it] is with feelings of profound gratitude, affection and respect that we say

God Bless You, Sir.
Nisi-Asibetu. Japan. August 1945.

Before evacuation, the former POWs were requested to make statements (as affidavits) against the conduct of any Japanese officer or guard during their three-and-a-half years of captivity. The majority of those were rounded up, tried by military and civilian tribunals and punished by hanging or prison sentences.

The following is a summary of the statement made by Frank Murray for the war crimes trial undertaken by the General HQ/Supreme Commander for the Allied Powers:

On the 11 January 1946 Major Francis Joseph MURRAY R.A.M.C. executed an affidavit, the original of which is on file with Criminal Registry Division. MURRAY stated in substance, that he was captured by the Japanese at Singapore 15 February 1942, and was in Changi Prison until May 1943, at which time he was taken to Hakodate P.O.W. Camp #1 located at Muroran. Murray stated that from 1943 until February 1944 Major R.R. STEWART was the senior British officer of the camp, and that after that time he (MURRAY) was the senior British officer, until June 1945. MURRAY stated that on 18 December 1943, Pvt. SUTTLE was sentenced to 10 days in the guard house for stealing a piece of fish and that SUTTLE was put in the guard house without any blankets or medical attention though the time was mid-winter.

MURRAY stated that on the 23 December SUTTLE was removed from the guard house in extremis – his feet were gangrenous and that SUTTLE literally froze to death and died one hour after entering the hospital. MURRAY stated that Sapper GLOVER died of acute Osteomyelitis owing to the refusal of the Japanese authorities to permit his being taken to the fully equipped Japanese hospital nearby or to supply MURRAY with the instruments. Murray stated that the camp commander and Sgt. Major ARAKI were responsible for GLOVER's death. MURRAY stated that there were beatings daily at the camp and that S/M ARAKI often beat sick men and sent them

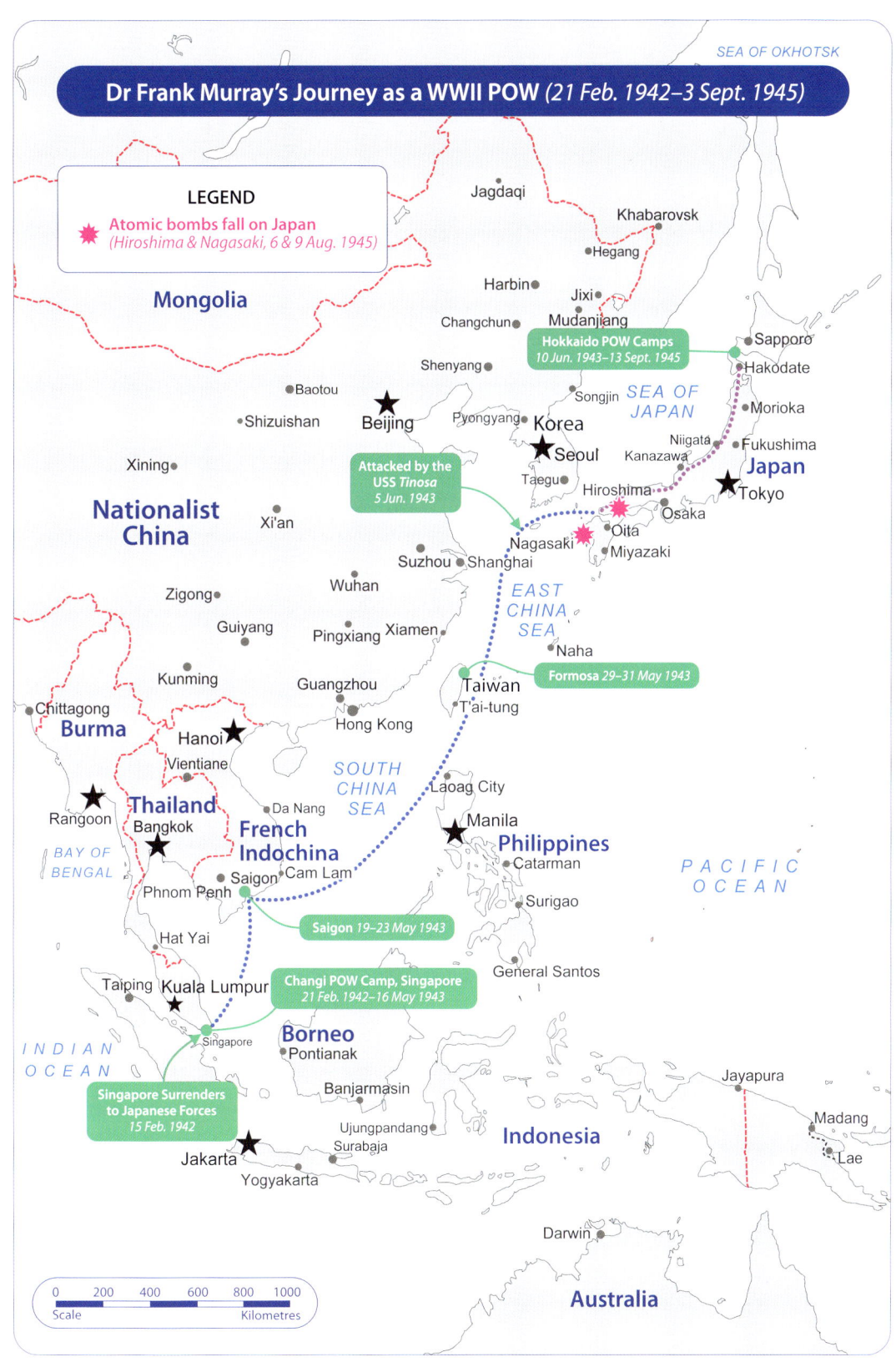

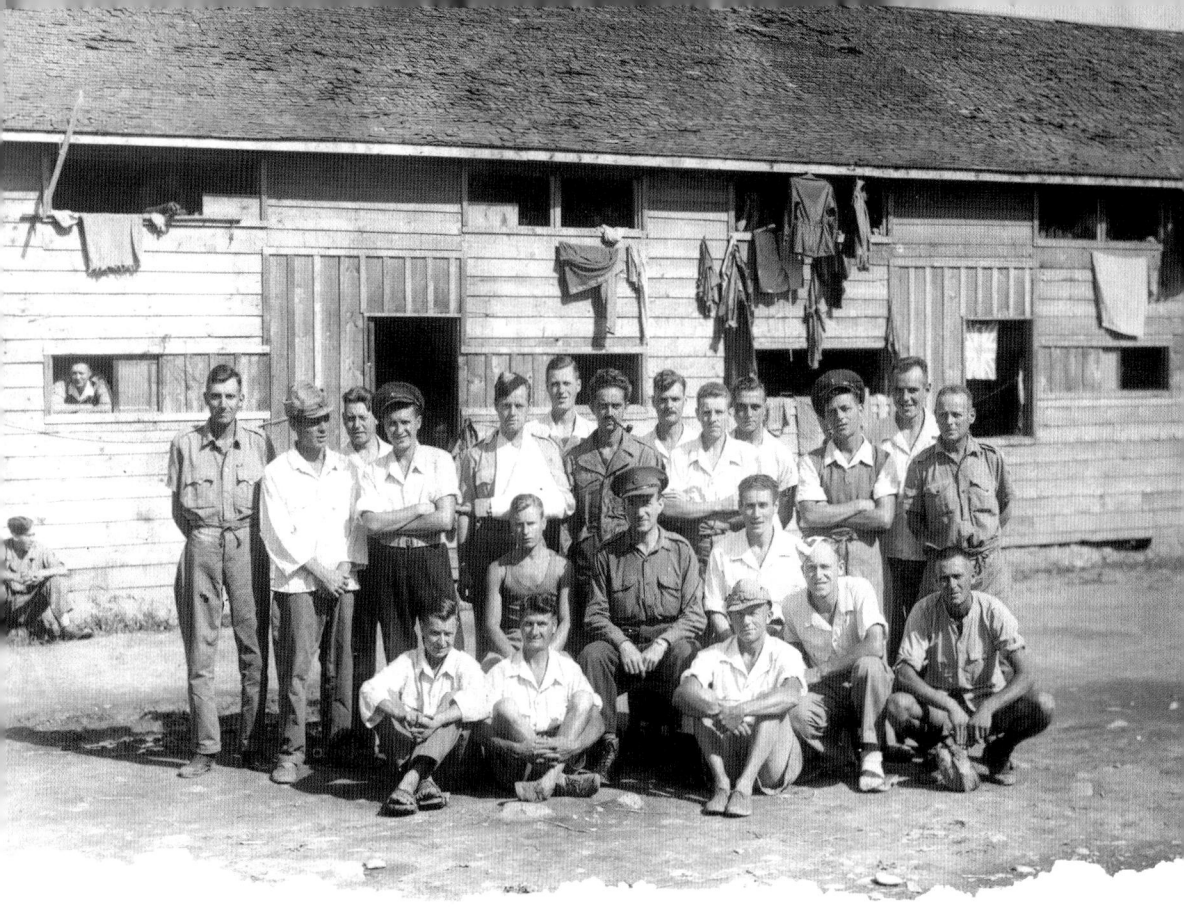

out to work. MURRAY stated that the Q.M. Sgt. (name unknown, but identified by P/Sgt. CAMPBELL as ASARI) made a point of beating someone every day, usually with his fist, and that on one occasion the Q.M. Sgt. split a man's head open with a sword scabbard. MURRAY stated that the camp guards were particularly brutal and that in spite of protests to the Camp Commander were never restrained. MURRAY stated that WATANABE was a particularly brutal guard and on one occasion lined 30 men up in a barracks room and knocked each man down with his fist. MURRAY stated that food was bad and entirely insufficient but that after the cessation of hostilities the Japanese produced every kind of food imaginable, butter, eggs, milk, meat, etc., which proved that they had the food available and that they could have provided better food had they wished. MURRAY stated that Dr. SHIBA a Japanese Military Doctor lined all sick men of the camp up in the snow and kept them on parade for two hours and beat every one across the face, and that Dr. SHIBA said that there were too many sick men in the camp and did this to discourage sickness. MURRAY stated that on 5 June 1945 Hakodate Camp #1 moved to Nishi Ashibetsu, and that at the new camp there were no special atrocities but that the general conduct of the camp officials was bad. MURRAY stated that on 5 June 1945 Hakodate Camp #1 moved to Nishi Ashibetsu, and that at the new camp there were no special atrocities but that the general conduct of the camp officials was bad. MURRAY stated that there was no water supply and that they had to rely on a stream outside the camp for water for 500 men quite inadequate. MURRAY stated that at this camp the food became really bad and that everyone grew thin but that fortunately they lost no one through starvation. MURRAY stated that as punishment the guards would stand a man outside the guard room for periods of 24 to 48 hours without food and that the prisoner would usually collapse after the end of 24 hours at which time they would be carried in to the guard room. MURRAY stated that authorities refused to allow any communication pass through to the Red Cross, so therefore no copies of any reports are available. MURRAY stated that H.F. PERRINS, W.P. BYRNE and W. COLLIER could give evidence of the facts which he had stated.

As a result of this and affidavits from other prisoners, the following were convicted after trials:

Kuniichi ARAKI; original verdict: hanged by the neck until dead (subsequently commuted to twenty years hard labour)

Eiji ASARI; original verdict: twenty-five years' confinement at hard labour

Kaichi HIRATE; original verdict: death by hanging

Tsutomi SHIBA; original verdict: five years' confinement at hard labour

Aidan MacCarthy

Dr Aidan MacCarthy from Castletownbere in County Cork qualified from UCC at the end of 1938. In common with many of his fellow medical graduates he moved to England in search of medical work and acted as a locum in general practice in both London and south Wales. By the outbreak of hostilities MacCarthy had joined the medical wing of the RAF on a short service commission. In December 1939 he was posted to France as part of the BEF and remained there until the German advance through Holland, Belgium and Luxembourg into France in May 1940. He was evacuated from Dunkirk along with the other 380,000 British and French troops who managed to escape the onslaught by the German Army.

In July 1940 Aidan MacCarthy was assigned as squadron leader at RAF Honington, a bomber command station on the Norfolk/Suffolk coast. Dr McCarthy was awarded the GM, the highest award for bravery in the British services for non-combat personnel, citing his actions in rescuing trapped airmen when a returning bomber crash-landed on

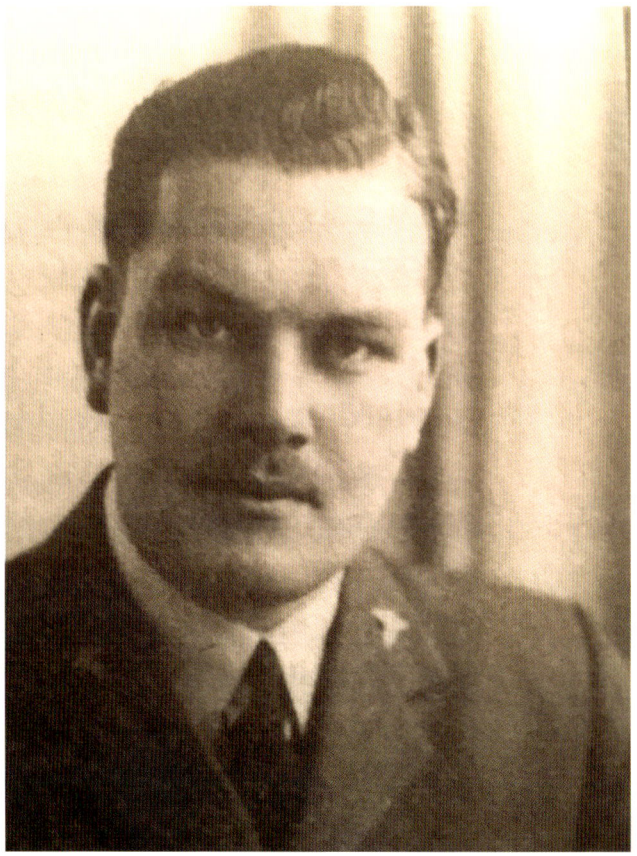

a bomb dump at Honington base. Along with Group Captain John Astley Gray he was presented with the GM by King George IV at Buckingham Palace in November 1941.

In December 1941 MacCarthy was appointed senior medical officer and was being posted along with a squadron of Spitfire and Hurricane fighter planes to North Africa. However, following the Japanese invasion of Malaya in December 1941, 116 Squadron was redirected to the Far East for the defence of Singapore.

MacCarthy's boat did not reach Singapore before it fell in February 1942. Instead, his convoy was diverted to the port of Batavia (now Jakarta) in Java, Indonesia, where they disembarked, unloaded their supplies, and assembled their planes. Java fell to the invading Japanese forces in March 1941 and the twenty-seven serving Allied doctors, of whom nineteen were Irish, became POWs. MacCarthy was initially interred in POW camps on Java, including Cycle camp, until May 1944, when he was transported to mainland Japan.

The Cycle camp, Batavia, was located in a former Dutch army barracks and was managed by a drug addict and sadist called Lieutenant Sonne who operated a particularly harsh regime. He was convicted at the end of the war and hanged for his treatment of Allied POWs.

The US fleet was active in the Pacific and was routinely attacking Japanese Navy and merchant shipping. And so, on 24 June 1944, as MacCarthy's ship the *Tamahoku Maru* approached mainland Japan, the American submarine USS *Tang* attacked the convoy, unaware that some of the ships were carrying POWs in their holds.

There was no escape for the prisoners below. In the ensuing chaos the survivors hung onto any floating wreckage and McCarthy recalls how the prisoners took vengeance on their former Korean guards as they too tried to seek safety out of the sea.

The POW survivors from the shipwreck were eventually picked up by a passing fleet of whaling boats, brought ashore and led to the Urakami Valley, the industrial centre of Nagasaki. There the POWs were incarcerated in Camp Fukuoka 14B where they were forced to work in the Mitsubishi Corporation shipyard until the end of the war.

In the autumn of 1944, the Japanese moved all the senior ranking POW officers to Manchuria, leaving doctors, dentists and clergymen as the senior Allied officers in the camps. MacCarthy suddenly found himself the senior ranking officer in POW camp 14B. From the time he became the senior ranking POW officer, McCarthy received the same punishment as each offender because they were his responsibility. Unfortunately for MacCarthy, his name sounded the same to Japanese ears as MacArthur, which was the surname of the commander of the American forces in the Pacific. His captors thought he must be related to General Douglas MacArthur and so they beat him on the head every time he was required to speak his name. These daily beatings took their toll many years later when he developed headaches and was thought to have a brain tumour. In fact, it turned out to be a benign brain cyst, which was excised, and he made a full recovery.

Amazingly, Aidan MacCarthy survived yet another explosion when the US air force dropped an atomic bomb onto Nagasaki on 9 August 1945. The sufferings that MacCarthy had already witnessed as a POW would be added to by the indescribable horrors that followed the explosion of the 'Fat Man' atomic bomb. Anyone within 1km of the blast was killed instantly or in the minutes after. MacCarthy and the rest of the POWs at 14B survived because they were some distance underground and around 1,600m from the epicentre of the explosion. MacCarthy, in *A Doctor's War*, described the moments before and after the explosion of the 'Fat Man' atomic bomb as follows:

In the shelters we prayed that there would not be a direct hit. A couple of POWs did not bother to go to the shelters, staying on the surface and crouching on the ground in the shadow of the barrack huts. They were gazing at the sky, watching the approaching vapour trails. One of them shouted to us that three small parachutes had dropped. Then there followed a blue flash, accompanied by a very bright magnesium-type flare which blinded them. Then came a frighteningly loud but rather flat explosion which was followed by a blast of hot air. Some of this could be felt by us as it came through the shelter openings, which were rarely closed owing to the poor ventilation.

Then an Australian POW stuck his head out of the shelter opening, looked around and ducked back in, his face expressing incredulity. This brought the rest of us scrambling to our feet and a panic rush to the exits.

The sight that greeted us halted us in our tracks. As we slowly surveyed the scene around us, we became aware that the camp had to all intents and purposes disappeared. Mostly of wooden construction, the wood had carbonized and turned to ashes. Bodies lay everywhere, some horribly mutilated by falling walls, girders and flying glass.

The gas mains had exploded, and those people still on their feet ran around in circles, hands pressed to their blinded eyes or holding the flesh that hung in tatters from their faces or arms.

But most frightening of all was the lack of sunlight – in contrast to the bright August sunshine that we had left a few minutes earlier, there was now a kind of twilight. We all genuinely thought, for some time, that this was the end of the world.

In 1948 MacCarthy married Kathleen Wall and was awarded the OBE for his medical work in the POW camps. He retired from the RAF in 1971, having attained the rank of air commodore, the highest rank attainable by non-combat personnel.

Dr Aidan MacCarthy OBE, GM, MB, BCh, BAL, Knight of Sylvester, Air Commodore RAF (retired), died in 1995 and is buried in Castletownbere, County Cork, where his grandfather had started MacCarthy's General Supply Store, which eventually became MacCarthy's Grocery and Bar. The high regard in which he is still held by the RAF is demonstrated by the fact that a new medical facility opened in 2017 at RAF Honington is named after him.

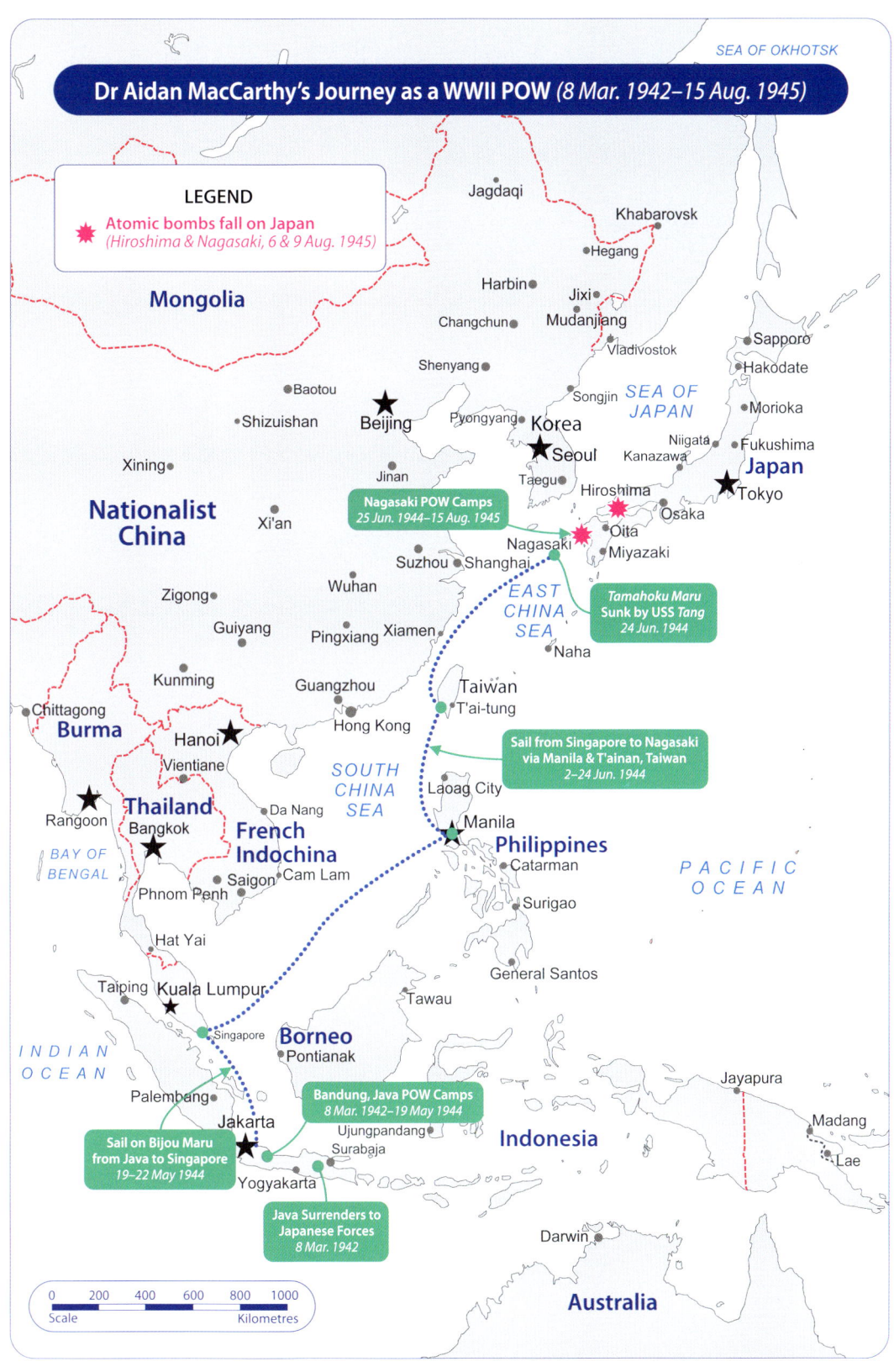

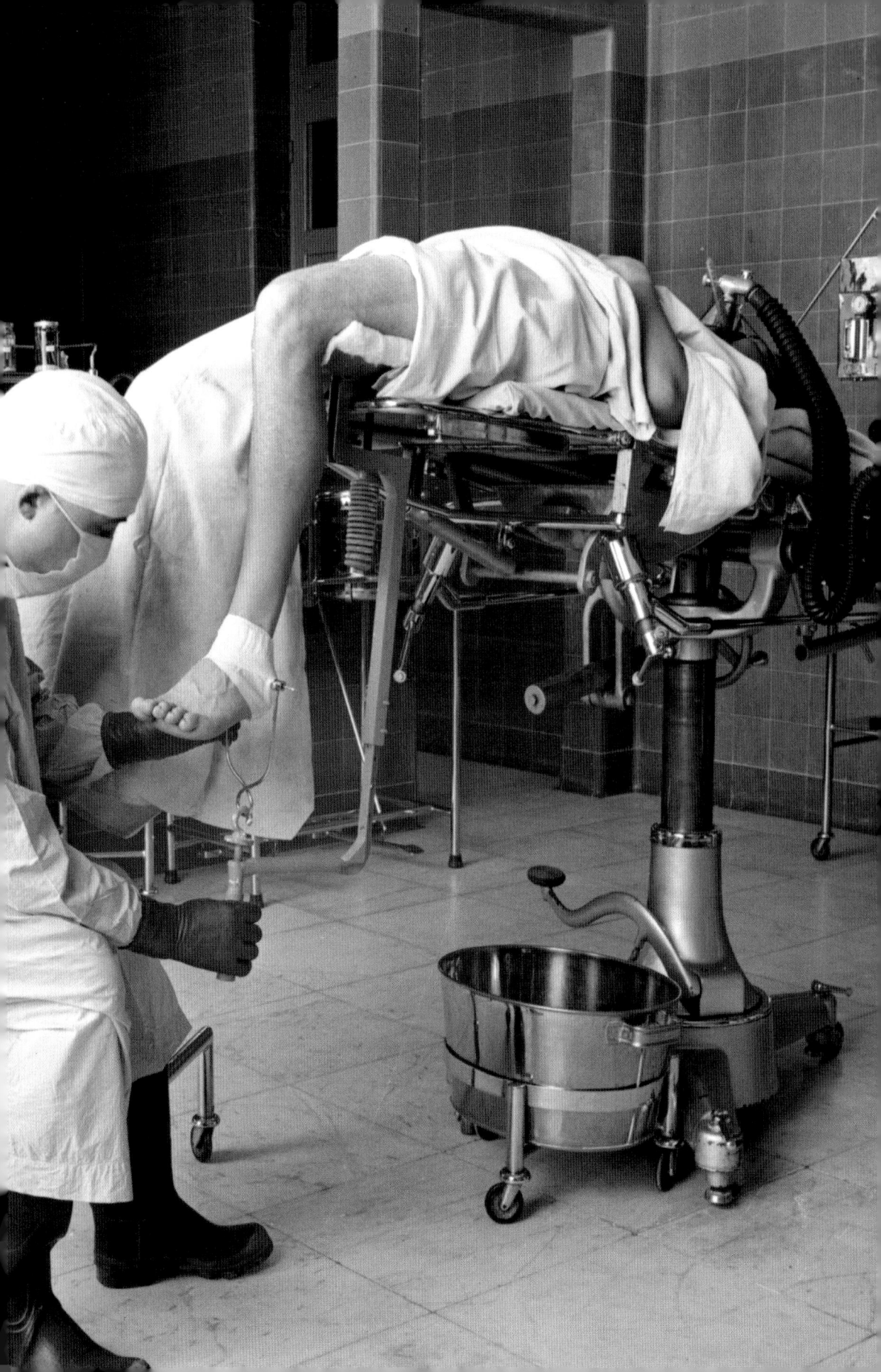

Chapter 6
PROFILES IN GALLANTRY AND PROFESSIONALISM BY IRISH DOCTORS

The statements that accompany the awarding of bravery and other decorations give an insight as to the range of circumstances encountered by doctors while they served with the fighting forces and in the planning of the health service delivered to the troops. The following are some examples.

Leslie Samuels

This officer has been employed as Regimental Medical Officer during several campaigns. His first consideration has always been the wounded and his succour has on many occasions been rendered with complete disregard to personal danger. During the attack across the river Trigno on October 27th, 1943, he tended the wounded under very heavy fire for five hours and there is no doubt he saved many lives. During this time he supervised evacuation across the river under continued enemy shell fire. His cheerfulness and courage under the worst conditions have been an inspiration and example to all.

Julius Summ

This officer has rendered invaluable services as my second-in-command throughout the whole period under review. The unit has on many occasions been 'straffed' from the air and bombed. Major Summ has invariably been the first to go round the leaguer completely regardless of his own personal safety to see if the patients are safe and reassure them; also to find and give medical treatment to the men of his own unit who have become casualties. Major Summ by his personal example and courage at all times has been an inspiration to the officers and men of this unit serving with a forward brigade throughout the battle since Alamein; he has been directly responsible for maintaining the morale of the unit at a high level during many difficult times.

Aiden Byrne

On the night of June 14th, 1942, this officer proceeded with his section and an ambulance car with an infantry column in an endeavour to break through the enemy lines to the west of the Brigade 'box'. Emerging through the 'Stanley Gap' which was then under heavy shellfire, the section under Captain Byrne picked up and attended wounded occasioned by the shelling and they were placed in the ambulance car which accompanied the section. Soon after this the ambulance car ran onto one of our own minefields in the dark. Captain Byrne who was travelling on another vehicle, immediately went into the minefield and assisted in extracting the patients from the vehicle, and he then marked a way out of the minefield along which patients could be brought, and led them to safety.

Kevin Patton

During the breakthrough of the enemy line towards El Hanna by an armoured division at first light on March 27th, 1943, the rear of the column was attacked by the enemy tanks at close range. Despite experiencing a broken ankle as a result of a fall from a portee, Captain Patton tended to, and evacuated all wounded from the scene of action in face of very heavy and accurate shellfire and machine-gun fire from the enemy tanks. During the approximate 30 minutes of the action, this officer not only showed complete disregard for his own personal safety, but also a very high standard of devotion to duty.

Terence Wilson

This officer established an ADVANCED Dressing Station in a gully on February 27th, 1942. This station is still in position. He was responsible for evacuation of casualties from the area around St. De Ksar Mezouar, and the high ground north and northwest of it. During this time he has handled his company with consummate skill, maintaining a close liaison with regimental aid posts and taking over responsibility from the regimental aid posts when they, of necessity, had ceased to function. He has inspired his men with zeal and devotion which has taken them beyond their normal role and pushed them forward to the limit of endurance with one intention, to get the wounded off the ground at all costs, and back quickly to skilled surgical hands. On the night March 4th–5th, 1943, he organised three of his stretcher squads to go forward to positions still held by a few platoons. These squads took up rations with them on open stretchers for the infantry and brought back casualties on the return journey. He has perfected his system of evacuation so well from that ground and has disposed his squads so well tactically, including a continuous staffing of the tunnel at St. Ksar Mezouar, that all casualties recoverable from our lines on that sector have been back at Beja on the operating table in three to four hours, a factor which has undoubtedly saved the lives and limbs of many badly wounded men and which has only been achieved by constant and tireless devotion to duty, carried out at times in face of heavy mortar and shell fire.

John Martin

On August 9th, 1943, the battery was in action south of Bronte. Captain Martin was with the battery. During the evening the road between the battery position and Bronte was very heavily and accurately shelled and mortared. This road was very congested with stationary guns and vehicles, and Captain Martin, realising that there were likely to be casualties, immediately proceeded to the place which was being most heavily shelled. A vehicle had been hit and there were a number of casualties, making it very dangerous to remain in the open. Captain Martin was quite undaunted by this heavy shellfire and attended to the wounded men without regard to his personal safety. By his brave action he undoubtedly saved some lives and his example had a steadying effect on all around him.

Peter May

As Officer Commanding a motor ambulance convoy, Major May has been responsible for the care and welfare of thousands of casualties from forward casualty clearing station to railroad or hospital ship port. It was due to his unbound enthusiasm that, although the distance involved was far greater than could have been anticipated, there was at no time any hitch and an even flow of casualties along the line of evacuation was always ensured. Major May's willing and intelligent co-operation with all concerned has earned the highest praise. A very high all-round standard was set by the unit, and by ensuring efficient and skilful maintenance it was at all times possible to call on 100 per cent of his ambulance cars for the evacuation; this is no small achievement when it is realised that these vehicles travelled over 190,000 miles in under two months.

Stephen Conway

On the morning of October 28th, 1942, the position to which he had advanced during the night was the object of heavy and intense enemy shellfire and numerous casualties were caused. For more than three hours Captain Conway made unceasing journeys rendering aid to wounded personnel in the locality. All ranks were forced by this shellfire to take cover either in their tanks or dug positions, but Captain Conway, without a thought for his personal safety, continued to carry out his duty even to the extent of visiting areas where casualties might have occurred. His coolness and courage were an example to all.

Arthur Odbert

During the period February to May 1943, Lieutenant Colonel Odbert has been indefatigable in the performance of his duties, and it has been largely due to his efforts that the phenomenally low sick rate of the Army has been attained. Over a vast area of difficult country he has supervised the hygiene arrangements with a complete disregard for anything else than the preservation of the health of the troops. He has personally investigated the important water supplies and arranged for their purification, while by prompt action and careful foresight he has prevented any outbreak of disease. Always one of the earliest on the spot in the many occupied towns and villages to anticipate and deal with hygiene problems, his preparation for the prevention of malaria was most comprehensive and machinery was immediately available should any epidemic have appeared likely. He is always cool and collected, ready with sound advice, while his devotion to duty has been an example and an inspiration to the whole hygiene tenor of the 8th Army and maintaining it fighting fit and at full strength.

Florence Joseph O'Driscoll

Landed with Corps Troops and immediately set about surveying the country and procuring information regarding malaria from local sources. As the troops advanced Lieutenant Colonel O'Driscoll and his men were never far behind and at great personal risk and under extraordinary difficult conditions brought back most valuable information showing details of malarial areas. Owing to the presence of numerous land mines, survey work along the banks of lakes, rivers and streams was extremely hazardous, and, in fact, two trucks were blown up and the occupants injured. In spite of this and due almost entirely to the leadership, drive and personal courage of Lieutenant Colonel O'Driscoll the work went forward. It is necessary to stress the importance of this work from the Army point of view, for it was on recommendations made by Lieutenant Colonel O'Driscoll that the whole fabric of anti-malaria work was built up. Had this information not been quickly obtained action would have been delayed and there is no question that malaria sick rates would have been much higher than they were.

Theobald Phelan

During the period under review Lieutenant Colonel Phelan has commanded a field ambulance attached to an armoured brigade. He has consistently shown a very high degree of vision, foresight and initiative – the results of which have been manifest in the work of his unit. His field ambulance has won for itself a reputation second to none in the 8th Army and Lieutenant Colonel Phelan and the team of doctors working under him have inspired the confidence and affection of everyone in the brigade. The medical record of this brigade and of Lieutenant Colonel Phelan's Field Ambulance is an impressive one, while the ratio of deaths to battle casualties dealt with by the main dressing station is most unusually low. The credit for the exceptionally fine work done by this unit must go to a large degree to its commanding officer.

Robert Walker

This officer, who is a Deputy Director of Medical Supplies in the Middle East, is mainly responsible to the Director of Medical Supplies for the many and difficult medical plannings to suit the 1,001 projects planned in the Middle East. Each plan necessitates the medical planning for the provision of the many large and small medical units required for the countries and climates through which the forces involved may pass. It also necessitates the planning of the type and quantity of medical stores required, special drugs, chemicals, clothing, medical and advance equipment, the provision and supply, and medical advice. It also necessitates the planning of the type of medical transport required in the different types of countries. Up to date, this officer's foresight, judgement and careful calculations based on his specialised knowledge have covered medical results in evacuation and nursing of casualties, which have brought nothing but praise from the highest authorities. His keenness, loyalty, devotion to duty and entire application to these many difficult problems have been an example to all.

Stanley Walsh

He dived from the deck of his ship the destroyer *Constance* to rescue a Naval Airman Ernest Leonard Lindsay of Newcastle on Tyne who fell overboard from the light fleet carrier *Theseus* during operations off Korea. The Admiralty stated that during an attack a Sea Fury aircraft unshipped a rocket when landing on the *Theseus* and the 80lb missile hurdled along the deck at 60 miles an hour. Lindsay jumped to avoid it and fell 40ft into the Yellow Sea. A lifebuoy was thrown to him but he was carried past it. Surgeon Lieutenant Walsh saw the rating was in difficulties and he dived in and supported him for several minutes until the destroyer's boat arrived.

Abbreviations and Acronyms

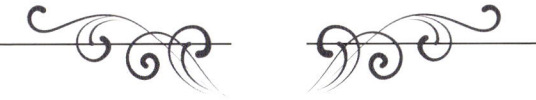

Note: The meaning of a few of the abbreviations recorded in Part 2 of the book have been lost to history.

A/	Acting
ADMS	Assistant Director of Medical Services
ADGMS	Assistant Director General of Medical Services
AFC	Air Force Cross
AFM	Air Force Medal
Amb	Ambulance
Anaes.	Anaesthetist
Armd	Armoured
ASC	Army Service Corps
ATS	Auxiliary Territorial Service
b.	Born
BAO	Bachelor of the Art of Obstetrics
BAOR	British Army of the Rhine
BCh	Bachelor of Surgery
BEF	British Expeditionary Force
BEM	British Empire Medal
BF	British Forces
BM	Bachelor of Medicine
BMH	British Military Hospital
BNAF	British North Africa Force
Brig.	Brigadier
BS	Bachelor of Surgery
BSH	British Station Hospital
Bt	Brevet
BTA	British Troops, Austria
BTE	British Troops, Egypt
BWM	British War Medal
Capt.	Captain
CB	Companion Order of the Bath
CBE	Commander Order of the British Empire
CCG	Control Commission Germany
CCS	Casualty Clearing Station

CDEE	Chemical Defence Experimental Establishment
Cdo	Commando
Cdr	Commander
CGH	Combined General Hospital
CGM	Conspicuous Gallantry Medal
ChB	Bachelor of Surgery
CIE	Commander Order of the Indian Empire
CIMH	Combined Indian Military Hospital
cl., cls	Clasp, clasps
CM, ChM	Master of Surgery
CMF	Central Mediterranean Force
CMG	Companion Order of St Michael & St George
CMH	Combined Military Hospital
CO	Commanding Officer
Combt	Combat
Comd	Command
Comdr	Commander
Comdt	Commandant
Comman	Commission
Comwel	Commonwealth
Con. Hosp	Convalescent Hospital
Cons.	Consultant
Coombe	Coombe Hospital Dublin
Corn	Coronation
CStJ	Commander Order of St John of Jerusalem
CVO	Commander Royal Victorian Order
d.	Died on Active Service
DADH	Deputy Assistant Director of Hygiene
DADMS	Deputy Assistant Director of Medical Services
DADP	Deputy Assistant Director of Pathology
DAH	Director of Army Health
Demobd	Demobilised
Dispatches	Mentioned in Dispatches
DFC	Distinguished Flying Cross
DDMS	Deputy Director of Medical Services
DGAMS	Director General of Army Medical Services
Dist.	District
Div.	Division
DM	Defence Medal
DOS	Death on Service

DPH	Diploma in Public Health
DSC	Distinguished Service Cross
DSM	Distinguished Service Medal
DSO	Companion Distinguished Service Order
dt	Daughter of
DTM&H	Diploma in Tropical Medicine & Hygiene
Edin.	Edinburgh University
Embkn	Embarkation
EMS	Emergency Medical Service
f.p.	Full pay
FARELF	Far East Land Forces
Fd Amb.	Field Ambulance
Fd Hosp.	Field Hospital
FDS	Field Dressing Station
FFA RCS	Fellow Faculty of Anaesthetists; Royal College of Surgeons
Flt Lt	Flight Lieutenant
Flt Offr	Flight Officer
FRCP	Fellow Royal College of Physicians
FRCS	Fellow Royal College of Surgeons of England
FRCSI	Fellow Royal College of Surgeons of Ireland
GC	George Cross
Gds	Guards
Gen.	General
Gen. Hosp.	General Hospital
GHQ	General Headquarters
Glas.	Glasgow University
GM	George Medal
Gordons	The Gordon Highlanders
GSM	General Service Medal
Hon.	Honorary
Hosp.	Hospital
h.p.	Half Pay
HQ	Headquarters
IAMC	Indian Army Medical Corps
IBGH	Indian Base General Hospital
IEF	Indian Expeditionary Force
IFS	Irish Free State
IG	Irish Guards
IGSM	Indian General Service Medal
IMS	Indian Medical Service

IOM	Indian Order of Merit
Ind	Indian
KBE	Knight Commander Order of the British Empire
KCB	Knight Commander Order of the Bath
KCMG	Knight Commander Order of St Michael & St. George
KGVI	King George VI
KHP	King's Honorary Physician
KHS	King's Honorary Surgeon
KIA	Killed in Action
KSA	King's South Africa Medal
KStJ	Knight Commander Order of St John of Jerusalem
Kt	Knight
LDS	Licentiate in Dental Surgery
LG	*London Gazette*
LM	Licentiate in Midwifery
L.LM	Licentiate and Licentiate in Midwifery
LRCPI	Licentiate Royal College of Physicians of Ireland
LRCP&S	Licentiate Royal College of Physicians and Surgery
LRCP&SI	Licentiate Royal College of Physicians and Surgery of Ireland
LRFPS	Licentiate Royal Faculty of Physicians and Surgeons
2Lt	Second Lieutenant
Lt	Lieutenant
Lt Col.	Lieutenant Colonel
Lt Gen.	Lieutenant General
(M)	Medical Branch Officer
Maj.	Major
Maj. Gen.	Major General
MAO	Military Administrative Officer
MB	Bachelor in Medicine
MBE	Member Order of the British Empire
MC	Military Cross
MCh	Master of Surgery
MD	Medical Doctor
Med.	Mediterranean
Med. Sch.	Medical School
Med. EF	Mediterranean Expeditionary Force
MEF	Middle East Force
MELF	Middle East Land Forces
MIA	Missing in Action
MID	Mentioned in Dispatches

Mil. Hosp.	Military Hospital
MMH	Military Maternity Hospital
MN	Merchant Navy
MO	Medical Officer
MOH	Medical Officer for Health
Mobd	Mobilised
MOD	Ministry of Defence
MRC	Medical Research Council
MRCOG	Member of the Royal College of Obstetricians and Gynaecologists
MRCPI	Member of the Royal College of Physicians in Ireland
MRCS	Member of the Royal College of Surgeons in England
MRCSI	Member of the Royal College of Surgeons in Ireland
MS	Master of Surgery
MSc	Master of Science
NAMC	Irish National Army Medical Corps
NUI	National University of Ireland
NWE	North West Europe
NWF	North West Frontier (India)
NZAMS	New Zealand Army Medical Service
O.	Order
OBE	Officer Order of the British Empire
OC	Officer Commanding
OCLF	Overseas Commonwealth Land Forces
Offr	Officer
OIC	Officer In Charge
OKW	High Command of the Armed Forces of Nazi Germany
OPS	Operations
OStJ	Order of St John of Jerusalem
Para	Parachute
Paiforce	Persia and Iraq Force
PMO	Principal Medical Officer
PRAC	Permanent Regular Army Commission
Prof.	Professor
POW	Prisoner of War
QA Mil. Hosp.	Queen Alexandra's Military Hospital
QEII	Queen Elizabeth II
QHP	Queen's Honorary Physician
QHS	Queen's Honorary Surgeon
QSA	Queen's South Africa Medal
QUB	Queen's University Belfast

r.	Religion
R. of O.	Reserve of Officers
RAF	Royal Air Force
RAFVR	Royal Air Force Volunteer Reserve
RAMC	Royal Army Medical Corps
RAMC (SR)	Royal Army Medical Corps (Special Reserve)
RAM College	Royal Army Medical College
RCPS	Royal College of Physicians and Surgeons (England)
RCPI	Royal College of Physicians in Ireland
RCSI	Royal College of Surgeons in Ireland
Regt	Regiment
Rempld	Re-employed
Retd	Retired
RMA	Royal Military Academy
RMO	Regimental Medical Officer
RN	Royal Navy
RNVR	Royal Navy Volunteer Reserve
Rot.	Rotunda Hospital, Dublin
r.p.	Retired Pay
RUI	Royal University of Ireland
RWAFF	Royal West Africa Frontier Force
S.	Star
s.	Son of
SAMC	South African Medical Corps
S/Capt	Staff Captain
Sch.	School
SEAC	South East Asia Command
Serv.	Service
SHAEF	Supreme Headquarters Allied Expeditionary Force
SHAPE	Supreme Headquarters Allied Powers in Europe
SMO	Senior Medical Officer
Sq. Ldr	Squadron Leader
Surg.	Surgeon
Surg. Cdr	Surgeon Commander
Surg. Lt	Surgeon Lieutenant
Surg. Lt Cdr	Surgeon Lieutenant Commander
T/	Temporary
T/Capt.	Temporary Captain
T/Col.	Temporary Colonel
TCD	Trinity College Dublin
TD	Territorial Decoration

ABBREVIATIONS AND ACRONYMS

UCC	University College Cork
UCG	University College Galway
USMC	United States Medical Corps
VC	Victoria Cross
W Comd	Western Command
W/	Wing
Wing Cdr	Wing Commander
WM	War Medal

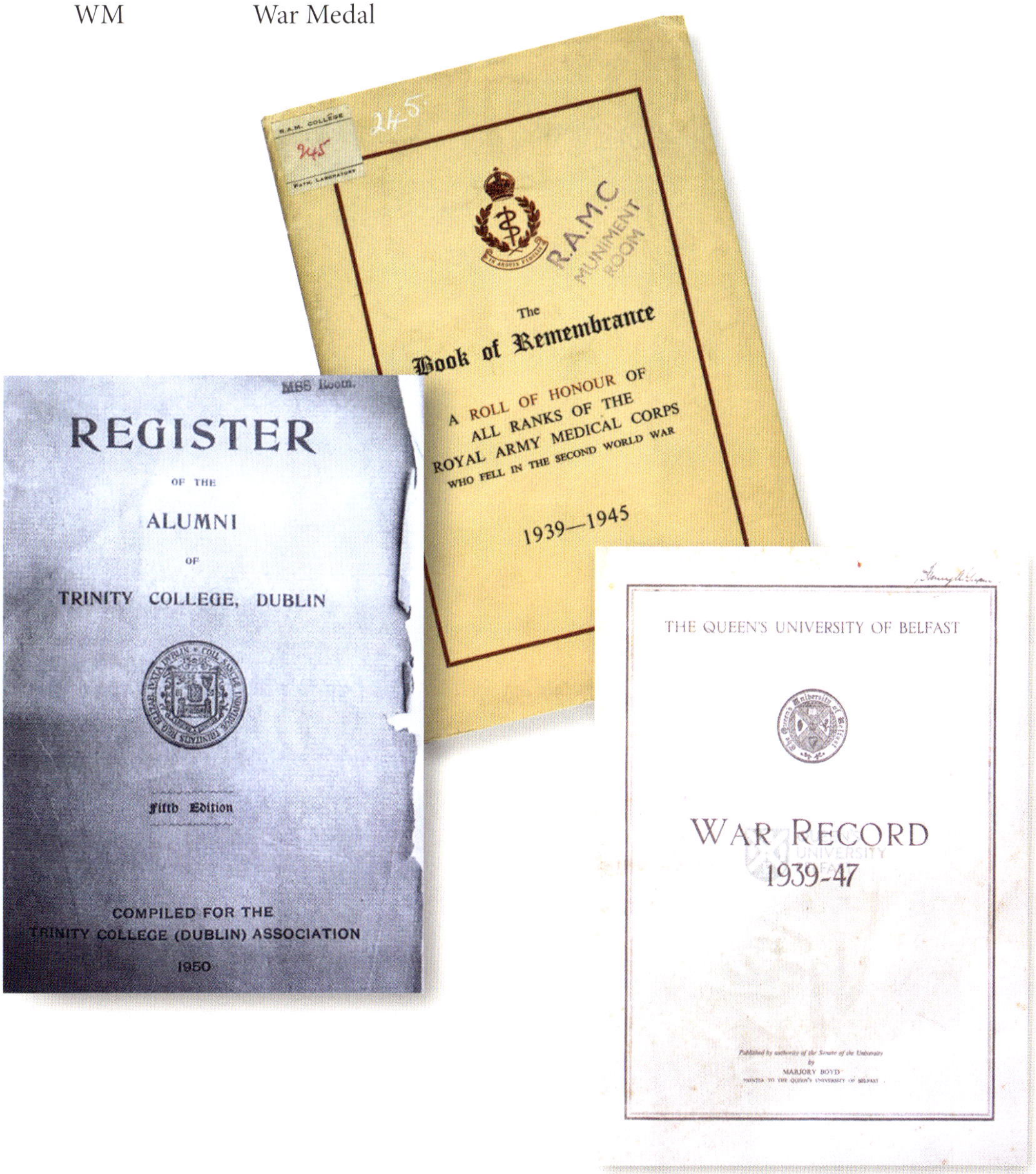

SELECT BIBLIOGRAPHY

Bennett, J.D. Courtnay and Young, J.R., 'Draffin and his Rods', *The Journal of Laryngology & Otology*, vol. 106, iss. 12 (1992), pp. 1035–6

Blake, John W., *Northern Ireland in the Second World War*, Blackstaff Press, 2000

Casey, P.J., Cullen, K.T., Duignan, J.P., *Irish Doctors in the First World War*, Merrion Press, 2015

Doherty, Richard, *Irish Men and Women in the Second World War*, Four Courts Press, 2021

Durnin, David, *The Irish Medical Profession and the First World War*, Palgrave McMillan, 2019

Ferguson, Ion, *Doctor at War*, Christopher Johnson, 1955

Gould, Robert W., *Campaign Medals of the British Army 1815–1972*, Arms and Armour Press, 1982

Jackson, Bob, *A Doctor's Sword*, The Collins Press, Cork, 2015

Lowry, Cecil, Frank *Pantridge MC: Japanese Prisoner of War and Inventor of the PortableDefibrillator*, Pen and Sword Military, 2022

MacCarthy, Dr Aidan, *A Doctor's War*, The Collins Press, Cork, 2005

Malone, Aubrey, *A Life in Medicine: A Biography of Malachy Smyth*, Web Publications, 2005

Mitchell, R. Keith, *Forty Two Months in Durance Vile*, R. Keith Mitchell 1997

Nott, David, *War Doctor: Surgery on the Front Line*, Picador, 2020

Purves, Alec A., *The Medals Decorations & Orders of World War II 1939–1945*, J.Hayward & Son, 1986

Russel, Lord of Liverpool, *The Knights of Bushido*, Cassell & Co. Ltd., 1958

List of Illustrations

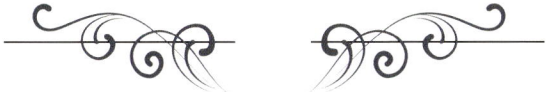

Plate 1	Colonel W.G. Luxford of Poplar, East London, a hospital technician, prepares the instrument table before an operation at a Field Surgical Unit in an Italian prison, December 1943. © IWM (NA10220)	x
Plate 2	Normandy medical evacuation. Public Domain.	3
Plate 3	Indian medical orderlies assisting wounded, Burma, February 1944, courtesy of the National Army Museum.	4
Plate 4	Surgical instruments. © Authors' collection	7
Plate 5	Bofors guns on the upper deck of a Landing Ship Tank, Sousse harbour, July 1943, courtesy of the National Army Museum.	8
Plate 6	Medical Officer Captain Parfitt and his orderly administer an emergency plasma transfusion to a serious casualty outside a tented Field Dressing Unit near Oostemalle in Belgium, October 1944. © IWM (B 10557)	11
Plate 7	A casualty being loaded into a motor ambulance at Ortona, Italy in December 1943. © IWM (NA 9923)	12
Plate 8	A Sister on her round chats with a soldier convalescing in a tented ward of a base hospital in the Middle East. © IWM (E 10657)	16
Plate 9	The scene at a Field Dressing Station during heavy fighting in the Western Desert in June 1942. © IWM (E 13325)	19
Plate 10	Field Surgical Unit performing an operation within a much-bombed Italian prison, December 1943 © IWM (NA 10223)	20
Plate 11	Collection of Second World War medals. © Authors' collection	22
Plate 12	Major Patton, RAMC, assisted by Private A. Haggard, removes a foreign body from a soldier's eye at No. 1 Mobile Ophthalmic Unit in Italy, March 1944. © IWM (NA 13013)	26
Plate 13	A Royal Army Medical Corps ambulance convoy moving forwards in the Western Desert. © IWM (E 13321)	28
Plate 14	Men of the Devonshire Regiment sign their autographs on Japanese flags captured at Nippon Ridge during the Battle of Imphal-Kohima, March–July 1944. © IWM (IND 3383)	30
Plate 15	West African casualties in Burma. Public domain.	33
Plate 16	War Memorabilia © Shutterstock	34
Plate 17	British prisoners in Dieppe, courtesy of the National Army Museum.	37
Plate 18	British and Canadian prisoners being guarded by German soldiers, Dieppe, 1942, courtesy of the National Army Museum.	39
Plate 19	A Sherman tank passing through the town of Francofonte 1943, courtesy of the National Army Museum.	42

Plate 20	Wounded being evacuated 1944, courtesy of the National Army Museum.	46
Plate 21	Wounded soldiers being loaded into a hospital train in Belgium, March 1945. © IWM (B15253)	49
Plate 22	A whaler bringing a patient from HMS Zulu approaching HMS *Hermione*. © IWM (A 6374)	50
Plate 23	Corpsmen wearing Red Cross Armbands look over a mixed load of casualties–American and German POWs. Public domain.	53
Plate 24	Troops wading ashore from landing craft, 6 June 1944, courtesy of the National ArmyMuseum.	56
Plate 25	Red Cross war poster, courtesy of Library of Congress LC-USZC4-8380.	59
Plate 26	A patient wounded in the leg is given a blood transfusion at a Field Transfusion Unit in Italy, 1944. © IWM (TR 2408)	60
Plate 27	Surgery in progress on board HMS Renown. Marine Thomas Quinn of Glasgow is being operated on for appendicitis. © IWM (A 24421)	62
Plate 28	Shell Dressing	63
Plate 29	War Memorabilia © Istockphoto	64
Plate 30	A Fijian medical orderly administers an emergency plasma transfusion during heavy fighting on Bougainville. © IWM (NZ 1445)	67
Plate 31	Old Medical and Surgical Instruments.© Shutterstock	69
Plate 32	A British sister instructs an Indian nurse how to adjust a doctor's mask at a first aid post in Calcutta, 1944. © IWM (IB 1869)	70
Plate 33	The Field Surgical Unit's recovery ward, based in a much-bombed Italian prison. © IWM (NA 10229)	73
Plate 34	A Reception Officer at an Advanced Dressing Station examines a casualty wounded in the leg to determine whether a blood transfusion is required. © IWM (TR 2406)	74
Plate 35	A patient wounded in the leg is given a blood transfusion in the Operating Theatre of an Advanced Dressing Station while a plaster bandage is applied to his leg. © IWM (TR 2410)	76
Plate 36	War Memorabilia © Shutterstock	79
Plate 37	Frank Murray Medical staff at a Japanese POW camp. Courtesy of Carl Murray	81
Plate 38	Major Frank Murray. Courtesy of Carl Murray	82
Plate 39	Frank Murray and fellow POWs at a Japanese POW camp. Courtesy of Carl Murray	86
Plate 40	Dr Aidan MacCarthy. Courtesy of Bob Jackson	88
Plate 41	A soldier with a fractured tibia and fibia having his leg placed in skeletal traction at a specialist orthopaedic centre in Cairo, Egypt. © IWM (E 17158)	92
Plate 42	Various publications recording the names of participants in the war. Authors' collection	105
Plate 43	A ward on No. 22 Hospital Carrier at Dieppe. © IWM (O 1841)	110
Plate 44	A ward on No. 22 Hospital Carrier at Dieppe. © IWM (O 1841)	111
Plate 45	Dennis Parsons Burkitt. © *British Medical Journal*, April 1993	135

Plate 46	Bob Collis, fourth left. © Holocaust Education Ireland	144
Plate 47	Dr David Alexander Draffin. © ENT & Audiology News, courtesy of Pinpoint Scotland Ltd	160
Plate 48	Michael Joseph Farrell. Courtesy of the family.	167
Plate 49	Thomas Ion Victor Ferguson. © Christopher Johnson, *Doctor at War*, 1955	168
Plate 50	Commander Surgeon Henry Hurst. © HMS *Hood* Rolls of Honour	194
Plate 51	Plaque for Frank Pantridge located at the Royal Victoria Hospital Belfast. Courtesy of Cecil Lowry.	250
Plate 52	Alfred Denis Parsons. Courtesy of the family.	251
Plate 53	Malachy Joseph Smyth. Courtesy of the family.	275

List of Maps

Map 1	Main Theatres of War – Europe	14
Map 2	Main Theatres of War – Pacific	17
Map 3	Battle of France	35
Map 4	Invasion of Yugoslavia & Greece	41
Map 5	North African Campaign (1942–43)	44
Map 6	Eastern Front	55
Map 7	Dr Frank Murray's Journey as a WWII POW (21 Feb. 1942–3 Sept. 1945)	85
Map 8	Dr Aidan MacCarthy's Journey as a WWII POW (8 Mar. 1942–15 Aug. 1945)	91

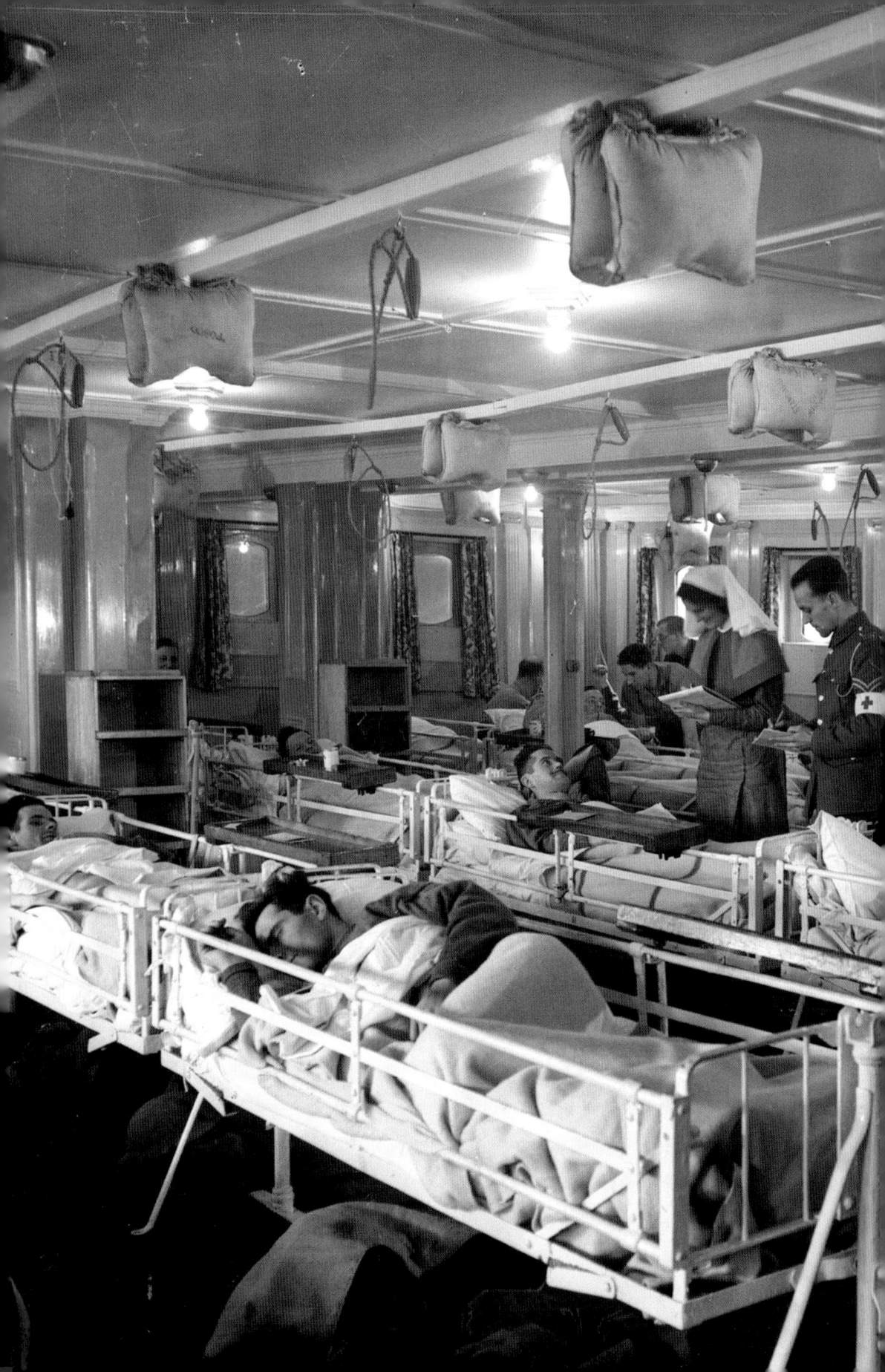

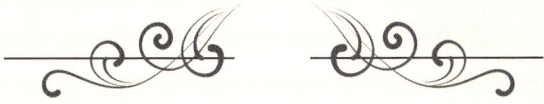

ROLL OF HONOUR OF IRISH DOCTORS
WHO SERVED IN THE
SECOND WORLD WAR

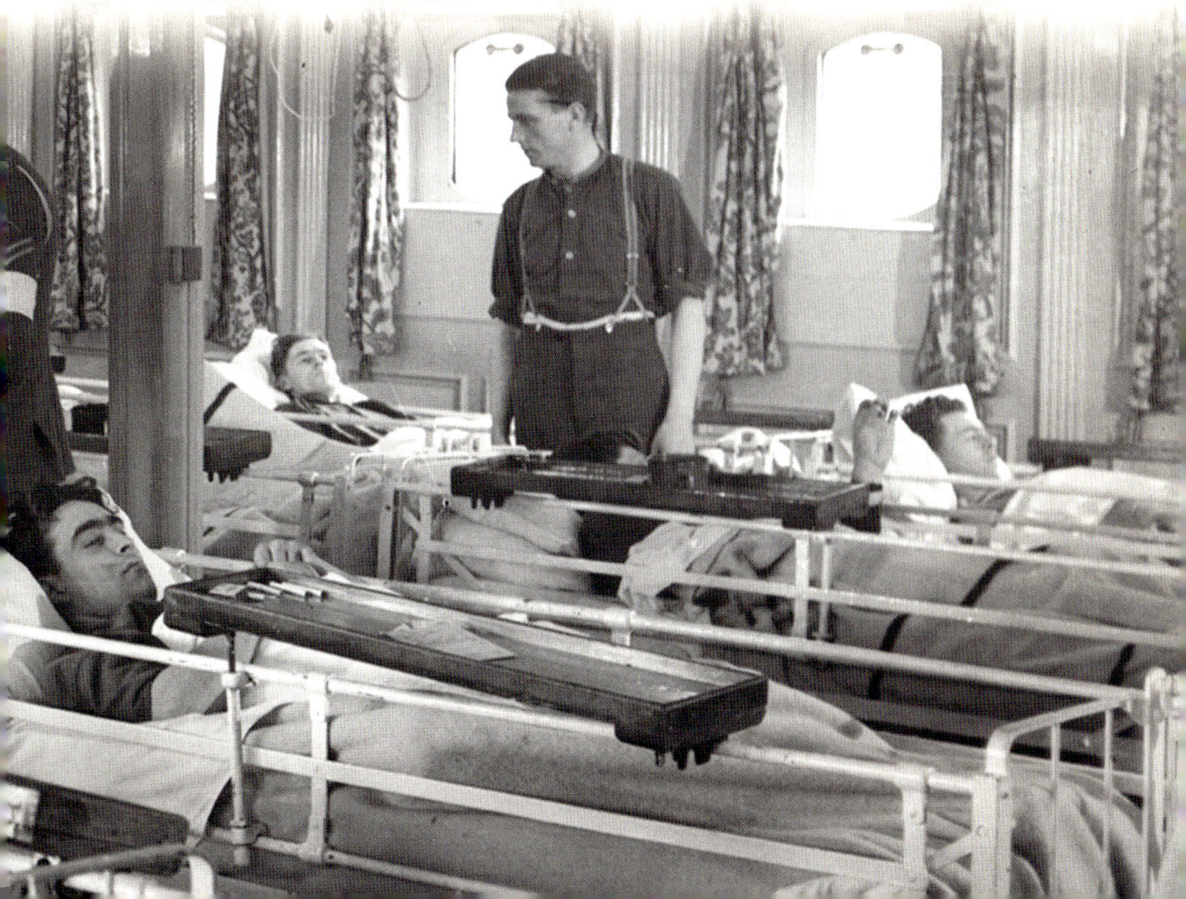

A

ABERNETHY Victor Alexander Address: Castle Avenue, Thurles, Co. Tipperary. L.LM (RCSI 1936), L.LM (RCPI 1936). Lt RAMC 26th Jun. 1941.

ACHESON Thomas Stafford (Achie) b. Ireland, 1st Nov. 1902. LRCP&SI (Dublin 1925), LM (Rot. Hosp. 1927), also TCD. At TCD was in the university XV and was later capped for Ireland. During WWII he was MO to the Home Guard and civilian medical practitioner to large military and air force establishments in his area.

ACTON John Harty Address: 10 Lr O'Connell St, Limerick. MB, BCh (TCD 1940) TCD. RAMC.

ACTON Kyrl Trysilian Address: 10 Lr O'Connell St, Limerick. MB, BCh (TCD 1940). RAFVR.

ADAM Walter Eustace b. 13th Apr. 1887, Dundrum, Co. Dublin. s. James Adam, 17 Merrion Row, Dublin, and Orwell Bank, Rathgar, Dublin. Educ. St Andrews Coll. (1896–1902). MB (TCD 1911), BCh, BAO, LM (Rot. Hosp.), MD (1913). R. Baptist. Lt RAMC 1st Dec. 1914. T/Capt. 1st Dec. 1915. A/Maj. 13th Feb. 1919–4th Jan. 1920. Maj. 1st Dec. 1926. Lt Col. 10th Nov. 1939. r.p. (ill health) 27th Nov. 1942. Rempld Maj. 27th Nov. 1942. Rempld 25th Sept. 1943. Served in 1914–18 War Greek Macedonia, Serbia, Bulgaria, European Turkey, islands of the Aegean Sea (Nov. 1915–Sept. 1917), Gallipoli (5th Aug. 1915–30th Sept. 1915), Egyptian EF (Sept. 1917–Oct. 18) inc. Palestine, CO 166th Fd Amb. (Jun.–Sept. 1919). India 1923–27. Burma 1927–29. China 1932–36. CO 131 Fd Amb. 1940–41. CO 46th Gen. Hosp. Aug.–Sept. 1941. PSMB W. Comd 1941–42. Medals: MC (19th Dec. 1916), 1915 S., BWM, VM, DM, WM. MID 5th Jun. 1919. d. 27th Nov. 1964. Commemorated on Roll of Honour Sir Patrick Dun's Hospital.

ADAMS George Fowler Address: 35 Kirkliston Drive, Belfast. MB, BCh (QUB 1938). Surg. Lt Comdr RNVR.

ADAMS John Hamilton Address: 21 Cranmore Gardens, Belfast. MD (QUB 1942). Capt. RAMC. MID.

ADAMS Maurice Henry Educ. Campbell College. MB, BCh (QUB 1930). Surg. Comdr RN.

ADAMSON Campbell Miller Taggart Address: Dromore St, Ballynahinch, Co. Down. MB, BCh (TCD 1935). Surg. Lt Comdr RN.

ADAMSON James Maurice Taggart Address: Northern Bank, Lurgan, Co. Armagh. MB (TCD 1941). Flt Offr RAF (1944).

ADAMSON John Edwin Address: Enniscrone, Co. Sligo. MB, BCh (TCD 1942). Flt Offr RAF (1943).

*****ADYE CURRAN** Francis George Address: 34 Harcourt St, Dublin. LRCP&S (RCSI 1940). Surg. MN. KIA 1944 SS Khedive.

ADYE CURRAN Gerald Francis Address: 34 Harcourt St, Dublin. LRCP&S (RCSI 1934). Lt IMS 23rd Apr. 1935. MC.

AHERN Donal Maurice MB, Bch, BAO (Dub. 1933), b. 30th Mar. 1911, Cork. Lt 27th Jul. 1933. Capt. 8th Jul. 1935. RAMC. A/Maj. 19th Apr. 1941. T/Maj. 19th Jul. 1941. Maj. 10th Jul. 1943. A/Lt Col. 1st Jan. 1942. T/Lt Col., 1st Apr. 1942. Lt Col. 9th Jun. 1948. A/Col. 13th Jul. 1945. T/Col. 13th Jan. 1948. Col. 25th Jul. 1957. T/Brig. 2nd Sept. 1963. Brig. 29th Oct. 1963. T/Maj. Gen. 9th Aug. 1960. Served India 1935–41. Fd Amb. 1943. NWE 1944–46. CO 8th Fd Amb. 1944–45. ADMS HQ 7th Armoured Div. 1945–46. MELF CO Base Depot RAMC 1946–48. BAOR DDMS Control Commission Germany 1948–50. Comdt Field Training School RAMC 1951–53. MELF ADMS HQ 1st Infantry Div. 1953–54. ADGMS War Office 1954–57. Norway Chief Med. Sec. Logistics Div. HQ 1958–60. Comdt HQ AER RAMC 1960–62. Comdt Depot and Training Estb. RAMC 1962–63. BAOR DDMS HQ 1 Br. Corps. 1964–66. DDMS HQ Eastern Comd 1966. Medals: CBE 2nd Jun. 1962, DSO 31st August 1944. Lieutenant Colonel Ahern was the first Field Ambulance Commander ashore having transhipped from a sinking craft. He rallied his party on the beaches, directed the collection of casualties, and then proceeded inland to establish an advance dressing station, which he set up with great speed. His unit was responsible for the evacuation of casualties from an Airborne Division. This task he carried out with complete success, going forward repeatedly to make contact, frequently under fire. Throughout the whole operation his cool conduct under fire was an inspiration to others. MID 16th Dec. 1943. IGMS and cl. NWF 1936–37, 1939–45 S., Burma S., France and Germany S., DM, WM, QEII Coronation M. 1953. d. 31st Oct. 1966, Woolwich, London.

AHERN Timothy Michael Richard b. 16th August 1908 at Kasauli, India. MB, BCh, BAO (TCD 1931). Lt RAMC 28th Jul. 1931. Capt. 1st May 1934. A/Maj. 27th Dec. 1940. T/Maj. 27th Mar. 1941. Maj. 28th Jul. 1941. A/Lt Col. 3rd Jun. 1941. T/Lt Col. 3rd Sept. 1941. Lt Col. 8th May 1947. A/Col. 29th Jun. 1945. T/Col. 29th Dec. 1945. Col. 30th Aug. 1955. T/Brig. 23rd Nov.

---

* Note: An asterisk before a name indicates that the individual died during the war.

1952. Brig. 6th Aug. 1960. Maj. Gen. 3rd May 1965. Served India 1933–37, Burma 1937–38, CO 19th Gds. Lt Fd Amb. 1941–42. ADMS HQ Combat Ops. 1943–44. Italy/MELF 1944–47. CO 13th Fd Amb. 1944. ADMS HQ 8th Army 1944–45. ADMS HQ 46th Div. 1945–46. ADMS HQ. 1st Armd Div. 1946–47. CO Mil. Hosp. 1947–48. ADMS HQ Northern Comd 1948–49. ADMS HQ British Mil. Mission Greece 1950–51. MRLF 1952–53. ADMS HQ 1st Infantry Div. 1952 and 1953. DDMS HQ BTE 1952–53. France: Chief Medical Plans and Ops SHAPE 1953–56. Comdt Fd Centre and HQ AER RAMC 1956–59. USA: Exchange Officer, Brooke Army Medical Centre, Houston, Texas, 1959–60. BAOR: DDMS HQ 1st Br. Corps. 1960–63. DDMS HQ Northern Comd 1963–65. DDMS HQ Eastern Comd 1965–66. DMS HQ BAOR 1966. CBE 13th Jun. 1959, OBE 26th Aug. 1945, OStJ 1958, MID 19th Jul. 1945, IGSM and cl. NWF Mohmand 1935, 1939–45 S., Italy S., DM, WM, GSM & cl. Palestine. QEII Corn Medal 1953.

AHERNE Richard John L.LM 1913, RCPI. L.LM 1913 RCS (Ire). Flt Offr RAF 30th Jul. 1940. Med. Serv. MC.

AIDIN Abgar Read MB, BCh (TCD 1919). Maj. RAMC (1943).

AINLEY John Francis MB, BCh (QUB 1917). Surg. Capt. RN. CBE.

*****ALARDYCE** Ransome McNamara MB, BCh (TCD 1926). b. IFS. Capt. 1942. RAMC. Bayonetted to death when the Japanese overran Alexandra Military Hosp., Singapore on 15 February 1942. Buried in Krangi War Cemetery, Singapore, Plot 7A 19.

ALDWELL Basil Ernest West MB, BCh (TCD 1935). Address: 25 Raglan Rd, Dublin. Capt.–Maj. RAMC. MC. 'Captain Aldwell, during the period of the Sicilian Campaign, as Medical Officer of his Regiment, has shown a complete disregard for his personal safety in his efforts to give the earliest possible attention to battle casualties. In particular on July 13th, 1943, he worked in the open under enemy fire for long periods. On July 20th the Battalion reached a very exposed position after a night attack in the Cardone area – which could only be reached by moving across open country. Having been hit by a piece of shrapnel he still came forward in daylight to the Battalion forward defence lines and brought additional stretcher bearers and some badly needed water. He continued to work in this area until another medical officer was able to relieve him to have his wound attended. On all occasions his firm determination and personal courage have contributed much to the morale of the troops and has sustained their confidence in the quick treatment and evacuation of casualties.'

ALEXANDER Hugh Moore b. 23rd May 1892, Co. Cavan. s. Hugh (Rector of Killinagh) and Louisa Harriett Alexander, Termon, Killinagh, Co. Cavan. Educ. R. Sch. Cavan. RCSI, LRCPI (1916), LRCSI, LM. R. C. of I. Lt RAMC SR 28th Aug. 1916. Capt. 28th Feb. 1917. PC Lt (T/Capt.) 1st May 1919. Capt. 28th Feb. 1920. Maj. 28th Aug. 1928. r.p. 25th Dec. 1948. Served Mesopotamia from 27th Nov. 1916–19. Salonika Feb.–Jun. 1919. N. Russia Aug.–Oct. 1919. Malta 1920–22. Constantinople 1922–23. Malta 1923–24. Egypt 1924–25. Shanghai 1927–29. India 1931–35 and 1938–44. Medals BWM, VM, 1939–45 S., Burma S., DM, WM.

ALEXANDER Kenneth Houston Address: 29 Villiers Rd, Rathgar, Dublin. L.LM (RCPI 1942), L.LM (RCSI 1942). Flt Lt RAF 15th Nov. 1940.

ALLEN George Vance MB, BCh (QUB 1917). King Edward VII College of Medicine, Singapore. POW.

ALLEN James Aloysius b. 26th Jun. 1913, Cork. Address: 4 Knocklaun, St Luke's, Cork. MB, BCh, BAO (NUI 1938). Lt 1st Feb. 1939. Capt. 4th Sept. 1940. A/Maj. 24th Aug. 1942. T/Maj. 25th Nov. 1942. PC Capt. 4th Sept. 1944. Maj. 4th Sept. 1946. T/Col. 1st Jun. 1949. Lt Col. 21st Sept. 1954. Col. 4th Sept. 1961. BEF France 1939–40. Hosp. Ships 1945–46. MELF 1948. E. Africa 1948–51. CO BMH MacKinnon Road 1949. ADMS GHQ E. Africa Comd 1949–50. BAOR 1952–54. CO 28th Fd Amb. 1952–54. CO BMH Hanover 1954. FARELF: CO 18th Fd Amb. Hong Kong 1954–57. BAOR CO BMH Rinteln 1957–61. N. Africa SMO Tripolitania area & CMO BMH Tripoli 1961–64. CO Mil. Hosp. Tidworth 1965. Medals 1939–45 S., DM, WM, QEII Corn Medal 1953. d. 12th Apr. 1965, Tidworth.

ALLEN Richard Francis William Kinkead MB, BCh (TCD 1928), MD (TCD 1936). IMS. Lt Col. and Civil Surgeon Raipura, India.

ALLEN Robert George Address: Allenton, Cregagh, Belfast. MB, BCh (QUB 1939). Surg. Lt RNVR.

ALLEN Sydney James MB, BCh (QUB 1935). Surg. Lt Comdr RNVR.

ALLEY George Oliver Fairclough b. 3rd Dec. 1892, Dublin. MB, BCh, BAO, DPH, MD (TCD 1922). Lt 17th Jul. 1915 RAMC, Capt. 17th Jul. 1916. T/Maj. 18th Sept. 1925. Maj. 17th Jul. 1927. A/Lt Col. 1st Sept. 1941. Lt Col. 13th Oct. 1941. A/Col. 29th Jul. 1942. T/Col. 29th Jan. 1943. Col. 24th Apr. 1946. r.p. 27th Apr. 1951. Served France 1916–19, Mesopotamia 1920–22, India 1923–24, Shanghai 1927, India 1929–34, Aneas Mil. Hosp., Catterick 1934–35, and 1936–37, Egypt 1935–36. Mil. Hosp. Hong Kong 1938–41, CO Mil. Hosp. Barming Heath 1941–42, MEF CO 93 General Hospital 1942–43, South Africa 1943–46, CO Oribi Mil. Hosp. 1943–44, CO 130 Mil. Hosp.

Baragwanath 1944–45 and Jan.–Feb. 1946, ADMS 203 British Military Mission Feb.–Nov. 1946, ADMS HQ Highland District 1947–49, ADMS HQ East Anglia District 1949–41 specialist in anaesthetics 1928. MC 4th Jun. 1917, bar 16th Sept. 1918, second bar 15th Feb. 1919. Order of St John 1949, BWM, BM, GSM cl. Iraq 1919–20, Africa S. and cl. 8th Army, DM, WM.

ALLISON George Frederick b. 22nd Apr. 1888, Monaghan. s. James Andrew (Presbyterian clergyman) and Florence Matilda Allison, Mullaghadun, Monaghan Town. Educ. Campbell Coll., Belfast, Sept. 1902–Jul. 1905. RCSI LRCPI (1910), LRCSI, LM (Belfast). R. Presbyterian. Married Mrs Allison, 8 Easton Crescent, Cliftonville, Belfast. Lt RAMC 26th Jul. 1912. Capt. 30th Mar. 1915. A/Maj. 2nd Jun. 1918–3rd Jan. 1919. Maj. 26th Jul. 1924. Lt Col. 26th Dec. 1934. A/Col. 6th Jan. 1940. Col. 11th May 1940. A/Brig. 14th Dec. 1941. T/Brig. 4th Jun. 1942–18th May 1943. r.p. disability Hon. Brig. 2nd May 1945. Deputy Director of Medical Services from December 1940. Served BEF France from 20th Aug. 1914–19. CO 150th Fd Amb. 1919. Germany Jul.–Sept. 1919. Egypt 1920–22. Constantinople 1922–23. Egypt 1923–24 and 26–30. India 1933–38. SMO Bordon/Longmoor area 1938–39. BEF France. OIC Med. Div. 2 Gen. Hosp. 1939–40. CO 27 Gen Hosp. 1940. MEF 1940–43. ADMS HQ Suez Canal Base and L of C area 1941–43. ADMS HQ E. Kent Dist. 1943. CO Gen. Hosp. 1943–44. NWE Jun. to Jul. 1944. d. 5th Oct. 1946. Medals: CBE (8th Sept. 1942), MC (2nd Apr. 1919), 1914 S., BWM, VM, BWM, VM, Africa S. MID 30th Dec. 1941. When he took over his appointment there was one hospital in the area. There are now eleven hospitals, three convalescent depots and five POW hospitals. He supervised the erection and organisation of all these, and with his wide medical experience, his advice and instructions were invaluable to less experienced officers commanding hospitals. MC and OBE (Kt Comdr). Commemorated on Roll of Honour RCSI.

ALLISON Richard Sydney b. 1899. Address: 27 University Sq., Belfast. Educ. R. Belfast Acad. Inst. and Queen's Uni. MB, BCh (QUB 1921). Surg. Capt. RNVR.

ALLISON Samuel Address: Drumnaha, Bellarena, Londonderry. MB, BCh (QUB 1940). Maj. RAMC.

ALLIT William Ernest Charlton Address: Lansdowne, Greystones, Co. Wicklow. MB, BCh (TCD 1943). Surg. Lt 1943 RNVR.

ALLMAN-SMITH Edward Percival b. 3rd Nov. 1886 at Balbriggan, Co. Dublin. MB, BCh, BAO (TCD 1910) and LM Rot (TCD 1910). Lt RAMC 26th Jan. 1912. Capt. 30th Mar. 1915. A/Maj. 4th Jan. 1918. Maj. 26th Jan. 1924. Lt Col. 1st Jul. 1934. Col. 1st Aug. 1939. A/Brig. 9th Mar. 1941. T/Brig. 9th Sept. 1941. r.p. (Hon. Brig.) 22nd Apr. 1947. Served India 1913–16. Mesopotamia 1916–20. Constantinople 1922–23. India 1923–

27. Shanghai 1927. Egypt 1931–35. SMO Bordon Area 1933–36 & 1937–38. Palestine CO 3 CCS 1936–37. India CO BMH Mahow 1938–40. ADMS HQ 2nd Armd Div. 1940. MEF: DDMS HQ BF in Palestine and Trans-Jordan 1941–42. CO Mil. Hosp. Catterick 1942–46. PSMB 1940–47. Medals: OBE 3rd Jun. 1919, MC 25th Aug. 1917, MID 15th Aug. 1917 & 5th Jun. 1919, 1914 S., BWM, VM, Africa S., DM, WM.

AMBROSE Charles Going s. Charles Ambrose LLD, Tramore St and Catherine Nicholson Ambrose (née Going). Married Maud Ambrose (née Kirk). MD (TCD). Surgeon. MN SS *Princess*, Liverpool. d. 28th Dec. 1947 aged 61. Remembered Thomastown New Catholic Cemetery Grave 225.

ANDERSON Adelaide Eleanor Address: 5 Knocklofty, Belfast. MB, BCh (QUB 1934). Capt. RAMC.

ANDERSON Cyril Arthur Nichol Address: 17 Gilford Drive, Sandymount, Dublin. LRCP&SI (RCSI 1940). Flt Lt RAFVR 8th Jun. 1944.

ANDERSON David Harry MB, DPH (QUB 1933). Surg. Lt Comdr RNVR.

ANDERSON Duncan McKenzie Address: 2 Winston Gdns, Knock, Belfast. MB, BCh (QUB 1939). Capt. RAMC.

ANDERSON George Alexander Address: Plum Hill, Turnaface, Moneymore, Co. Derry. MB, BCh (TCD 1939). Capt. RAMC. POW Italy 1942.

ANDERSON George Francis Nicholas Address: 4 Pembroke Pk, Ballsbridge, Dublin. MB, BCh (TCD 1939). Maj. RAMC. Served at Almaza Egypt.

ANDERSON Henry James b. 19th Nov. 1912 at Holywood, Co. Down. Address: Oakleigh, Alexander Pk, Holywood, Co. Down. MB, BCh, BAO (TCD 1935). DPH (England 1949). Lt 22nd Oct. 1937 RAMC. Capt. 22nd Oct. 1938. PC Capt. 11th Oct. 1941. A/Maj. 1st Feb. 1941. T/Maj. 7th Mar. 1942. Maj. 1st Jul. 1946. Lt Col. 26th Jun. 1951. T/Col. 9th Jan. 1956. Col. 29th Feb. 1960. r.p. disability 7th Aug. 1963. Served India 1938–41. Malaya 1941–42. POW Singapore 1942. MELF 1949–52. ADMS HQ British Mil. Mission to Greece 1952. DDAH HQ N. Comd 1956–58. MELF 1958–61. ADAH GHQ 1958. DDAH HQ MELF/NEARELF 1959–61. ADAH HQ Scottish Comd 1961–63. Medals: 1939–45 S., Pacific S., DM, WM, GSM (with Cyprus cl.).

ANDERSON James Eric MB, BCh (TCD 1939). 2nd Lt Royal Inniskilling Fus. Invalided out 1942.

ANDERSON Kenneth Harold Address: The Rectory, Lisnaskea, Co. Fermanagh. MB, BCh (TCD 1942) Capt. RAMC.

ANDERSON Norman James Address: Cooley, Bernagh, Co. Tyrone. MB, BCh (TCD 1941). RAFVR.

ANDERSON Patrick St George b. 8th Nov. 1918 at Nottingham. MB, BCh, BAO (TCD 1942). FRCS (Edinburgh 1948). Lt RAMC 13th Mar. 1943. PC Capt. 3th Feb. 1953. T/Maj. 2nd Feb. 1953. Maj. 13th Aug. 1957. T/Lt Col. 10th Jan. 1954. Lt Col. 13th Aug. 1962. r.p. 1st Dec. 1965. Served NWE 1944–46. BAOR 1953. FARELF CIC Surg. Div. BMH Singapore 1954–57. BAOR: OIC Surg. Div. BMH Iserlohn 1961–65. Snr Spec. Surg. 1953. Consultant 1963. Medals: OBE (8th May 1956), 1939–45 S., France and Germany S., WM, GSM (cl. Malaya). MID 22nd Mar. 1945, 1946.

ANDERSON Robert Alexander b. 3rd Jan. 1891, Portadown, Co. Armagh. s. Robert (Draper) and Margaret Ann Anderson, 38 High St, Portadown, Co. Armagh. Educ. Dublin. MB (TCD 1914), BCh, BAO, LM (Rot. Hosp.), DPH (Belfast), DTM&H (Camb.), MA, FRFP and S (Glasgow), FRIPHH. R. C. of I. Lt RAMC SR 10th Nov. 1914. Mobd 16th Dec. 1914. Capt. 16th Jun. 1915. PC Lt (T/Capt.) 1st Jan. 1917. Capt. 16th May 1918. T/Maj. 20th Feb. 1919–18th Sept. 1920. Maj. 10th Nov. 1926. Lt Col. 7th Jul. 1939. A/Col. 16th Feb. 1941. T/Col. 16th Aug. 1941. r.p. Hon. Col. 21st Aug. 1947. Served Gallipoli from 23rd Jun. 1915–16. Egypt Jan. and Feb. 1916. India 1916–21 (Afghan. 1920) and 1923–29. DADH Wessex area 1929–31 and 1935–36. China: DADH/DADMS HQ Hong Kong 1931–34. India 1936–40: ADH & P HQ DADH/ DADMS HQ Hong Kong 1931–34. India 1936–40: ADH & P HQ E. Comd 1939–40. ADH HQ N. Comd Apr.–Jul. 1940. CO 217th Fd Amb. 1940–41. CO 25th Gen. Hosp. 1041. MEF 1942–43: ADMS 25 Corp/Tps. Cyprus 1942. DDH GHQ 1942–43. India/ALFSEA 1943–47: CO BMH Lahore & Ferozepore 1943, CO 74th IGH (C) 1943–45, HQ & L. of C. area A/ADMS Jul.–Aug. 1944. ADMS 1945–46, CO 139 IBGH Apr.–Jun. 1946, CO CMH Ranchi 1946–47. Medals: OBE (6th Feb. 1945), 1915 S., BWM, VM, 1939–45 S., Africa S., Burma S., DM, WM. MID 19th Sept. 1946. d. 2nd Apr. 1955.

ANDERSON Samuel Campbell College MB, BCh (QUB 1928), DPH (QUB 1931). Maj. RAMC.

ANDERSON William Maurice Eyre b. 31st Aug. 1908, Dublin. Address: 4 Mountjoy Sq., Dublin. Eldest s. the late Rev. William Anderson, Mountjoy School. MB, BCh, BAO (TCD 1933). MD (TCD 1941). Lt RAMC 7th Jun. 1934. Capt. 7th Jun. 1935. PC Capt. 7th Jun. 1939. A/Maj. 1st May 1940. T/Maj. 1st Aug. 1940. Maj. 7th Jun. 1943. A/Lt Col. 18th Nov. 1941. T/Lt Col. 18th Feb. 1942. Resigned 2nd Aug. 1946. Served India 1934–40. CO 206th Fd Amb. 1941–43. CO 105th AL Fd Amb. 1943–45. NWE 1944–45. CO 171 Fd Amb 1945. CO 2 Medical LT CDO 1945. Wounded at Normandy Jun. 1944 first Allied Airborne Army. DSO. Medals DSO (24th Jan. 1946), IGSM (with cl. NWF and Mohmand 1935), 1939–45 S., France and Germany S., CM, WM. d. 13th Dec. 1986. Cremated England.

ANDREWS Samuel Address: Fern Hill, Annaclone, Banbridge, Co. Down. BSc, MB, BCh (QUB 1921). Maj. RAMC.

ARCHER Gilbert Thomas Lancelot b. 6th Apr. 1903. Dublin. MB, BCh, BAO 1926 LM Coombe 1926 MRVPI 1953 FRCPI 1958 (TCD). Lt 26th Jan. 1928. Capt. 26th Jul. 1930. Maj. 26th Jan. 1937. A/Lt Col. 26th Jun. to 17th Sept. 1940 and 1st to 2nd Jul. 1943. T/Lt Col. 3rd Jul. 1943. Lt Col. 4th Sept. 1945. T/Col. 18th Feb. 1949. Col. 7th Feb. 1950. T/Brig. 25th Oct. 1953. Brig. 16th Apr. 1956. Maj. Gen. 2nd May 1958. r.p. 27th Jan. 1961. Ceased R/O 6th Apr. 1963. India 1929/34. China 1937/40. CO Emergency Vaccine Lab 1940. Madagascar 1942–43. ADP West Africa 1943/45. ADP Northern Comd 1945. ADP War Office 1945/46. Assistant Prof. of Path. RAM College 1946–49. MELF DDP and CO COMD Path Lab 1949/52. CO David Bruce Lab 1952/53. D Path. and Cons. Path. To the Army 1953/60. QHS 30th Nov. 1953. Specialist in Path. 1935. CB 11th Jun. 1960, 1939–45 S., DM, WM.

ARMSTRONG Brian MB. Capt. RAMC. POW.

ARMSTRONG Harold Kenneth Brian Address: 11 Deramore Pk, Malone Rd, Belfast. LRCP (Edinburgh 1937), LRCS (Edinburgh 1937). LRFPF (Glasgow 1937). Capt. RAMC.

ARMSTRONG Herbert Capper s. Councillor Hugh Armstrong, 11 Deramore Pk, Malone Rd, Belfast. MB, BCh (QUB 1930), DPH (QUB 1933). Maj. RWAFF, Ethiopian Campaign.

ARMSTRONG James Rowan Address: Audley Lodge, Ballymena, Co. Antrim. MB, BCh (QUB 1933). Wing Comdr RAFVR.

ARMSTRONG John Hunter Address: Claremont Rd, Sandymount, Dublin. LRCP&S (RCSI 1934). Lt British Army 4th Jan. 1941. Served Burma.

ARMSTRONG John Killen MB, BCh (QUB 1933). Surg. Lt Comdr RNVR.

ARTHUR James Lynn LAH (Dublin 1941), L.LM (1941 RCPI), L.LM (RCSI 1941). Lt RAMC 7th Nov. 1942.

ARTHUR Thomas Neil MB, BCh (TCD 1939). Sq. Ldr RAF.

ASHE Edward Samuel Armstrong MB, BCh (TCD 1933). Lt Col. RAMC (1939). OC 62 Indian Fd Amb.

ASHFORTH Eric Stanley L.LM (RCPI 1936), L.LM (RCSI 1936). Lt RAMC 9th Sept. 1939.

ASHTON Eric George Address: Cooleveen, Athlone, Co. Westmeath. MB, BCh (TCD 1933). Surg. Lt Comdr RN.

ATCHINSON Robert William Rupert Address: Loy, Cookstown, Co. Tyrone. MB, BCh (QUB 1939). Capt. RAMC.

ATKINS Robert Ringrose Gelston b. 29th Apr. 1891, Cork City. s. Thomas (Surg. Physician) and Rose Margaret Atkins, 20 St Patrick's Pl., Cork. Educ. TCD. BA, MB (1914), BCh and BAO (1914), MD (1918), LM (Rot. Hosp.). R. C. of I. Lt RAMC SR 31st Aug. 1914. Mobd 23rd Sept. 1914. Capt. 1st Apr. 1915. A/Maj. 4th Sept.–27th Dec. 1918. PC Capt. 1st Sept. 1910. Maj. 28th Aug. 1926. Lt Col. 22nd Apr. 1937. A/Col. 17th Jun. 1940. T/Col. 17th Dec. 1940. Col. 27th Apr. 1943. A/Brig. 6th Oct. 1941. T/Brig. 6th Apr. 1942. Hon. Brig. 12th Aug. 1946. Served in France from 21st May 1915 and 1916–18. Wounded Jul. 1917. Mesopotamia 1920–22. Egypt 1922–25. Cyprus 1923–24. Mil. Hosp. Edinburgh 1927–28. India 1928–34. BMH Calcutta 1928–30. BMH Lahore & Dalhousie 1931–33. Mil. Hosp. Tidworth 1934–37. Malaya: CO Mil. Hosp. Tanglin, Singapore 1937–39 invalided. Comdt 11th Depot & 50 Gen. Hosp. May–Jun. 1940. CO 40 Gen. Hosp. Jun.–Aug. 1940. CO 3 Gen. Hosp. 1940–41. MEF/CMF 1941–43. ADMS HQ 7th Armd Div. Aug.–Oct. 1941. DDMS HQ 30th Corps. 1941–42. CO 9th Gen. Hosp. 1942–43. DDMS Feb.–Jul. 1943 invalided. ADMS HQ Hants. & Dorset Dist. 1943–44. ADMS HQ NI Dist. 1944–45. DDMS 1945–46. Medals: OBE (9th Sept. 1942), MC (18th Oct. 1917) 1915 S., BWM, VM, GSM (cl. Iraq), 1939–45 S., Africa S., ITS, DM, WM. MID 1st Jan. 1916 and 23rd Mar. 1944.

AUSTIN Frederick Cecil Kyle b. 11th Dec. 1889, Londonderry. s. George S. (Draper) and Bessie Austin, Hillmount, Victoria Pk, Londonderry. Educ. Foyle Coll. Londonderry. Edinburgh Uni. MB (1913), ChB, MD (Edin. 1925), DTM&H (Eng. 1929). R. Methodist. T/Lt 18th Aug. 1914. Capt. 18th Aug. 1915. PC Lt 1st Jan. 1917. Capt. 18th Feb. 1918. Maj. 18th Aug. 1926. Lt Col. 2nd Feb. 1937. Col. 2nd Jul. 1942. r.p. 17th Feb. 1950. Served BEF France 21st Sept. 1914–18. India 1918–22. E. Persia 1918–19. NWF 1919–22. Malaya 1926–29 and 1933–36. Med. Special Mil. Hosp. Shorncliffe 1936–37. OIC Med. Div. Cambridge Hosp. Aldershot 1937–38. India 1938–47. Med. Spec. Meerut 1939–40. CO BMH Chatrata 1939. BMH Nowshera 1940–42. CO BMH Calcutta 1942. CIMH Barrackpore 1942–44. ADMS HQ Sind Dist. 1944–45. ADMS HQ 110 L of C area 1945–46. PSMB London Dist. 1947–49. Spec. In Med. 1933. Medals: 1914 S., BWM, VM, IGSM (cl. Afgh. 1919), Burma S., DM, WM. d. 18th Oct. 1966, Gilford, Surrey.

AUSTIN Richard Andrew b. 25th Oct. 1892, Londonderry. s. Richard Andrew (Pharmaceutical Chemist) and Marjory Jane Austin, 1 Goldsmith Tce, Bray, Co. Wicklow. Educ. RCSI LRCPI (1914), LRCSI, LM. R. Presbyterian. Lt RAMC SR 9th Sept. 1914. Mobd 23rd Sept. 1914. Capt. 1st Apr. 1915. PC. Capt. 1st Jun. 1918. A/Maj. 4th Sept. 1918–17th Jan. 1919. Maj. 9th Sept. 1926. Lt Col. 30th Sept. 1937. A/Col. 18th Oct. 1941. T/Col. 18th Apr. 1942. Col. 16th Oct. 1943. A/Brig. 26th Feb. 1942. T/Brig. 12th Sept. 1942. r.p. Hon. Brig. 29th May 1955. Served Gallipoli 5th Jul. 1915–16. Egypt Feb.–Jun. 1916. France 1916–19. India 1919–22. W. Afr. (Sierra Leone) 1925–26 and 1927–28. Chief Instructor and 2 IC Depot RAMC 1938–41. MEF 1941–45. DDMS HQ N. L of C Dist. 1941–42, DDMS HQ 10 & 30 Corps. 1942–43. ADMS HQ 16 Area 1943–45. ADMS HQ N.W. Dist. 1946–47. PSMB London Dist. 1947–49. E. Comd 1949–55. Medals: MC (25th Nov. 1916), 1915 S., BWM, VM, IGS (Waz. 1919–21), Africa S. with 8th Army cl., WM. d. 28th Dec. 1968 in hospital after sustaining severe injuries from a motorcycle on 9th Dec. Commemorated on Roll of Honour RCSI.

B

BAILIE Hugh William Cochrane Address: Seabank, Waterloo, Larne, Co. Antrim. Campbell College. MB, BCh (QUB 1938). Major RAMC. MID.

BAILIE Thomas Harold Campbell College. MB, BCh (QUB 1928). Maj. RAMC.

BAIRD Robert Hamilton Address: 46 Ravenhill Pk, Belfast. MB, BCh (QUB 1939). Lt Col. RAMC. MID.

BAIRD Thomas Terence Address: The Rectory, Strabane, Co. Tyrone. MB, DPH (QUB 1939). Surg. Lt RNVR.

BAKER Abraham Sydney BSc, MB (QUB 1934). Maj. RAMC.

BAKER Robert Ruckley MB, BCh (TCD 1922). Surg. Comdr Mediterranean Fleet 1939–41. RN Hosp. Portland 1942–44. Bermuda 1944–45.

BAMBER David Murrough MB, BCh (TCD 1943). Capt. RAMC.

BAMBER William Address: Farm Lodge, Ballymena, Co. Antrim. MB, BCh (QUB 1936), DPH (QUB 1939). Maj. RAMC.

BAMFORD Frederick Edward Address: Lisnaroe House, Clones, Co. Monaghan. LRCP&S (RCSI 1937). Lt IMS 4th May 1937.

BAMFORD William Earls Address: Lisnaroe House, Clones, Co. Monaghan. MB, BCh (TCD 1939). Sq. Ldr RAF (1941).

BANNERMAN Walter Biggar MRCS (England 1900), LRCP (London 1900), DPH (RCPI&S 1910). OBE.

BANNIGAN Charles Address: Edenville, Strabane, Co. Tyrone. MB, BCh (NUI 1913). MC.

BANNISTER Muriel Address: 1 Grosvenor Sq., Rathmines, Dublin. MB, BCh (TCD 1939). Capt. RAMC.

BARBER Alfred Desmond MB, BCh (TCD 1931). Maj. IMS.

BARBER Harold Stuart MB, BCh (TCD 1938), MD (TCD 1938), FRCPI (1941) W/Cmdr RAF.

BARBER John Morgan Address: 28 Ballyholme Esplanade, Bangor, Co. Down. Eldest s. J. G. Barber. Married 2nd dt. William Moore, Demesne House, Bangor, Co. Down. Educ. Bangor Grammar School. MB, BCh (QUB 1939). Maj. RAMC. Captured by the Germans on the island of Leros,

Greece and POW for a month before being rescued by the RN while en route to a POW camp on the mainland.

BARDON Desmond Terence Address: Glenaros, Dartry Rd, Rathmines, Dublin. MB, BCh (TCD 1936). RAMC.

BARLAS Alexander Richard b. 17th Jul. 1895, Dublin. s. Alexander Richard (Civil Service Sec.) and Mabel Evelyn Barlas, 16 Bushy Park Rd, Rathgar, Dublin. Educ. TCD, MB (1917), BCh, BAO (1917). R. Presbyterian. T/Lt RAMC 4th Oct. 1917. T/Capt. 4th Oct. 1918. PC Lt 1st Apr. 1919. Capt. 4th Apr. 1921. Maj. 4th Oct. 1929. A/ Lt Col. 23rd Feb. 1940. Lt Col. 30th Jan. 1944. A/Col. 25th Jan. 1943–12th Jan. 1946. r.p. Hon. Col. 11th Nov. 1948. First served in the theatre of war Mesopotamia Nov. 1917 until 1921. RMO 1st/10 GR 1918–20. India 1921. Malta Sept.–Nov. 1922. Constantinople 1922–23. India 1926–29. Shanghai 1927. Bermuda 1933–36. BEF France 1939–40. CO 4th Fd Amb. Feb.–Oct. 1940. India/SEAC 1942–45: CO CIMH Quetta 1942–43. ADMS HQ 39 Indian Div. 1943–44. CO 38 Gen. Hosp. 1944–45. CO 35 Gen. Hosp. 1945. Scottish Comd Med. Pool 1946–47. CO Mil. Hosp. Shaftsbury Feb.–Jul. 1947. ALFSEA/FARELF 1947–48: CO 2 CMH Malaya 1947–48. ADMS HQ Johore Sub Dist. Apr.–Jun. 1948. Medals: BWM, VM, IGSM (3 cls Iraq, NW Persia, Kurdistan), 1939–45 S., Burma S., DM, WM. MID 20th Dec. 1940. Commemorated on Roll of Honour Sir Patrick Dun's Hosp.

BARNETT Norman Selig Address: 62 Cliftonville Rd, Belfast. MB, BCh (QUB 1938). Capt. RAMC.

BARNSLEY Alan Gabriel MRCS (England 1942), LRCI (London 1942). TCD (1940). RAMC.

*****BARRETT** Anthony Richard b. 1915. Educ. at St Muirdeach's College, Ballina, Co. Mayo. Younger s. John Barrett of Ballybeg Lodge, Bangor Erris, Co. Mayo. MB, BCh (1938 UCC). Ship's surgeon and in 1939 joined the staff of Westham Mental Hospital. Married Madge McDonagh of Ballymote, Co. Sligo. T/Surgeon Lt RNVR. Missing presumed KIA 10th Dec. 1942, HMS *Stanley*.

BARRETT Daniel Francis MB, BCh, BAO (UCD 1927).

BARRETT St Clair Edward John MRCSI & LACP (London). (QUB 1919). Lt Col. RAMC. MID.

BARRY David Martin Address: Gracefield, Waltham Tce, Blackrock, Dublin. MB, BCh (TCD 1938). Sq. Ldr RAF.

BARRY James Harding L.LM (1912 RCPI), L.LM (1912 RCSI). Address: Inver, The Grove, Burnham-on-Sea. Medals: DSO, MC.

BARRY Michael Joseph Address: 1 Victoria Villas, Old Blackrock Rd, Cork. MB, BCh, BAO (UCC 1936). Lt IMS.

BARRY Phillip Cahill b. 19th Jan. 1918, Dublin. Address: Thurles, Co. Tipperary. LRCP&SI (RCSI 1944). Lt RAMC 26th May 1945. Capt. 26th May 1946. T/Maj. 20th Mar, 1950. Maj. 25th May 1953. PC Lt 14th Apr. 1955. Capt. 14th Apr. 1955. Maj. 14th Apr. 1955. T/Lt Col. 10th Aug. 1956. Lt Col. 12th Dec. 1960. retd 1st Feb. 1962. Served India 1945–47, MELF Egypt/Palestine 1947. FARELF 1949–52. BAOR 1952–55. CO 36th Fd Amb. 1956–58. Malta 1956. Cyprus 1956–59. CO 4rd Bde. Gp. Med. Coy. 1958–59. CO 19th Bde. Gp. Med. Coy. 1959–60. 19th Fd Amb. 1961. S. Cameroons 1961. CO 2 Bde. Gp. Med. Coy. 1961–62. Medals: WM, GSM (with Palestine 1945–48 cl.), Malaya cl., Cyprus cl.

BARRY Richard Garrett George Address: Greenville, Carrigtwohill, Co. Cork. MB, BCh, BAO (UCC 1937). Lt RAMC.

BARRY Stephen James b. 25th Apr. 1885 at Carrigtwohill, Cork. LRCP&SI LM 1909 (Cork). Lt 26th Jan. 1912. Capt. 30th Mar. 1915. T/Maj. 25th Feb. 1918. Maj. 26th Jan. 1924. Lt Col. 29th May 1934. Col. 15th Jul. 1939. r.p. 10th Jul. 1942. Served India 1913–14. Mesopotamia 1914–16. India 1916–22 and 1924–30. China SMO Tientsim 1934–37. CIC Surg. Div. Royal Victoria Hosp. Netley 1938–39. ADMS HQ Lancs Area Jul.–Sept. 1939. HQ Southern Area 1939–40. HQ S. Midland Area 1940–41. HQ 1 Div. 1941–42. d. 10th Nov. 1959. Medals: Dispatches 13th Jul. 1916, 1915 S., BWM, VM, WM.

BARRY-WALSH M.H. Capt. RAMC.

BARTER Richard Wade MB (TCD 1942) Flt Lt RAFVR (1945) Merchant Service 1947–48.

BARTON Michael Address: Co. Kerry. L.LM (RCPI 1921), L.LM (RCSI 1921). Flt Offr RN & RAF 8th Jun. 1944.

BATESON William George Address: Mullowoud, Balmoral, Belfast. MB (QUB 1934). Col. RAMC. Served India NWF. Dunkirk: minesweeper on which he was escaping was bombed for two-and-a-half hours and set on fire and he was the sole survivor. MID (2).

BEAMISH Desmond William, b. 13th May 1891, Datchet, Bucks., England. Educ. RCSI L.LM (1913), RCPI, L.LM (1913), RCSI, LM (Rot. Hosp). R. C. of I. T/RAMC 21st Jan. 1915. T/Capt. 21st Jan. 1916. PC Lt 1st Jan. 1917. A/ Maj. 21st Oct. 1918. Maj. 21st Jan. 1927. A/ Lt Col. 4th Jan. 1940. Lt Col. 29th Jun. 1940. Col. 10th Aug. 1945. r.p. 12th Oct. 1948. Served 1914–18 War Western Europe from 19th Sept. 1915. Salonika & Danube 1915–19. India 1919–24. Hong Kong 1927–31. Pathology Spec. Experimental station Porton 1931–35. Egypt DADP BTE 1935–39. ADP N. Comd Jan.–Jul. 1940. MEF 1940–45. Physiologist GHP MEF 1940–41. 63 Gen. Hosp. 1941–42. PMO Cyrenaica 1942–43. NWE/Germany 2 CA Pool

1945–48. Medals: MC (3rd Jun. 1918), 1915 S., BWM, VM, Africa S. with 8th Army cl. WM. MID 28th Nov. 1917. Commemorated on Roll of Honour RCSI.

BEARE Abraham Seftel b. 1st Feb. 1916. Address: Sheares St, Cork City, Co. Cork. MB, BCh, BAO (NUI 1938), DTM&H (England 1954). Lt RAMC 19th Jan. 1940. Capt. 19th Jan. 1941. A/Maj. 22nd May 1946. T/Maj. 22nd Aug. 1946. PC Capt. 15th Jan. 1948. Maj. 19th Jan. 1948. T/Lt Col. 1st Jul. 1954. Lt Col. 4th Sept. 1958. r.p. 16th May 1960. India 1941–45. Trooping Duties 1946–48. MELF 1948. E. Africa 1948–52. CDEE/MRE Porton 1954–55. BAOR 1955–57. ADP Scottish Comd & OIC Comd Lab. 1957. Demonstrator in Serology RAM Coll. 1957–59. FARELF 1959–60: Path Lab. Singapore 1959. BMH Kinrara 1959–60. Medals: DM, WM.

BEARE John Martin Address: Linenhall Street, Ballymoney, Co. Antrim. MB, BCh (QUB 1942). Surg. Lt RNVR.

BEATTIE John MB, BCh (QUB 1923). Col. RAMC. Legion D'Honneur. MID (2).

BEATTIE Myra Kathleen Address: 6 Ravenhill Tce, Ravenhill Rd, Belfast. MB, BCh (QUB 1924), MD (1927). IMS Maj. IMC.

BECKETT Donal Park Address: Caragh, Gordon Avenue, Foxrock, Dublin. MB, BCh (TCD 1937). Maj. RAMC.

BELL Robert James Edwin Address: 11 Broughton Gdns, Ravenhill Rd, Belfast. MB, BCh (QUB 1939). Lt Col. RAMC.

BELTON William MB, BCh, BAO, DPH (UCD 1924). Lt RAMC. First enlisted 7th Oct. 1939.

BENNET Edward Armstrong b. 21st Oct. 1888, Co. Armagh. s. Mrs Marion Bennet, Ardstrathan, Richmond. Educ. Campbell Coll. Belfast from Sept. 1901. TCD BA (1910), MB (1925), BCh, BAO, MD (1930), MA (1930), DPH (Eng. 1926). R. C. of I. Brig. CF 4th class AC Dept. 21st Nov. 1914. Served 1914–18 War France from Jul. 1915. CF 1914–19. Served in WWII India. Medals: MC (25th Nov. 1916), 1915 S., BWM, VM.

BENNETT David Address: 80A Church St, Newtownards, Co. Down. MB, BCh (QUB 1936). Surg. Lt Comdr RNVR.

BENNETT Harry Milne Address: Ballinrees, Macosquin, Coleraine. MB, BCh (QUB 1940). Capt. RAMC.

BENNETT James Henderson b. 2nd May 1915. Address: 236 Chestnut Gdns, Belfast, Co. Antrim. MB, BCh, BAO (QUB 1941), DPH (England 1953), DIH (1964). Lt 15th Aug. 1942. Capt. 15th Aug. 1943. A/Maj. 7th Dec. 1945. T/Maj. 4th Mar. 1946. PC Capt. 15th Aug. 1947. T/Maj. 14th Mar. 1949. Maj. 15th Aug. 1950. T/Lt Col. 4th Aug. 1956. Lt Col. 26th Nov. 1959. Col. 15th Aug. 1965. Paiforce 1943. Egypt/Syria 1943–44. CMF 1944–45. RMO 15th FA 1943–45. NWE 1945. Italy

1945–47. FARELF 1949–52. MELF: ADAH HQ 2nd Corps. 1956. FARELF Singapore 1958–59. SMO RMA Sandhurst 1960–64. FARELF Hong Kong 1964–67. Sen. Spec. Army Health 1949. Medals: 1939–45 S., Italy S., DM, WM, GSM with cls Malaya and Near East, OStJ 1966. MID 19th Jul. 1945, 23rd May 1946, 27th Apr. 1951.

BENNETT Morris TCD 1937. Surg. Lt RNVR.

BENNETT Vincent Address: Highfield Villa, Highfield Ave., College Rd, Cork. MB, BCh, BAO (UCC 1936). Lt RAMC.

BENSON Wallace b. 14th Jun. 1878 at Bouqueron, Isire, France. MB, BCh, BAO (TCD). Lt RAMC 31st Jul. 1905. Capt. 31st. Jan. 1909. Maj. 15th Oct. 1915. T/Lt Col. 1st Jun. 1916. Bt. Lt Col. 3rd Jun. 1918. Lt Col. 11th May 1929. Bt.Col. 1st Jan. 1932. Col. 1st May 1934. r.p. 14th Jun. 1935. Rejoined 24th Aug. 1939. Reverted to r.p. ill health 18th Apr. 1944. Served India 1907–12. Gallipoli 1915. Egypt 1915–16. E. Africa 1916–19. CO 14th CCS 1916–17 and 1918–19. ADMS GHQ GB. Egypt 1924–29. SMO & CO Mil. Hosp. Ras-el-Tin 1929. CO QA Mil. Hosp. 1939–43. Medals: CBE (3rd Jun. 1935), DSO (1st Feb. 1917). IGSM (with cl. NWF 1908). 1914–15 S., BWM, VM, DM, WM, KGV Silver Jub. Medal 1935.

BEREEN James Frederick Joseph Address: Rathcoole, South Parade, Belfast. MB, BCh (QUB 1937). Maj. RAMC.

BERGIN, Francis Patrick Thomas MB (TCD 1933). RAFVR.

*****BERGIN** Matthew Donald Murrough Address: Beechgrove, Kildare, Co. Kildare. L.MED, LCh (TCD 1938), MB, BCh (TCD 1939). Capt. 188636 RAMC. KIA. 15 Sept. 1944. Italy. Buried in Gradara War Cemetery, Plot 11F4.

BERMINGHAM Patrick Xavier Address: 32 Harcourt Street, Dublin. MB, BCh, BAO (UCD 1936). Lt RAMC.

BERMINGHAM William Thomas MB, BCh (TCD 1933). Capt. RAMC. Invalided 1940.

BERRY Sydney Lurton TCD 1936. Lt RAMC.

BETTY Brendan Ernest Address: Fort Lodge, Enniskillen, Co. Fermanagh. L.LM (RCPI 1935), LM (RCSI 1935). Flt Offr RAF 9th Jul. 1942.

BEVERIDGE Arthur Joseph b. 21st Mar. 1893, Rathgar, Dublin. s. John F. (Town Clerk of Dublin) and Jane Beveridge, 33 Belgrave Sq., Rathmines, Dublin. Educ. Belvedere Coll. Dublin. NUI MB (1915), BCh, BAO, LM, MSc (NUI 1929), DPH (QUB Belfast 1926). R. RC. Married 1928 Sheila McNamara. Lt RAMC SR 27th Jul. 1914. Mobd 19th Jul. 1915. Capt. 19th Jan. 1916. A/Maj. 4th Jan. 1918–15th Feb. 1919 and 16th Feb–26th Apr. 1919. PC Capt. 1st Apr. 1919. Maj. 19th Jul. 1927. A/Lt Col. 27th Feb.–1st Jun. 1940. Lt Col. 21st Oct. 1941. A/Col. 13th Oct. 1941.

T/Col. 11th Apr. 1942. Col. 1st May 1946. A/Brig. 17th Aug.–2nd Sept. 1947. T/Brig. 12th Feb.–14th Aug. 1948 and 11th–27th Nov. 1949. Brig. 28th Nov. 1949. T/Maj. Gen. 1st Nov. 1950. Maj. Gen. 8th Nov. 1951. r.p. 24th Apr. 1953. Served France 5th Jun. 1916–19 and 1919–20. Mesopotamia 1920–23. India 1923–25. BAOR 1925–27. Jamaica DADH and P 1928–31. Malaya 1935–38. DADH and P 1935–36. DADP E. Anglia area 1938. Physiologist Antigas lab 1939–40. BEF France 1939–40. Norway Apr.–May 1940. ADMS HQ 146 Inf. Brig. Feb.–Mar. and Apr.–May 1940. CO 197 Fd Amb. Mar.–Apr. 1940. CO 23rd CCS May–Oct. 1940. CO 221 Fd Amb. 1940–41. ADMS HQ 55 Inf. Div. 1941–43. W. Africa 1943–45. CO 6 (WA) Gen. Hosp. Nov.–Dec. 1943. CO 36 (WA) Gen. Hosp. Dec. 1943–Jan. 1944. ADMS HQ Sierra Leone area Feb.–Oct. 1944. CO 37 (WA) Gen. Hosp. 1944–45. ADMS HQ 1AA Gp. 1945. E. Africa 1945–46. CO 6th E. (EA) Gen. Hosp. Dec. 1945–Mar. 1946. CO 1 BMH Apr.–Sept. 1946. 1946–48. ADMS HQ S. area 1946–47. ADMS/DDMS HQ BT and Trans Jordan 1947–48. ADMS HQ Aldershot Dist. 1948–49. DDMS HQ Scottish Comd 1949–50. DMS GHQ MELF 1950–53. KHP 2nd Oct. 1951. QHP 1st Apr. 1952. Medals: CB (1st Jan. 1953), OBE (3rd Jun. 1935), MC (4th Feb. 1918), BWM, VM, GSM (cl. Iraq), Palestine (1946–48), 1939–45 S., DM, WM, Norwegian Mil. Cross (11th Aug. 1942) for bravery and devotion to duty during the Norwegian Campaign. MID 24th Dec. 1917, 20th Dec. 1940, 7th Jan. 1949. d. 25th Sept. 1959, Venice.

BEW Kenneth Address: Nalleen, Hawthornden Rd, Knock, Belfast. MB, BCh (QUB 1942). Flt Lt RNVR.

BIGGART Hugh Gault Address: 64 Kings Rd, Knock, Belfast. MB, BCh (QUB 1942). Maj. RAMC.

BIGGER Joseph Warwick b. 1892, Belfast. s. Edward Cory (Med. Insp. Local Gov.) and Maud Coulter Bigger, 104 Palmerston Rd, Rathmines, Dublin. Address: Ardrigh, Temple Rd, Dartry, Dublin. Educ. St Andrews Coll. 1901–10, TCD (1915) MA, MB, BCh (1919), DPH (1918), MD (TCD 1918), FRCP (London 1943). R. Presbyterian. Lt Col. RAMC. Served 1914–18 War. d. 17th Aug. 1951.

BINGHAM Edward William MB, BCh (TCD 1926). Surg. Comdr RNVR. OBE.

BINGHAM John Alexander Address: 482 Lisburn Rd, Belfast. MB, BCh (QUB 1934), FRCS (England 1938). Maj. IMS.

BINGHAM William Address: Lacken, Ballyroney, Banbridge, Co. Down. MB, BCh (QUB 1941). Surg. Lt RNVR.

BINGHAM William George Ashleigh MB, BCh (QUB 1933). Capt. RAMC.

BLACK David Address: 11 North Circular Rd, Belfast. MB, BCh (QUB 1937). Surg. Lt Comdr RNVR.

BLACK Duncan McCallum Address: 12 Cliftonville Rd, Belfast. Campbell College. MB, BCh (QUB 1936). Maj. IMS.

BLACK James Knowles Address: 630 Antrim Rd, Belfast. MB, BCh (QUB 1941). Surg. Lt RNVR.

BLACK John Joseph Address: Ballintoy, Ballycastle, Co. Antrim. MB, BCh (QUB 1939). Flt Lt (M) RAFVR.

*****BLACK** Thomas Alexander Hamilton Address: Leardin, Gortin, Co. Tyrone. s. William Samuel and Margaret Hamilton. MB, BCh (TCD 1942). Flt Offr 160654 RAF (Medical Branch). d. 1st Apr. 1944 aged 26. Buried in Blackpool (Carleton) Cemetery, grave section 2.

*****BLACKHAM** Charles Hubert Address: Ballymount, Clondalkin, Co. Dublin. s. Rachel Kathleen. Husband of Idrys Mary Griffith-Blackham of Brenockshire. MB, BCh (TCD 1937). Capt.127673 RAMC (1943). KIA Italy 4 Jun. 1944 aged 29. Buried Casino War Cemetery, Plot I.B.1.

BLACKHAM George Cecil Address: 10 Nutley Pk, Stillorgan Rd, Dublin. Only s. the late Richard Blackham of Ballymount, Clondalkin, Dublin. MB, BCh (TCD 1936) Surg. Lt RNVR. SEAC (1945).

BLACKSTOCK Arthur Millar MD, ChB (QUB 1939). Surg. Lt RNVR.

BLAIR James William McCloy Address: Pine Hill Manse, Knockanollet, Co. Antrim. MB, BCh (QUB 1941). Capt. RAMC.

BLAIR John Norman Address: 8 St Jude's Avenue, Ormeau Rd, Belfast. MB, BCh (QUB 1940). Capt. RAMC. MID. Kt of the Order of Orange Nassau with Swords.

BLAIR Joseph Lindsay Address: Innis, Ballycastle Rd, Coleraine. MB, BCh (QUB 1941). Capt. RAMC.

BLAND Ronald Haywood MB, BCh (TCD 1928). MD (TCD 1937). MRCPI (1938). Maj. (Temp. Lt Col.) RAMC. from Bray, Co. Wicklow. PMO Eritrea. OBE. This officer was in charge of the civilian medical work in Eritrea from the occupation in April 1941. He showed remarkable ability in organising and maintaining the civil medical service of Eritrea with very limited resources and in the face of considerable apathy on the part of the local Italian officials and the Italian and native population. His resolute and efficient handling of the situation was the means of securing the confidence of the local population on the medical and sanitary side of the administration, and materially contributed to the success of the British Military Government in this territory.

BLEWETT Basil b. 4th Sept. 1904, Belfast. MB, BCh, BAO (QUB 1931), DTM&H (England 1950). MD (QUB 1951). Lt 17th Aug. 1931. Capt. 1st May 1934. A/Maj. 25th Nov. 1939. T/Maj. 25th Feb. 1940. Maj. 17th Aug. 1941. A/Lt Col. 12th Aug. 1943. T/Lt Col. 12th Nov. 1943. Lt Col. 15th Jun. 1947. A/Col. 5th Jan. 1946. T/Col. 5th Jul. 1946. r.p. Hon. Col. 1st Feb. 1953. Served India 1932–38, BEF France 1939–40, West Africa (Nigeria) 1941–43. CO 180th Fd Amb. 1943–45. CMF 1944–45. CO 2nd Mobile CCS, 1st Fd Amb, 140th Fd Amb., 6th Lt Fd Amb. India 1945–47. ADMS HQ 26th Indian Div. 1946. CO CMH Dinapore 1947. ADP W. Comd 1949–52, A/ADMS HQ W. Comd 1951–52, MELF: ADP and CO Central Path Lab. 1952–53. Medals: 1939–45 S., Italy S., DM, WM, GSM with SE Asia cl. 1945–46. MID 26th Jun. 1947.

BLUETT Douglas b. Delgany, Co. Wicklow. MB, BCh (TCD 1926). A/Col. RAMC. Brig. OBE. O. of Leopold, Croix de Guerre 2 MIDs. 'As officer Commanding 14th Field Ambulance in the Western Desert until May 28th 1942, Colonel Bluett showed exceptional efficiency and devotion to duty, being quite imperturbable under fire and an example to all ranks, thereby welding together a unit which was a model field ambulance in every way. Selected as Assistant Director of Medical Services on May 28th 1942, his work in co-ordinating the reception and evacuation of thousands of casualties under circumstances of extreme difficulty and danger was beyond praise. He remained at his post until the day before the fall of Tobruk, when to his regret he was ordered to another responsible appointment elsewhere.'

BLUMBERG Louis MB, BCh (TCD 1914). SAMC 1940.

BOAL Robert Basil Address: Brigadee, Ballymena. MB, BCh (QUB 1934). Maj. RAMC.

BOHN Joseph Francis MB, BCh (NUI 1938). Flt Lt RAF 4th Jun. 1940. Address: Glenesk, Claremont Rd, Ballsbridge, Dublin.

BOLAND John Wilfred Address: 21 Templemore Avenue, Rathgar, Dublin. MB, BCh (TCD 1938). Surg. Lt Comdr RNVR. HMS *Birmingham*. Medals: DSC.

BOLTON Samuel Ernest MB (QUB 1926). Maj. RAMC.

BOND Ronald Alexander b. 10th May 1911 at Mountmellick, Queen's County. MB, BCh, BAO (TCD 1936), MC Path (1965). Lt RAMC 22nd Oct. 1937. Capt. 22nd Oct. 1938. PC Capt. 22nd Oct. 1942. Maj. 1st. Jul. 1946. T/Lt Col. 21st Jan. 1952. Lt Col. 16th Feb. 1953. Served India 1938–44. NWE/BAOR 1944–46. BAOR 1949–52. ADP W. Comd 1952. MELF: CO Stationery Hosp. Tel-el-Kebir 1952–54. OIC Path. Lab. E. Anglia Dist. 1954–55. CO 6th Fd Amb. 1955. ADP Scottish Comd 1955–57.

BAOR 1957–59. ADP Southern Comd and OIC Leishman Lab. 1960–62. E. Africa 1962, 1963–64 invalided. ADP Northern Comd and OIC Comd Lab. 1965. Medals: France and Germany S., DM, WM.

*BONNAR William McKee s. Samuel and Elizabeth Ellen Bonnar. Address: Ballycraigy House, Carnmoney, Co. Antrim. MB, BCh (QUB 1939). Sq. Ldr 10881 (M) RAFVR. Killed on active service 25th Feb. 1946, aged 28. Buried in Kirkee War Cemetery India, Plot 4C8.

BONUGLI Frederick Silvester Address: Waverley House, Larne, Co. Antrim. MB, BCh (QUB 1937). Capt. RAMC.

BOOTH Frederick John Address: Glenall, Ballygawley, Co. Tyrone. MB, BCh (QUB 1931). MD (1935.) Maj. Aus. AMS.

BOUCHER Charles Maxwell Address: Donaghcloney, Co. Down. MB, BCh (QUB 1940). Capt. RAMC.

BOURNS Herbert Kitchener Address: Lisbeg House, Eyrecourt, Co. Galway. MB, BCh (TCD 1940). Maj. RAMC.

BOWDEN James William MB, BCh (TCD 1925.) Col. IMS (1932), 4th Indian Corps (1942), 14th Army, SEAC (1943) Indian Comd (1944), O/C 141 B.G.H.

BOWE James Coleman Address: 25 Nutsford Drive, Cliftonville, Belfast. MB, BCh (QUB 1933), MD (1942). Wing Comdr (M) RAF.

BOYCE Hubert Stanley Address: St Mary's, Ashdale Rd, Terenure, Dublin. MB, BCh (TCD 1939). Flt Lt RAF.

BOYD Arthur Malin MB, BCh (QUB 1937). Capt. RAMC. MID.

BOYD Arthur Stanley Address: Roden House, Hillsborough, Co. Down. MB, BCh (QUB 1942). Capt. RAMC.

BOYD Clarence James MB, BCh (QUB 1924). Malaya Medical Service. POW.

BOYD Douglas Herbert Stuart MB, BCh (TCD 1932). Col. Med. Serv. Gibraltar.

BOYD John Stewart Address: Ballyhenry, Carnmoney, Co. Antrim. MB, BCh (QUB 1941). Flt Lt (M) RAFVR.

BOYD Matthew Walter John Address: Fair View, Causeway St, Portrush, Co. Antrim. MB, BCh (QUB 1941). Capt. RAMC.

BOYD Ringland Gilmore Address: Finvola, Garvagh, Co. Tyrone. MB, BCh, DPH (QUB 1941). Lt Col. RAMC. MC.

BOYD Robert Benjamin Address: Lough View House, Kircubbin, Co. Down. MB, BCh (QUB 1942). Capt. RAMC.

BOYLE Henry Aloysius b. 16th Jan. 1891, Ballymoney, Co. Antrim. Educ. MB (Edinburgh 1913), ChB. T/Lt RAMC 14th Feb. 1916. T/Capt. 14th Feb. 1917. PC Capt. 1st Jun. 1920. Maj. 14th Feb. 1928. A/Lt Col. 7th Jul. 1941. T/Lt Col. 7th Oct. 1941. Lt Col. 15th Aug. 1942. A/Col. 18th Mar. 1944. T/Col. 18th Sep. 1944. r.p. Hon. Col. 24th Sep. 1948. Served in France 1916–17 and 1917–18. Salonika and Trans Caucasia 1918–21. Black Sea (Constantinople) 1921–23. BAOR 1923–25. India 1927–32. Jamaica 1934–37. India 1938–44, Paiforce 1941–44, CO 32 CGH 1941–44. CO 61 GH 1944. CO 36 CCS Jan.–Feb. 1945, CO 32 CGH 1941–44, CO 61st Gen. Hosp. 1944, CO 36th Gen. Hosp. 1945. ADMS HQ S. Iraq area 1946. PSMB 1947. CO Mil. Hosp. Waringfield 1948. Medals: BWM, VM, DM, WM.

BRADBURY Eric Blackburn Address: Ulster Bank, Armagh. MB, BCh (QUB 1934). Surg. Comdr RN. MID.

BRADBURY Samuel MB, BCh (QUB 1906), DPH RCPS (England 1914). Surg. Capt. RN.

BRADBURY William MB, BCh (QUB 1908). Surg. R. Admiral RN. DSO, CBE.

BRADFIELD Claude Wilfred TCD 1936. Lt Col. RAMC.

BRADLAW Albert Stanley MB, BCh (TCD 1921). Surg. Comdr RNVR (1939).

BRADLEY John Laurence Address: 21 Eglington St, Portrush, Co. Antrim. MB, BCh (QUB 1924), DPH (QUB 1931). Capt. RAMC.

BRADSHAW Desmond Burton MB, BCh (TCD 1932), DPH (TCD 1935). Maj. RAMC.

BRADSHAW Harold Joseph Address: 28 Bawnmore Rd, Belfast. MB, BCh (QUB 1939). Surg. Lt RNVR.

BRADSHAW John Russell MB, BCh (TCD 1924). Capt. RAMC.

BRADY Terence Address: Cormaddyduff, Virginia, Co. Cavan. MB, BCh, BAO (UCD 1937). Lt RAMC. Capt. IMS 23rd Mar. 1943.

BRADY Victor Alexander Address: St Andrew's Rectory, 39 Malone Ave., Belfast. MB, BCh (QUB 1940). Capt. RAMC.

BRAIDWOOD Walter Standish Address: Willowbank, Keady, Co. Armagh. MB, BCh (QUB 1938). Maj. RAMC.

BRANDON Richard Ernest Address: Beechfield, Abbeyleix, Co. Laois. L.LM (RCPI 1940), L.LM (RCSI 1940). Wing Comdt RAF 23rd Apr. 1940.

BRASS Ronald Address: 78 Chaworth Pl., South Circular Rd, Dublin. MB, BCh (TCD 1939). Capt. RAMC.

BRASS Sydney MB, BCh (TCD 1932), MD (TCD 1936). Maj. RAMC.

BREAKEY William James Jellicoe Address: Lisdrum House, Newry, Co. Down. MB, BCh (QUB 1940). Surg. Lt RNVR.

BRENNAN Richard Brownell Address: The Croft, Adelaide Rd, Dun Laoghaire, Dublin. MB, BCh (TCD 1942). Surg. Lt RNVR.

BRENNAN Joseph Roland MB, BCh. Surg. Capt. RN retired. d. 2nd March 1953 at home, Anacloon, Oughterard, Galway.

BRENNAN Terence Nigel Norman Address: 5 Upr Crescent, Belfast. MB, BCh (QUB 1940). Sq. Ldr (M) RAF.

BRENNAN William Brian Francis Address: 5 Upr Crescent, Belfast. b. 23rd May 1907 at Belfast. MB, BCh, BAO (QUB 1930). PC Lt 28th Jul. 1931. Capt. 28th Mar, 1934, A/Maj. 18th Jan. 1940. T/Maj. 18th Apr. 1940. Maj. 28th Sept. 1940. A/Lt Col. 17th Feb. 1942. T/Col. 17th May 1942. Lt Col. 12th Jan. 1947. Col. 12th Sept. 1952. Brig. 29th Feb. 1960. T/Maj. Gen. 10th Jun. 1963. Maj. Gen. 29th Oct. 1963. r.p. 23rd May 1967. Served India 1932–37. MEF 1941–43. CO 9th Lt Fd Amb. 1942. POW 1942–43. Chief Instructor Officers Wing Depot RAMC 1943–44. ADMS War Office Liaison Staff HQ Etousa France 1944–45. India 1945–48. Comdt Depot RAMC India. CO BMH Deolali 1947–48. CO Mil. Hosp. Chepstow 1948–49. Mil. Hosp. Leominster 1949–50. West Africa SMP Gold Coast and CO Mil. Hosp. Accra 1950–52. BAOR: ADMS HQ Lubbecke Dist. 1952–56. FARELF 1956–57. DDMS HQ Malaya Comd 1956–57. DDMS 17th Gurkha Div./OCLF 1957. ADMS HQ E. Anglia Dist. 1958 & HQ London Dist 1958–60. DDMS HQ Scottish Comd 1960–62. FARELF: DDMS HQ 17th Gurkha Div./OCLF 1962–63. QHP 2nd May 1962. DDMS HQ Southern Comd 1963–67. Medals: CB 11th Jun. 1966, IGSM 1908 with cl. NWF Mohand 1933 and Mohand 1935, IGSM & cl. NWF 1936–37, 1939–45 S., Africa S., France and Germany S., DM, WM, GSM and cl. Malaya, QEII Corn Medal 1953, USA Legion of Merit (Offr) 26th Jan. 1948.

BREW Kenneth MB (QUB 1942). Maj. RAMC.

BREWSTER Howard, Address: 11 Richmond Pk, Stranmillis, Belfast. MB, BCh, DPH (QUB 1938). Flt Lt (M) RAFVR.

BREWSTER James Heron Address: 11 Richmond Pk, Stranmillis, Belfast. MB, BCh, DPH (QUB 1937). Sq. Ldr (M) RAFVR.

BRIDGE George Allman b. 12th Mar. 1890, Dungar Pk, Roscrea, Co. Tipperary. s. Henry Powell (Land Agent) and Elizabeth Maria Bridge. Educ. St Columba's Coll., Rathfarnham, Dublin 1905. BA, MB, BCh, BAO (TCD 1914), LM (Rot. Hosp. 1914). R. C. of I. Lt RAMC SR 28th Aug. 1914. Capt.

28th Feb. 1918. PC Capt. 1st May 1919. Maj. 28th Aug. 1926. Lt Col. 30th Jun. 1937. Col. 30th Jun. 1940. r.p. 15th Apr. 1947. Served in 1914–18 War France and Belg. from 6th Nov. 1914. MO 8th Div. Train 11th Fd Amb. India 1919–24 and 1927–31. Egypt 1935–36. India 1938–44. CO BMH Jullundur Apr.–May 1938. BMH Sialkot 1938–42. BMH Rawalpindi and Murree Apr.–Jun. 1942. A/ADMS HQ Meerut Dist. Jun.–Sept. 1942. CO 126 IBGH Poona 1942–43. ADMS HQ S. Army 166 L of C sub area and 197 L of C area 1943–44. CO 38 Gen. Hosp. Feb.–Mar. 1944. CO Royal Victoria Hosp. Westbury 1944–45. NWE 1945–46. ADMS HQ 12 & 11 L of C areas Feb.–Oct. 1945. CO 108 Gen. Hosp. 1945–46. ADMS HQ S. Western Dist. 1946–47. Medals: MC (16th Sept. 1918), 1914 S., BWM, VM, IGSM (cl. Waz 1921–24), France and Germany S., DM, WM.

BRITTAIN Herbert Alfred s. the late J.W. Brittain of Dublin. Educ. Sedbergh School and TCD. MB, BCh (1926) & MCh & FRCS (1921). Lt Col. RAMC (1941). During the 2nd WW served in the RAMC obtaining the rank of Lt Col. Medals: MC, OBE. d. 4th Mar. 1954, suddenly, leaving a widow formerly Ms Sonya Barclay, and two daughters.

BROADWOOD Walter Standish MB (QUB 1938). Maj. RAMC.

BROSNAN Martin Joseph Address: Lough Rd, Lurgan, Co. Armagh. MB, BCh, DPH (QUB 1942). Surg. Lt RNVR. MBE.

BROSNAN Michael Joseph MB, BCh, BAO (NUI 1928). Surg. Lt RN.

BROUGH Maurice Cresswell MB, BCh (TCD 1937), MD (TCD 1943). RAMC.

BROWN Samuel Stuart Address: 297 Newtownards Rd, Belfast. MB, BCh (QUB 1923). Sq. Ldr (M) RAFVR.

BROWN Valentine Vincent Address: 159 Rathgar Rd, Dublin. L.LM (RCPI 1922), L.LM (RCSI 1922). Flt Lt RAF 23rd Sept. 1944.

BROWN Wilfred Maurice Address: 32 Knockbreda, Belfast. MB, BCh (QUB 1936), DPH (QUB 1939). Surg. Lt RNVR.

BROWNE Harold Jackson Address: Latharna, Whiteabbey, Co. Antrim. MB, BCh (QUB 1932). Capt. RAMC. MC.

BROWNE James MB, BCh (QUB 1938). Maj. RAMC.

BROWNE John Alphonsus Address: Castle Pl., Strabane, Co. Tyrone. MB, BCh, BAO (NUI 1927). Surg. Lt RN 15th Dec. 1931.

BROWNE John Henry Address: 7 High Street, Galway. MB, BCh (NUI 1936). Flt Lt RAF 8th Oct. 1940.

BROWNE John Woodburn Address: 25 Donaghadee Rd, Bangor, Co. Down. MB, BCh (QUB 1928). Capt. RAMC.

BRUCE-HAMILTON William b. 23rd Aug. 1905, Dublin. s. Bruce and Cornelia Mary Bruce-Hamilton of Dublin. Husband of Aileen Bruce-Hamilton of Dublin. MB, BCh, BAO (TCD 1929), MD. Lt RAMC 25th Apr. 1935. Capt. 25th Apr. 1936. PC Capt. 25th Apr. 1940. A/Maj. 24th Dec. 1939. T/Maj. 24th Mar. 1940. Maj. 65317 RAMC 25th Apr. 1944. A/Lt Col. 17th Dec. 1944. T/Lt Col. 17th Mar. 1945. Served Egypt 1936–43. MEF 1944–45 with 8th Army. Medals: 1939–45 S. Africa S. (with cl. 8th Army), DM, WM. d. 16th Dec. 1947 aged 42. Buried in Brookwood Mil. Cemetery, plot 33 AD5.

BRYSON John Millard Address: 31 Villiers Rd, Rathgar, Dublin. MB, BCh (TCD 1936). Maj. RAMC.

BUCHANAN Georgina (née Wallace) Address: Co. Antrim. L.LM (RCPI 1937), L.LM (RCSI 1937). Lt RAF 31st Oct. 1942.

BUCHANAN Harry McVey MB, BCh (TCD 1938). RAMC.

BUCHANAN Joan (née MacAuley) MB, ChB (QUB 1942). Flt Lt (M) RAFVR.

BUCKLEY Charles Dudley Maybury b. 10th Dec. 1890, Glenageary, Co. Dublin. s. Frederick (Civil Servant/Rates Office) and Amy Buckley, 76, Northumberland Rd, Dublin. Educ. TCD MB (1914), BCh, BAO. R. C. of I. Lt RAMC SR 5th Aug. 1914. Capt. 1st Apr. 1915. A/Maj. 4th Jan. 1918. PC Capt. 1st Apr. 1919. Maj. 5th Aug. 1926. Lt Col. 20th Mar. 1936. Col. 13th Oct. 1942. r.p. 15th Feb. 1947. Served 1914–18 War France from 8th Oct. 1914. Italy 1917–19. Somaliland 1919–20 (Colonial Office). India 1920–24 & 1928–33: DADP Baluchistan Dist. 1928–30. Enteric Lab. Kasauli 1930–32. Path Spec. Royal Victoria Hosp. Netley 1933–36. India 1936–43: DADP Madras Dist. 1936–38, ADP S. Comd Feb.–Dec. 1938. ADH & P GHQ (I) 1938–41. CO 111 Gen. Hosp. 1945. CO Cambridge Hosp. Aldershot 1945–46. Medals: MC (1st Jan. 1918), 1914 S., BWM, VM, 1939–45 S., France and Germany S., DM, WM. d. 17th Jun. 1961, London.

BUCKLEY John MB, BCh, BAO (UCC 1930). Lt RAMC.

BUCKLEY Patrick MB, BCh, BAO (UCC 1933). Lt RAMC.

BULMER Maurice Edward Carson Address: Glenshane, Ranfurly Ave., Bangor, Co. Down. MB, BCh (TCD 1938). Maj. RAMC. (1942) BLA. Burma.

BUNTING John Address: 24 Napier St, Belfast. MB, BCh (QUB 1938). Capt. RAMC.

BURDEN Alexander James MB, BCh (TCD 1928) Surg. Lt RN. HMS Ajax during the Battle of the River Plate.

BURGESS Denis John Address: 17 Gillabbey Tce, Cork. MB, BCh, BAO (UCC 1935). Lt RAMC.

BURKE Edmund MB, BCh (NUI 1939). Lt RAMC 5th May 1945.

BURKITT Dennis Parsons b. Enniskillen, Co. Fermanagh 1911. Educ. Dean Close School, Cheltenham. Address: Laragh, Ballinamallard, Co. Fermanagh. Lost an eye as a child. MB, BCh (TCD 1938). RAMC 1941. Major in East Africa until 1946. Pioneer in epidemiological assessment. Professionally he wrote 'citation classics' in two different medical fields. Burkitt's lymphoma was the first cancer proved to be caused by a virus. His realisation of the importance of dietary fibre was to change the breakfast tables of the Western World. Many discoveries and honours. Died following a stroke in 1993.

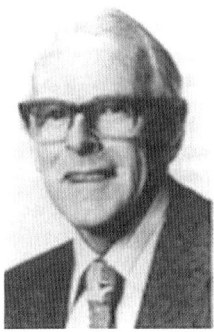

Dennis Parsons Burkitt. His realisation of the importance of dietary fibre was to change the breakfast tables of the Western World.

BURKITT Robert Townsend Address: Laragh, Ballinamallard, Co. Fermanagh. MB, BCh (TCD 1938). Capt. RAMC. Served in Burma.

BURNS George Address: The Mullagh, Maghera, Co. Derry. MB, BCh (QUB 1938). Maj. RAMC.

BURNS Gerard Vincent Address: 9 Victoria Rd, Rathgar, Dublin. L.LM (RCPI 1940), L.LM (RCSI 1940). Lt RAMC 18th Oct. 1941.

BURNS Joseph Patrick John Address: 45 The Mount, Belfast. MB, BCh, DPH (QUB 1941). Maj. RAMC.

BURNS Leopold Francis L.LM (1926 RCPI), L.LM (1926 RCSI). Indian Medical Services. d. Jan. 1942.

BURNS Robert MB, BCh, BAO (UCD 1922). Lt RAMC.

BURROWES William Lewson, Address: 272 Upr Newtownards Rd, Belfast. MB, BCh (QUB 1943). Sq. Ldr (M) RAFVR.

BURTON Erroll Fitzgerald MB, BCh (TCD 1931). Sq. Ldr RAF.

BUSHE Charles Kendal b. 1878, Dublin. s. the late Charles Percy Bushe, Queen's Bench, of Clonskeagh and grandson of the late Charles Kendal Bushe, Lord Chief Justice. Educ. TCD. BA, MB (1900), BCh, MD (1901). R. C. of I. Surg. RN 9th Jun. 1902. Staff Surg. 9th Dec. 1909. Surg. Cmdr 9th Dec. 1917. Surg. Rear Adm. Occupation House Surg. Meath Hosp. Served in 1914–18 War. Led an expedition to Bathurst to establish a base and was returning to England when his boat was torpedoed and he drifted in a small boat for a few weeks. At the outbreak of WWII he was put in charge of the Royal Naval Hospital at Great Yarmouth. Retired in 1947. Medals: OBE (1st Apr. 1919), CBE (1919). d. 19th

Aug. 1950, suddenly at Winchester. Survived by his son and daughter.

BUTLER Edward Gerald Robert Address: The Rectory, Thomastown, Co. Kilkenny. MB, BCh (TCD 1940). Lt Col. IMF. Served in Burma.

BYRN Francis MacDermot, b. 15th Aug. 1912, Dublin. Address: The Rectory, Kilternan, Co. Dublin. MB, BCh, BAO (TCD 1936), DA RCPI (1950), FFA RCSI (1960). Lt IMS 31st Oct. 1936. Capt. 2nd Feb. 1938. Maj. 31st Aug. 1946. PC Maj. RAMC 18th Aug. 1948. Lt Col. 2th Jun. 1951. Col. 14th Jan. 1960. India 1938–41. Malaya 1941–42. India 1942–47. MELF: Anaes Spec. BMH DHEKELIA 1960–62. ADMS HQ Cyprus & CO BMH Dehekelia 1962–63. 1939–45 S., Pacific S., WM, India Service M.

BYRN Maureen Nancy (née Mason) MB, BCh (TCD 1936). RAMC.

BYRNE Aiden Asquith Address: 429 North Circular Rd, Dublin. LM (1939), RCP & s (RCSI 1939), LM (1939 RCSI), MB, BCh (TCD). Lt RAMC 23rd Oct. 1939). Capt. b. Dublin. MC. 'On the night of June 14th, 1942, this officer proceeded with his section and an ambulance car with an infantry column in an endeavour to break through the enemy lines to the west of the brigade "box". Emerging through the "Stanley-Gap", which was then under heavy shellfire, the section under Captain Byrne picked up and attended wounded occasioned by the shelling and they were placed in the ambulance car which accompanied the section. Soon after this the ambulance car ran onto one of our own minefields in the dark. Captain Byrne, who was travelling on another vehicle, immediately went into the minefield and assisted in extracting the patients from the vehicle. He then marked a way out of the minefield along which patients could be brought, and led them to safety'.

BYRNE Edward Aloysius Joseph Address: St Leonard's, Warrenpoint, Co. Down. MB, BCh (QUB 1932), MD (QUB 1935), MRCP (London 1938). Maj. RAMC.

BYRNE Gerald Address: 15 Kelvin Parade, Cliftonville, Belfast. MB, BCh (QUB 1938). Capt. RAMC.

BYRNE John Walter Address: 16 St Patrick's Hill, Cork. MB, BCh, BAO (UCC 1939). Lt RAMC.

BYRNE Patrick Joseph Address: Cork St, Dublin. L.LM (RCPI 1931) L.LM (RCSI 1931). Lt RAMC 1st Sept. 1943.

BYRNES James Munchin Francis Address: Glebe House, Bruree, Co. Limerick. L.LM (RCPI 1933), L.LM (RCSI 1933). Lt IMS 1st Feb. 1936.

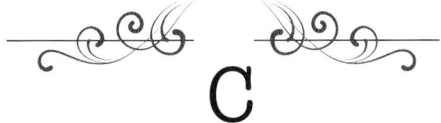

C

CAITHNESS George Sinclair b. 19th Mar. 1912, Lisnaskea, Co. Fermanagh. Address: St Margaret's Vicarage, Fivemiletown, Co. Tyrone. MB, BCh, BAO (TCD 1936). Lt 17th Jun. 1940. Capt. 27th Jun. 1941. A/Maj. 8th Dec. 1944. T/Maj. 8th Mar. 1945. PC Capt. 27th Jun. 1945. Maj. 27th Jun. 1948. A/Lt Col. 24th Jan. 1945. T/Lt Col. 31st Oct. 1945. r.p. disability Hon. Lt Col. 2nd Apr. 1959. India 1942–47. RMO 2nd Welch 1942–43. CO & OIC Med. Div. CMH 1945. CO CMH Wellington 1946. FARELF 1955–58. BAOR: CO 28th Fd Amb. 1958–59. Invalided. Medals: DM, WM, GSM with cl. Malaya.

CALDWELL John McCormick Address: 14 Harcourt St, Dublin. MB, BCh (TCD 1937). Maj. Kings A. Rifles. MID.

CALDWELL William Gordon Dickson Address: 76 Frankfort Avenue, Rathgar, Dublin. MB, BCh (TCD 1941). Lt RAMC.

CALLAGHAN Alfred William Address: Ahascaragh. Ballinasloe, Co. Galway. MB, BCh (TCD 1933). RAF.

CALLAGHAN Alphonsus MB, BCh, BAO (UCC 1926). Lt RAMC.

CALVERT Cecil Armstrong Address: 8 University Sq., Belfast. MB, BCh (QUB 1922). Lt Col. RAMC.

CALVERT Frederick Charles Address: Sunnymount, Portadown, Co. Armagh. MB, BCh (QUB 1942). Capt. RAMC.

CALVERT George Edgar Address: Glenburn, Green Rd, Ballyclare, Co. Antrim. LRCP (Edinburgh 1939), LRCS (1939), LRFPS (Glasgow 1939). Capt. RAMC.

CALVERT Mary Address: 13 Tower Hill, Armagh. MB, BCh (QUB 1936). Sq. Ldr (M) RAF.

CAMPBELL Alfred Edward b. 21st May 1901, Dublin. MB, BCh, BAO (QUB 1923), DPH (Dublin 1924), MD (Belfast 1931). PC Lt 30th Jul. 1924 RAMC, Capt. 30th Jan. 1928, Maj. 30th Jul. 1934, A/Lt Col. 10th Jan. 1942, T/Lt Col. 10th Apr. 1942, Lt Col. 2nd Feb. 1945, A/Col. 1st Oct. 1943, T/Col. 27th Jul. 1945, Col. 14th Jan. 1949, T/Brig. 7th May 1953, Brig. 4th Jun. 1953, A/Maj. Gen. 27th Feb. 1950, T/Maj. Gen. 26th Mar. 1956, Maj. Gen. 10th Apr. 1956. r.p. Apr. 1956. India 1925–30 & 1934–39, DDH HQ 21st Army Group 1943–44, CO 54 Hosp. Ship 1944, NWE: ADMS HQ Force 135 1944–45, DDH HQ 21st Army Group/BAOR 1945–46, DDH GHQ ALFSEA/FARELF 1946–49, Prof. of AH RAM Coll. 1949–53, DAH War Office 1953–56. QHP 5th Jun. 1953, DDGAMS War Office 1956–60. Col. Comdt RAMC 1961–64, Rep. Col. Comdt 1962–63. Medals: CB

1st Jan. 1957, MID 13th Dec. 1949, CStJ 1958, OStJ 1943, 1939–45 S., France and Germany S., DM, WM, GFM (with Malaya cl.).

*CAMPBELL Archibald Norman s. Archibald and Anna Campbell of Limavady. Husband of Margaret Campbell. Address: Main St, Limavady, Co. Derry. MB, BCh (QUB 1942). Flt Lt 156465 RAFVR. Killed on active service 10th Dec. 1944 aged 26. Buried in Drumachose Pres. Cemetery, Grave 132.

CAMPBELL Charles Finbarr Address: 15 East Bridge St, Belfast. MB, BCh (QUB 1935), DPH (QUB 1938). Flt Lt (M) RAFVR.

CAMPBELL John Francis Jennings Address: 115 Fitzroy Ave., Ormeau, Belfast. MB, BCh (QUB 1943). Capt. RAMC.

CAMPBELL John Shaw Address: Enfield, Drumard, Co. Down. MB, BCh (QUB 1938). Capt. RAMC.

CAMPBELL Margaret Stanton (née Burns) MB, BCh (QUB 1942). Capt. RAMC.

CAMPBELL Robert Francis Cassidy McDowell Address: 84 Ardenlee Ave., Ravenhill Rd, Belfast. MB, BCh (QUB 1941). Surg. Lt RNVR.

CAMPBELL Stephen Address: 32 Cabinhill Pk, Belfast. MB, BCh (QUB 1936). Capt. RAMC. MID.

CAMPBELL Wilfred Ayre Boyd Address: 38 Wellington Pk, Belfast. MB, BCh (QUB 1941). Surg. Lt RNVR.

CAMPBELL William Kealty b. 12th Nov 1889, Belfast. MB, BCh, BAO (QUB Belfast 1915). Lt SR 8th Aug. 1914. Mobilised 7th Feb. 1915. Capt. 6th Aug. 1915. PC Lt 1st Jan. 1917. Capt. 7th Aug. 1918. A/Maj. 4th Jan. 1918. T/Maj. 7th Nov. 1920. A/MAj. 21st. Jul. 1921. Maj. 7th Feb. 1927. Lt Col. 10th Jul. 1940. A/Col. 1st May 1941. T/Col. 1st Nov. 1941. A/Brig. 29th Nov. 1942. T/Brig. 29th May 1943. r.p. Hon Brig. 12th May 1947. Served France 1915–19. India 1919–24. China 1927–30. Malaya 1931–34. Egypt 1935–36. Palestine 1936 & 42–43. India 1937–44. ADMS HQ 31st Indian Armd Div. 1941–42. DDMS HQ 21st Ind. Corps. 1942. 43. DDMS HQ Spec. Forc. 1943–44. CO Mil Hosp. Drymen Jul.–Aug. 1944. ADMS HQ 6th and 5th AA Groups 1944–45. CO Mil Hosp. Naburn Yorks. 1945–46. BAOR: CO 77 (Wuppertal) BMH Aug.–Dec. 1946. Medals: MBE 30th May 1924, DSO 22nd Dec. 1916, MC 18th Jan. 1918 and bar 16th Sept. 1918, MID 1st Jan. 1916, 4th Jan. 1917 and 24th Dec. 1917, Panama Medal la Solidaridad 3rd class 17 Feb. 1920, French Silver Medal de la Reconnaissance 31 Mar. 1925.

CAMPBELL William Stewart Address: Culloden, Craigavad, Co. Down. MB, BCh (QUB 1932). Maj. RAMC.

CANTON Nathaniel Anthony MB, BCh (UCD 1922), DPH (UCD 1922). Health Singapore. POW.

CAPLIN Jacob Address: 2 Raymond St, South Circular Rd, Dublin. L.LM (RCPI 1935), L.LM (RCSI 1935). Lt RAMC 6th Jan. 1940.

CARAHER Edward Francis More MB, BCh, BAO (NUI 1932). Lt RAMC. MC. 'Capt. Caraher was in command of the advanced dressing station, 150 Field Ambulance, and under command of the late Officer Commanding 150 Brigade. During the period 29th May–1st Jun. 1942, the brigade box was surrounded by the enemy and communication with M.D.S. some miles to the north-east was severed. This box was the left flank of the Gajala position, Western Desert. No evacuation of the wounded could take place. Throughout the above period enemy fire came from all quarters, and he continually attacked with armour, infantry and from the air, gradually whittling away the defences, shortening his range, improving his observation, and increasing the accuracy of his fire. Casualties were heavy, but although now only the more severe cases were sent to the A.D.S., it quickly became full to overflowing. Captain Caraher and his small staff worked day and night operating, bandaging, giving such blood transfusions as were possible, improvising beds and stretchers preparing hot drinks and food as best they could, while all the time enemy fire continued and the wounded came streaming in. It was under these trying conditions that Captain Caraher set an example of courage, cheerfulness and devotion to duty which will rank high in the annals of the corps, and it is not too much to say that in his skill, ingenuity, and untiring care, many of the wounded owe their lives. In the early afternoon of 1st June the enemy finally overran the area, and found Captain Caraher carrying on'.

CARBONI Augustus William MB, BCh, BAO (UCD 1939). Lt RAMC 11th Jul. 1940.

CAREY Charles Francis MB, BCh, BAO (UCD 1926). Lt RAMC 8th Feb. 1929.

CARNEY Philip b. 18th Jan. 1890, Cootehill, Co. Cavan. MB, BCh, BAO (NUI) Hons. M.Sc. (TCD). Lt RAMC 1st Mar. 1915, Capt. 1st Mar. 1916, A/Maj. 20th Mar. 1918, A/Lt Col. 15th Jul. 1919, Retd. and granted the rank of Maj. 27th Aug. 1923. Rejoined 8th Sept. 1939. A/Lt Col. 2nd Jan. 1941, T/Lt Col. 2nd Apr. 1941. R. of O. 27th Oct. 1945. Served France 1917–18, Germany 1919, India 1920–23, BEF France 1939–40, CO 12th Light Field Ambulance 1941–42, MEF/CMF 1941–45, 53 General Hospital 1942–45. Medals: MC 16th Sept. 1918, MID 6th Apr. 1944, 1939–45 S., Africa S., Italy S., DM, WM, Croix de Guerre 22nd Nov., 1918. d. 8th Nov. 1953.

CARNWATH John Thomas Educ. Foyle College, Derry and QUB and University of Berlin. MB, BS (1903 RUI), DPH (Cambridge). Married Margaret Ethel, dt. A. McKei.Address: Whitehead, Co. Antrim. Medals: DSO (LG 1st Jan. 1918), 1914 S., BWM, VM. MID.

CARPENTER Walter Francis Address: Irishtown, Rathfeigh, Co. Meath. MB, BCh (TCD 1939). Capt. RAMC. Served in N. Africa. Wounded.

CARREY John MB, BCh (QUB 1922). Lt Col. IMF.

CARROLL Brendan Benedict Address: Whitehall, Westminster Rd, Foxrock, Co. Dublin. MB, BCh, BAO (UCD 1940). Lt RAMC.

CARROLL Edward Patrick Address: High Street, Tuam, Co. Galway. L.LM (RCPI 1927), L.LM (RCSI 1927). Flt Offr RAF 17th Sept. 1940.

CARROLL James Desmond Address: Bundoran, Co. Donegal. MB, BCh, BAO (UCD 1939). Lt RAMC.

CARROLL John Donal MSc, MB, BCh, BAO, DPH (UCD). Lt RAMC. First Enlisted 14th Aug. 1914.

CARROLL John Vincent Address: Bank Pl., Mallow, Co. Cork. MB, BCh (1922), MC (1931 TCD), DPH (RCFS England 1925). Lt Irish Army 1944.

CARSON Andrew Albert George Address: Hillhead House, Dromore, Co. Down. MB, BCh (QUB 1942). Surg. Lt RNVR.

CARSON David McMurry, Campbell College. MB, BCh (TCD 1928). Maj. RAMC.

CARSON Henry Montgomery MB, BCh (TCD 1937). Sq. Ldr RAF.

CARSON James Address: Ballybay, Co. Monaghan. Campbell College. MB, BCh (QUB 1930), MD (QUB 1934), DPH (QUB 1935). Lt Col. RAMC.

CARSON Thomas Desmond Address: Ballybay, Co. Monaghan. Campbell College. MB, BCh (QUB 1935). Lt Col. RAMC.

CARVER James MB, BCh (UCC 1920), MRCS (1924), FRCS (1928) (England), LRCP (London 1924). Lt RAMC.

CASEMENT Francis b. 29th Oct. 1881, Dublin. s. Roger (Landowner. DL) and Charlotte Casement, Magherintemple, Ballycastle, Co. Antrim. Educ. TCD. MB (1906), BCh, BAO. R. C. of I. Lt RAMC 28th Jan. 1907. Capt. 28th Jul. 1910. Maj. 28th Jan. 1919. A/Lt Col. 17th Nov. 1917–27th Jan. 1918. T/Lt Col. 20th Jun. 1931. Lt Col. 1st Jul. 1931. Bt. Col. 1st Jul. 1934. Col. 18th Aug. 1935. Maj. Gen. 15th Apr. 1938. r.p. Remained employed. 29th Oct. 1941. r.p. 28th Nov. 1941. India 1908–14. DADMS France, Oct. 1914. Gallipoli 1915–16. France and Belg. 1916–19. Mauritius 1920–24. DADP Home Cos. Area (East) 1924–27. DADP Malta 1927–31. ADH and P Western Comd 1931–35. ADGAMS War Office 1935–37. DDGAMS War Office 1937–38. DDMS HQ S. Comd 1938–41. KHS 21st Feb. 1940. Medals: DSO (4th Jun. 1917), bar (26th Jul. 1918), 1914 S., BWM, VM, LdeH (CdeCav) French (24th Feb. 1916). MID 1st Nov. 1916, 29th May 1917, 30th Dec. 1918.

CASEY Kathleen Mary Address: 1 Adare Villas, Highfield Ave, College Rd, Cork. MB, BCh (UCC 1942). Lt RAMC.

CASSIDY Anthony Denis MB, BCh (NUI 1938). Lt RAMC 15th May 1940.

*****CASSIDY** James Gerard b. IFS. s. James and Ellen Cassidy, Rathfriland, Co. Down. MB, BCh (NUI 1938) Lt RAMC 19th Dec. 1939. Capt. 114828 RAMC attached HQ Parachute Regt. d. 10th Mar. 1943, aged 28, Tunisia. Buried Tabarka Ras Rajel War Cemetery, Plot 3.C.7.

CASTLES Wilfred Address: Nevara, Chichester Pk, Belfast. MB, BCh, DPH (QUB 1942). Surg. Lt RNVR.

*****CAVANAGH** William Anthony Address: Drumaweir House, Greencastle, Co. Donegal. L.LM (RCPI 1934), L.LM RCSI (1934). Surgeon Lt RNVR. Drowned when HMS *Repulse* was sunk by the Japanese off Malaya on 10th Dec. 1941. He chose to remain with the injured instead of abandoning ship. Commemorated on the Plymouth Naval Memorial Devon, Panel 61 Column 3, and on a maritime memorial in Greencastle, Co. Donegal.

CHAMBERLAIN George Harry Amyrald b. 1920. s. Canon George Ashton Chamberlain and Rebecca Elsie Chamberlain. The Mariners Church Rectory, Adelaide Rd, Dun Laoghaire, Co. Dublin. Educ. Monkstown Park School, Monkstown, Co. Dublin, Campbell College Belfast and Bloxham School, Oxfordshire. MB, BCh (TCD 1943). Awarded the Connolly Norman Medal and a Gold Medal for Medicine. Capt. RAMC. POW Italy.

CHAMBERS Charles Perceval b. 17th Feb. 1894, Sligo. MB, BCh, BAO, LM (Rot. Hosp), TCD (1917). Lt RAMC 26th Feb. 1918, Capt. 26th Feb. 1919, PC/Lt 1st Sept. 1919, Capt. 26th Aug. 1921, Maj. 26th Feb. 1930, A/Lt Col. 28th Feb. 1942, T/Lt Col. 28th May 1942, Lt Col. 21st Feb. 1944, A/Col. 25th Jun. 1945, T/Col. 25th Dec. 1945, Col. 1st Mar. 1948, r.p. disability 17th Feb. 1951. Served France Mar.–Jun. 1918, Egypt 1920–24, Royal Herbert Hosp. Woolwich 1928–29, India 1929–34: Connaught Mil. Hosp. Poona 1929–32, Mil. Hosp. Thimbleberry 1932–34, Mil. Hosp. Tidworth 1934–38, Burma 1938–42, Mil. Hosp. Maymyo 1938–42, CO 3rd Burma Gen. Hosp. Feb.–Aug. 1942, CO Mil. Hosp. Bangor 1945–46, Royal Mil. Hosp. Waringfield 1946–48, FARELF: CO BMH Singapore 1948–50, PSMB S. Comd 1950–51. Medals: MID 24th Oct. 1950, BWM, VM, 1939–45 S., Burma S., DM, WM, GSM with cl. Malaya.

CHAPMAN Robert William b. 7th Feb. 1891, Athlone, Co. Westmeath. s. Thomas (newspaper editor) and Eleanor Chapman, 7, Athlone Villas, Athlone, Co. Westmeath. Educ. TCD MB (1914), MD (1919), BCh, BAO (1914). T/Lt RAMC 14th Mar. 1916. Capt. 14th Mar. 1917. PC Capt. 1st Jun. 1920. Maj. 26th Mar. 1928. r.p. 9th Apr. 1932. Rempld 9th Jun. 1941. A/Lt Col. 20th Jan. 1944. T/Lt Col. 20th Apr. 1944. r.p. 15th Dec.

1948. Served France Aug.–Sep. 1916. Egypt Feb.–Jun. 1920. Black Sea 1920–21. Constantinople 1922–23. BAOR 1925–26. India 1926–28 invalided, and 1929–32. East Africa 1942–46, CO 53 (EA) CS 1944, CO Stat. Hosp. Suarez 1944–45, CO Stat. Hosp. Gilgil 1945, OC Mil. Hosp. Fort George 1946–48.

CHARNEY William MB, BCh (TCD 1935). Capt. USAMC. Served in N. Africa, Italy and France.

CHESNEY George MB, BCh, DPH (1920), MD (QUB 1927). Maj. RAMC.

CHESNEY William McMeekin b. 10th Apr. 1892, Ahoghill, Co. Antrim. MB, BCh, BAO (QUB 1914). SR. Lt RAMC 30th Apr. 1914, Mob. 9th Aug. 1914, Capt. 1st Apr. 1915, A/Maj. 4th Jan. 1918, PC Capt. 1st Oct. 1919, retired and granted the rank of Maj. 16th Jul. 1921. Rejoined 1st Sept. 1939, A/Lt Col. 19th Aug. 1942, T/Lt Col. 19th Nov. 1942, Hon. Lt Col. 21st Jun. 1949. BEF France 1914–15, 1916–17, 1918–19, Salonika 1915–16, Italy 1917–18, Germany 1919–20, India 1920–21, ADMS Med. Embkm. HQ 1942. Medals: MC 23rd Jun. 1915 and bar 19th Nov. 1917. MID 22nd Jun. 1915, VM, WM.

CHOMSE Herbert Donald MB, BCh (TCD 1939). Capt. SAMC.

CHRISTIE David Edward Address: Coorang, Prospect Rd, Portstewart. MB, BCh (QUB 1938). Sq. Ldr (M) RAFVR.

CLAHANE Daniel Patrick Address: St Patrick's, Collins Ave., Drumcondra, Dublin. MB, BCh, BAO (NUI 1932). Lt RAMC.

CLANCY Martin Address: Ennis Rd, Kilrush, Co. Clare. L.LM (RCPI 1927), MB (RCPI 1934), L.LM (RCSI 1927). Flt Lt RAF 1st Apr. 1944. Belsen concentration camp.

CLARKE Denis Mervyn Patrick Rae Address: Castle Villa, Easkey, Ballina, Co. Mayo. MB, BCh, BAO (UCD 1939). Lt RAMC.5. AD RAF.

CLARKE Patrick James Holland MB, BCh, BAO (UCD 1935), DPH (NUI 1937). Lt RAMC.

CLARKE Robert Edward John Address: Claremont, Galgorm Rd, Ballymena, Co. Antrim. MB, BCh (QUB 1940). Flt Lt (M) RAFVR.

CLARKE Robert Hugh Address: Lisnastrean House, Lisburn, Co. Antrim. MB, BCh (QUB 1939). Maj. RAMC.

CLARKE William Aylmer Address: 9 Lodge Rd, Coleraine, Co. Derry. MB, BCh (TCD 1933). Surg. Lt RNVR.

CLARKE William Norman James b. 12th Sept. 1908, Staffordstown, Co. Antrim. MB, BCh, BAO (QUB 1934). Lt RAMC 24th Oct. 1935, Capt. 24th Oct. 1936, A/Maj. 2nd Mar. 1940, T/Maj. 2nd Jun. 1940, PC Capt. 24th Oct. 1940, Maj. 24th Oct. 1944, A/Lt Col. 28th Jun. 1943, T/Lt Col. 28th Sept. 1943,

Lt Col. 14th Jan. 1949, d. 7th Oct. 1952, Millbank London. Served Malaya 1936–39, BEF France 1939–40, MEF/CMF 1943–45, CO 6th Light Fd Amb. 1943–45, CO 140 Fd Amb. 1945, CO 133 Gen. Hosp. 1945–46, W. Africa 1946–48: CO 44 Kaduna Mil. Hosp. 1946, 68th Lagos Mil. Hosp. 1946–48, CO Hosp. Ship El Nil 1949–50, FARELF 1950–52, A/ADMS HQ Singapore Base Dist. 1950, CO BMH Kamunting 1950–52. Medals: OBE 20th Sept. 1945, MID 4th Apr. 1952, 1939–45 S., Africa S. with cl. 1st Army, Italy S., DM, WM, GSM with cl. Malaya.

CLEIN Arthur Israel MB, BCh, BAO (UCD 1925). Lt RAMC 28th Nov. 1940.

CLERKIN Peter Alphonsus MD (QUB 1912). Capt. WAMS.

CLYNE Michael Henry Address: East Hill House, Athlone, Co. Westmeath. MB, BCh, BAO (UCD 1935). Lt RAMC.

COAKLEY Thomas Joseph MB, BCh, BAO (UCC 1920). Brother OStJ.

COCHRANE Ernest McGregor MB, BCh (TCD 1937). Surg. Lt RNVR.

COCHRANE Sarah Isobel Address: The Inch, Downpatrick, Co. Down. MB, BCh (QUB 1942). Capt. RAMC.

COEN Stella Mary MB (TCD 1936). RAMC.

COFFEY Cornelius William Address: Ballyard, Birdhill, Co. Tipperary. L.LM (RCPI 1925), L.LM (RCSI 1925). Flt Offr RAF 3rd Mar. 1940.

COGAN Jeremiah Address: Ballybodane, Donoughmore, Co. Cork. MB, BCh, BAO (UCC 1935). Lt RAMC.

COGHLAN Bernard Augustine b. 1899. MB, BCh, BAO (UCD 1922). Lt RAMC. 'Married Eileen Bennett, a librarian. Drilling with wooden rifles in the grounds of the Royal College of Surgeons, he was arrested by the police and imprisoned in Crumlin Prison Belfast and later in Wales. Following his release, he completed his medical examinations and was installed with the Irish National Army as Superintendent of Military and Civilian Hospitals during the Civil War. Because of his affiliations he could not find employment. He studied tropical medicine and joined the British Colonial Service and was posted to Tanganyika and Uganda. During WWII he became an A/Maj. and Field Surgeon in the Kings African Rifles. Lt RAMC. Enlisted 8th Jan. 1940. After the war he moved to South Africa and became Chief Officer of Health inGrahamstown and died in 1990.'

COHEN Michael MB, BCh (QUB 1924). Capt. RAMC.

COLE James Owen Young Address: 13 Ravenhill Pk, Belfast. MB, BCh (QUB 1935). Maj. RAMC.

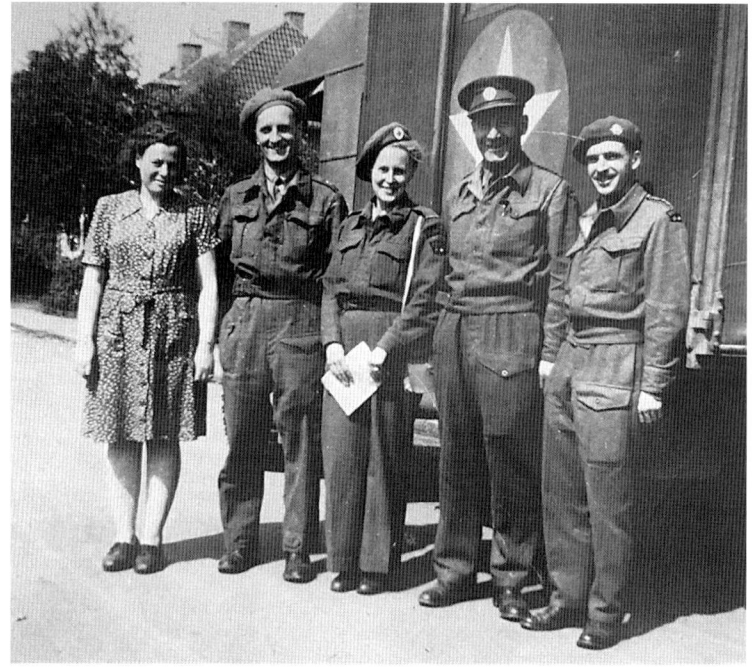

Bob Collis, fourth left, was among the first medics to attend the Belsen concentration camp after its liberation by Allied troops.

COLE John McMurray Address: Fernlea, Balmoral, Belfast. MB, BCh (QUB 1940). Flt Lt (M) RAFVR.

COLHOUN James Hamilton Address: Milebush, Carrickfergus, Co. Antrim. MB, BCh (QUB 1928). Maj. RAMC.

COLLIER Hugh Herbert Address: 62 Donaghadee Rd, Bangor, Co. Down. MB, BCh (QUB 1928), DPH (QUB 1938). Maj. RAMC. MID.

COLLIER Terence Desmond Address: Co. Dublin. L.LM (RCPI 1937), L.LM (RCSI 1937). Lt RAMC 15th Jan. 1940.

COLLINS Michael Joseph Address: Teachers Residence, Baltimore, Co. Cork. MB, BCh, BAO (UCC 1943). Flt Offr RAF.

COLLIS Robert b. 16th Feb. 1900 Address: Fitzwilliam Sq., Dublin. Educ. Rugby, Warwickshire, Kings Hospital. Joined the British Red Cross and was among the first medics to attend the Belsen concentration camp after its liberation by Allied troops.

CONAN Arthur Robert TCD (1931) Capt. RA.

CONCANNON John Noel b. 25th Dec. 1910 at St Vincent, British West Indies. LM, LCh (TCD 1932). PC Lt 27th Feb. 1933. Capt. 1st May 1934. A/Maj. 12th Jan. 1940. T/Maj. 12th Apr. 1940. India 1934–39. BEF France 1939–40. KIA 1st Jun. 1940.

CONLON Patrick Joseph MB, BCh, BAO (UCD 1921). Lt RAMC. Enlisted 22nd Mar. 1940.

CONNOLLY George Rankin Address: Lisnaskea, Co. Fermanagh. MB, BCh (TCD 1942). Lt RAMC.

CONNOLLY Jeremiah MB, BCh, BAO (UCC 1931). Lt RAMC.

CONNOLLY John Francis TCD (1933). Lt Col. RAMC. Served in Abyssinia and Burma.

CONNOLLY John James Bernard Address: Forthill, Ballymote, Co. Sligo. MB, BCh, BAO (1939 NUI). Enlisted 19th Oct. 1939. Lt RAMC.

CONNOLLY Patrick Joseph Address: Boyle Sq., Clonakilty, Co. Cork. L.LM (RCPI 1935), L.LM (RCSI 1935). Flt Offr RAFVR 8th Nov. 1940.

CONNOR George Haslett Address: Seaview Cottage, Warrenpoint, Co. Down. MB, BCh (QUB 1942). Capt. RAMC.

CONNOR Herbert Lionel Address: 23 Hawthorn Rd, Knock, Belfast. MB, BCh (TCD 1934). Lt Col. RAMC. Served in Dunkirk. MID.

*****CONNOR** James Lawrence Address: Newry Rd, Banbridge, Co. Down. MB, BCh (QUB 1940). Flt Lt (M) RAFVR. d. Dec. 1945. Buried in Hereford C. of E. (Grove), Grave 5658.

CONRAN Thomas Joseph Address: 13 Dunedin, Connaught Ave., Cork. MB, BCh (UCC 1937). Flt Offr RAF.

CONROY Martin Patrick Address: MB, BCh, BAO (UCD 1923). Lt IMS. First Enlisted 3rd Mar. 1925. MC.

CONWAY Stephen Martin Patrick b. 4th Aug. 1916, Dublin. Address: 112 Pembroke Rd, Ballsbridge, Dublin. L.LM (1939 RCSI), L.LM (1939 RCSI). LRCP&SI (1939), LM Coombe Hosp. 1940. Lt 11th Mar. 1940. Capt. 11th Mar. 1941. PC Capt. 11th Mar. 1945. A/Maj. 13th Nov. 1945. T/Maj. 13th Feb. 1946. WS/Maj. 12th Sept. 1946. A/Lt Col. 12th Jun. 1946. T/Lt Col. 12th Sept. 1946. Lt Col. 4th Sept. 1958. Col. 11th Mar. 1963. BEF France 1940. MEF 1941–44. RMO The Queens Bays 1942–44. Italy 1944–45. MELF 1946–47. CO BMH Benghazi 1946–47. ADMS HQ Cyrenaica area 1947. CO BMH Salonika 1947. E. Africa PMO Brit. Mil. Admin. Somalia 1947–49. FARELF: CO 16th Fd Amb. 1952–55. CO Mil. Hosp. Tidworth 1955–59. BAOR CO 28th Fd Amb. 1959–60. FARELF CO BMH Kamunting 1961–63. BAOR: ADMS HQ Rhine area 1963–65. ADMS HQ 1st

Div. 1965. Medals: OBE 25th Oct. 1955. MC 25th Feb. 1943. 1939–45 S., Africa S. with cl. 8th Army, Italy S., DM, WM, GSM with cl. Malaya, QEII Corn Medal 1953. MC. 'On the morning of October 28th, 1942, the position to which he had advanced during the night was the object of heavy and intense enemy shellfire and numerous casualties were caused. For more than three hours Captain Conway made unceasing journeys rendering aid to wounded personnel in the locality. All ranks were forced by this shellfire to take cover either in their tanks or dug positions, but Captain Conway, without a thought for his personal safety, continued to carry out his duty even to the extent of visiting areas where casualties might have occurred. His coolness and courage were an example to all.'

CONYNGHAM Robert Henry Cecil Address: c/o Provincial Bank of Ireland, Belfast. MB, BCh (TCD 1943). Flt Offr RAF.

COOKE Albert Frederick Address: Kingstown, Co. Dublin. LRCP&S (RCSI 1924). Flt Offr RAF 30th May 1938.

COOKE Eric Robert Nathaniel MB, BCh (TCD 1937). s. Herbert Cooke, Gorey, Co. Wexford. Married Elizabeth G. Wolfe only child of Mr William and Mrs Wolfe, The Corner House, Skibbereen. Capt. Kings A. Rifles.

COOKE Michael James MB, BCh, BAO (UCD 1924). Lt RAMC. First enlisted 29th Jan. 1940.

COOKE Rowland Chaloner Hoffe Address: 16 North Circular Rd, Dublin. MB, BCh (TCD 1939). Flt Offr RAF.

COOPER William James Douglas Address: 9 High St, Antrim. MB, BCh, DPH (QUB 1940). Capt. RAMC.

COPE Joseph Victor b. 25th Jun. 1892, Dublin City. s. George Patrick (MD) and Mary Maud Cope, 36 Harcourt St, Dublin. Educ. St Andrews Coll. Dublin 7th Sept. 1900–31st Mar. 1910. TCD/RCSI MB (1915), BCh, MD (1919), FRCSI (1919). R. C. of I. T/Lt RAMC 10th Jul. 1915. T/Capt. 10th Jul. 1916. First entered a theatre of war on 29th Sept. 1915 Gallipoli. Wounded Dec. 1917. In 1941 he joined the Home Guard and was Battalion Medical Officer with the rank of major when it was disbanded. Medals: MC (4th Feb. 1918), 1915 S., BWM, VM. d. 13th Feb. 1977. Commemorated on Roll of Honour RCSI.

COPPINGER Charles Joseph MB, BCh, BAO (TCD) 1904. b. 5th Nov. 1880, Dublin. IMS Lt 1st Feb. 1905, Capt. 1st Feb. 1908, Capt. RAMC 31st Mar. 1911, Maj. 15th Oct. 1915, Lt Col. 15th Sept. 1928, r.p. 5th Nov. 1905. Rempld 25th Sept. 1939. Reverted to r.p. 13th Oct. 1940. India 1905–11, BEF France 1914 invalided, India 1919–23, ADP War Office

1927–31, India 1931–33, Emergency Vaccine Lab. Tidworth 1939–40, Spec. Bacteriology 1913. Medals: OBE 3rd Jun. 1831, 1914 S., VWM, VM.

COPPINGER Francis Romney b. 10th May 1883, Dublin. Brother of Charles Joseph above and son of Valentine J. Coppinger. Educ. TCD. BA, MB, BCh, BAO, DPH (1912). Lt IMS 1st Feb. 1908. Capt. 1st Feb. 1911. Capt. RAMC 15th Jul. 1914. Maj. 1st Feb. 1920. Lt Col. 9th May 1932. Col. 15th Apr. 1936. Rtd and remained employed 15th Apr. 1940. r.p. 4th Feb. 1942. First entered a theatre of war 4th Aug. 1914, Aden. IC of vaccine dept. RAMC Coll. Grosvenor Rd, London SW. India 1911–18, Aden 1914–16, Burma 1916–18, DADP Jamaica 1923–25. DADP S. Comd 1926–29. India 1929–34. DADP Baluchistan Dist. 1929–31. ADH & P E. Commd. 1931–34. OIC Med. Div. R. Herbert Hosp. Woolwich 1935–36. SMO CLED 1936–38. ADMS HQ S. Area 1938–39. BEF France. DDMS HQ 2 Corps. 1939–40. ADMS HQ E. Midland Area 1940–42. Specialist in bacteriology. Medals: OBE (12th Sept. 1919), 1915 S., BWM, VM. MID 4th Jul. 1916, 20th Jan. 1920.

CORBETT Mary Address: Kenneigh, Montenotte Pk, Cork. MB, BCh, BAO (UCC 1938). Flt Offr RAF.

CORCORAN John Patrick Address: 15 St Patrick's Tce, Magazine Rd, Cork. Younger son of Mrs Corcoran and the late Cornelius (Overseer of Cork GPO). Married Angela Attwood, only dt. Mr and Mrs Benjamin Attwood, Glenbeg, St Clare's Avenue, Cork. MB, BCh, BAO (UCC 1935). Lt RAMC. Reported to have saved the lives of many Allied prisoners of war held in Sumatra and later transferred to Singapore.

CORR James Patrick MB, BCh (QUB 1924). Capt. RAMC.

CORRIDAN Maurice Address: Ballyhorgan House, Lixnaw, Co. Kerry. MB, BCh (NUI 1941). Lt 5th Jun. 1942. Surg. Lt RNVR 1st Mar. 1943.

CORRIGAN Philip Joseph Address: 8 Orchard Tce, Enniskillen, Co. Fermanagh. L.LM (RCPI 1941), L.LM (RCSI 1941). Flt Offr RAFVR 6th Aug. 1938.

*****CORRY** Samuel David MB (QUB 1938). Capt. RAMC (Cdo) b. NI. s. Samuel and Anna Corry (née Stoupe) Bangor, Co. Down. MID (LG 3rd Apr. 1942). Reported missing after the Dieppe raid. d. 20th Aug. 1942 of wounds in France while a POW. Buried in St Sever Cemetery ext. Rouen, Block 'S', Plot 4, Row R, Grave 14.

COSGRAVE Patrick Address: Borrisnoe, Templemore, Co. Tipperary. MB, BCh (NUI 1938). Lt RAMC 18th Oct. 1941.

COSGROVE Joseph Patrick Address: 34 Kings Street, Belfast. MB, BCh (QUB 1935). Lt RAMC 9th Jan. 1941.

COTTER William Joseph MB, BCh, BAO (UCC 1928). Flt Offr RAF.

COUNIHAN Francis Harold Address: Bellevue, Kilrush, Co. Clare. MB, BCh (TCD 1938). Maj. RAMC.

COUNIHAN William Edward Address: Bellevue, Kilrush, Co. Clare. MB, BCh (TCD 1936). Maj. RAMC.

COURTNEY John Christopher Address: The Green, Killaloe, Co. Clare. L.LM (RCPI 1942), L.LM (RCSI 1942). Sq. Ldr 1st Jun. 1942 RAFVR.

COWAN Jacob Address: Brighton House, Brighton Sq., Rathgar, Dublin. L.LM (RCPI 1939), L.LM (RCSI 1939). Lt RAMC 17th Jul. 1941. MC.

COWAN William Saunderson Address: 102 Belmont Rd, Belfast. MB, BCh (QUB 1938). Capt. RAMC.

CRAIG Catherine Eleanor Address: The Grove, Newry, Co. Down. MB, BCh (TCD 1942). RAMC.

CRAIG David Hanna Address: 3 Ben Madigan Pk South, Antrim Rd, Belfast, MB, BCh (QUB 1931). Maj. RAMC.

CRAIG Eric William MB, BCh (TCD 1914). PMO RAMC. PMO Fighter Comd. MC.

CRAIG George Archibald MB (QUB 1935). Maj. RAMC. MBE.

CRAIG James MB, BCh (TCD 1926). Lr. Col. RAMC.

CRAIG James Kenneth Address: Adelaide Tce, Bailieboro, Co. Cavan. MB, BCh (TCD 1939), MD. Sq. Ldr RAF (1940).

CRAIG John Gray MB, BCh (1929), MD (QUB 1932). Maj. RAMC.

CRAIG John Quentin Address: Victoria St, Ballymoney, Co. Antrim. MB, BCh (1936), DPH (QUB 1938). Sq. Ldr (M) RAFVR.

CRAIG John Victor Address: Manor Tce, Cregagh Rd, Belfast. MB, BCh (QUB 1929). Capt. RAMC.

CRAIG Wilhelmina Mary Address: 171 Malone Rd, Belfast. MB, BCh (QUB 1937), DPH (QUB 1937). Flt Lt (M) RAFVR.

CRAIG William Johnston Address: 18 Merrion Sq., Dublin. MB, BCh (TCD 1932). Sq. Ldr RAFVR (1941).

CRAWFORD David Johnston Address: Drumakeely, Clarryford, Co. Antrim. MB, BCh (QUB 1942). Maj. RAMC.

CRAWFORD Thomas George Brown MB, BCh (TCD 1925). Surg. Comdr RN.

CREAGH Edward Philip Nagle b. 29th Feb. 1896, Fermoy, Co. Cork. Educ. NUI (UCC). MB (1917), BCh, BAO,

MRCP (London 1931). Lt RAMC SR 6th Dec. 1917. Capt. 6th Dec. 1918. PC Lt (T/Capt.) 1st Apr. 1919. Capt. 6th Jun. 1921. Maj. 6th Dec. 1929. A/Lt Col. 8th Nov. 1939. T/Lt Col. 8th Feb. 1940. WS Lt Col. 15th Jan. 1943. Lt Col. 7th Feb. 1944. A/Col. 15th Jul. 1942. T/Col. 15th Apr. 1943. Col. 21st Feb. 1948. T/Brig. 31st Oct. 1949. Brig. 26th Jun. 1951. T/Maj. Gen. 1st Jul. 1952. Maj. Gen. 16th Feb. 1953. r.p. 6th Mar. 1956. Served in France 5th Jan. 1918–19. India 1919–24. BAOR 1924. India 1924–29. Med. Spec. Mil. Hosp. Catterick 1931–32. India 1932–37: CMH Poona 1932–35, Surg. to HE C in C 1936–37. Royal Victoria Hosp. Netley 1937–39. BEF France 1939–40. 7 Gen. Hosp. Spet. No. 1939. OIC Med. Div. 6 Gen. Hosp. Nov. 1939–Feb. 1940. CO 144 Fd Amb. 1940–41. OIC Med. Div. 1936 (WA) Gen. Hosp. 1941–42: W. Africa 1941–43. CO 46 (WA) Gen. Hosp. 1942–43. CO Mil. Hosp. York May–Aug. 1943. CO 77 Gen. Hosp. 1943–45. NWE 1944–45. Gibraltar: CO Mil. Hosp. 1945–57. CO Mil. Hosp. Chepstow 1947–48. CO R. Herbert Hosp. Woolwich 1948–49. DDMS HQ W. Comd 1952–56. QHP 5th Mar. 1953. Col. Comdt RAMC 1956. Medals: CB (1st Jan. 1954), BWM, VM, 1939–45 S., DM, WM, KGV Silver Jub. Medal 1935, QEII Corn Medal 1953, OStJ (5th Jul. 1955). MID 20th Dec. 1940.

CREALEY John b. 5th Jul. 1902, Belfast. MB, BCh, BAO (QUB 1925). PC Lt 30th Jan. 1929, Capt. RAMC. Served India 1930–32, resigned 19th Apr. 1932.

CREAN Gerrard Patrick b. 8th Nov. 1912, Dublin. MRCS (England), LRCP (London 1939). Lt 1st Feb. 1939. Capt. 2nd Jun. 1940. PC Capt. 1st Feb. 1944. T/Maj. 18th Jun. 1948. Maj. 5th Aug. 1948. T/Lt Col. 10th Nov. 1953. Lt Col. 10th Oct. 1962. BEF France 1939–40. MEF 1940–44. RMO 1940–43. NWE/BAOR 1944–50. E. Africa 1952–53. OIC Con. Wing, Royal Victoria Hosp. Netley 1953–55. BAOR 1956–61. FARELF Hong Kong 1961–64. BAOR: CO and Snr Partner GP practice Dortmund 1966. Medals: 1939–45 S., Africa S. with 8th Army cl., Italy S., France and Germany S., DM, WM, AGSM with cl. Kenya.

CREAN Thomas Francis Address: 3 Douglas St, Cork. L.LM (RCPI 1924), L.LM (RCSI 1924). Flt Lt RN and RAF 26th May 1940.

CREERY Robert Desmond Gibson Address: 26 North Circular Rd, Lisburn, Co. Antrim. MB, BCh (QUB 1943). Surg. Lt RNVR.

CREIGHTON Patrick Address: Westacre, Cultra, Co. Down. MB, BCh (QUB 1942). Surg. Lt RNVR.

CROGHAN Hubert Joseph MB, BCh, BAO (UCD 1923). Lt RAMC. First enlisted 8th Sept. 1939.

CROKER William Pennefather b. 26th Oct. 1889, Clondalkin, Co. Dublin. s. Edward James O'Brien (railway manager) and Henrietta Emily Croker,

Gweebarra, 99, Palmerston Rd, Rathmines, Dublin. Educ. St Andrew's Coll. Dublin 30th Aug. 1905–31st Oct. 1906. TCD. MB (1912), BCh, BAO, LM (Rot. Hosp. 1912). R. C. of I. Lt RAMC 24th Jan. 1913. Capt. 30th Mar. 1915. Maj. 24th Jan. 1925. Lt Col. 12th Jul. 1935. Col. 17th Nov. 1940. r.p. Hon. Brig. 27th Apr. 1947. Served in 1914–18 War from 15th Aug. 1914, France. POW Oct. 1914–Jul. 1915. France and Belgium 1916–19. India 1919–21. Afghanistan 1919. Gibraltar 1925–27. Shanghai 1927–28. SMO R. Arsenal Woolwich 1937–39. CO 30 Gen Hosp. 1939–40. Iceland Jul.–Nov. 1940. ADMS HQ W. Sussex Area 1940–41. DDMS FHQ Gibraltar 1941–42. MEF/CMF 1942–44. DDMS HQ Corps 1943–44. CO 99 Gen Hosp. 1944. CO Royal Victoria Hosp. Netley 1945–47. Medals: 1914 S., BWM, VM, IGSM (1908) cl. Afghanistan, 1939–45 S., Africa S. and cl. 8th Army, ITS, DM, WM. French L de H. War Cross 6th Nov. 1918. MID 24th Aug. 1944.

***CROMIE** Robert Stevenson s. Samuel James and Sarah Morton Cromie of Ballymoney, Co. Antrim. Husband of Mable of Coulson, Surrey. MD (QUB 1931). Flt Lt 90485 (M) R. Aux. AF (615 Sq.). Killed on active service 18th Aug. 1940, aged 32. Buried in Ballymoney Cemetery, Section 3, Grave 37.

CRONE William Plunkett Address: 10 Kings Rd, Knock, Belfast. MB, BCh (QUB 1942). Flt Lt (M) RAFVR.

CRONIN Columba MB, BCh, BAO (NUI 1936). Lt RAMC 1942.

CROOK Alfred Frazer Address: The Willows, Newry, Co. Down. MB, BCh (QUB 1939). Capt. RAMC.

CROSBIE John Henry Breuell MB, BCh (TCD 1920). Surg. Capt. RN.

CROSBIE Pierce Desmond L.LM (RCPI 1941), L.LM (RCSI 1941). Flt Lt RAF 14th Jan. 1944.

CROUCH Henrietta Elizabeth (née Hunter) MB (QUB 1942). Capt. RAMC.

CROUCH Hubert Andrew MB (QUB 1933). Maj. RAMC.

CROWE John Address: Galbally, Co. Tipperary. LRCP&S (RCSI 1934). Lt IMS 23rd Apr. 1936.

CROWLEY Alan Fergus Address: 3 Eglington Pk, Kingstown, Co. Dublin. MB, BCh (TCD 1941). Surg. Lt RNVR.

CROWLEY Christopher MB, BCh, BAO (UCC 1925), DPH (RCPSI England 1938). Flt Lt RAF.

CROWLEY Matthew Address: Ardmore, Youghal, Co. Cork. MB, BCh, BAO (UCC 1936). Flt Offr RAF.

CROWLEY Timothy Finbarr MB, BCh, BAO (UCC 1926). Lt RAMC.

CROZIER Thomas Howard Address: 3 University Sq., Belfast. MD, BSc, DPH (QUB 1921). Lt Col. RAMC. MID (2).

CSONKA George William MB, BCh (QUB 1941). Capt. RAMC.

CUBITT George Rowland Address: Waterville, Co. Kerry. MB, BCh, BAO (UCC 1938). Lt RAMC.

CULLEN Edward Address: Rose Hill, Newport, Limerick. MB, BCh (TCD 1939). Maj. RAMC. Chindit Force. MID.

CULLENAN John b. 12th Nov. 1889, Lurgan, Co. Down. MB, BCh, BAO (QUB 1916). Lt RAMC SR 4th Jun. 1914. Mobd 1st Jul. 1916. Capt. 1st Jan. 1917. PC Capt. 1st Jun. 1920. Maj. 1st Jul. 1928. A/Lt Col. 14th Feb. 1940. T/Lt Col. 14th May 1940. Served Mesopotamia 1916–18. India 1918–20. Aden 1920–22. India Gynae. Spec. BSH Meerut 1925–30, OC Gynae Spec. MFH Chatham 1930–37, Malta OC MFH Imtarfa 1937–40, CO 180th Fd Amb. 1940–41, CO 9th CCS 1941, PSMB W. Scotland area 1942, N. Comd 1942–46, 101st Mil. Con. Dep. 1946–47. Medals: BWM, VM. d. 6th Mar. 1947.

CUMMINS Cecil Stratford MB (TCD 1941). Capt. RAMC (1944). Egypt and Palestine 1945–47.

CUNNINGHAM Charles Address: Culloville House, Crossmaglen, Co. Armagh. MB, BCh (TCD 1937). RAMC.

CUNNINGHAM John Gerard Address: Culloville House, Crossmaglen, Co. Armagh. MB, BCh (TCD 1937). RAMC.

CUNNINGHAM Joseph Irwin Address: 14 Eglington St, Portrush, Co. Antrim. MB, BCh (QUB 1938). Surg. Lt RNVR. MBE.

CUNNINGHAM Thomas Arthur Address: Culloville, Crossmaglen, Co. Armagh. MB, BCh (TCD 1935). Lt Col. IMS.

CUPPLES Samuel Eric Address: Loughbrickland, Banbridge, Co. Down. MB, BCh (QUB 1941). Flt Lt (M) RAFVR.

CURRAN Edward Joseph b. 18th Feb. 1906, South Glanmire, Cork. MB, BCh, BAO (NUI 1928), DPH (London 1938). PC. Lt RAMC 23rd Oct. 1929, Capt. 23rd Apr. 1933, A/Maj. 3rd Sept. 1939, Maj. 23rd Oct. 1939, A/Lt Col. 6th Dec. 1945, T/Lt Col. 6th Mar. 1946, Lt Col. 5th Sept. 1946, Col. 28th Dec. 1951, T/Brig. 11th Mar. 1958, Brig. 14th Jan. 1960. r.p. 1st Jan. 1963. Served India 1931–36, Hong Kong 1939–41, POW 1941–45, Asst Comdt AS of HYG 1945–47, ADH HQ Scottish Comd 1947–51, DDAH GHQ FARELF 1953–54, CO Mil. Hosp. Chester 1955–57, ADMS HQ Northern Comd 1961–62. Medals: CBE 31st May 1953, IGSM with cl. Burma 1930–32, 1939–45 S., Pacific S., DM, WM, GSM with cl. Malaya, QEII Corn Medal 1953.

CURRAN Hubert Joseph MB, BCh, BAO (UCG 1924). Lt RAMC & IMF.

CURRY James Terence MB, BCh, BAO (NUI 1939). Lt RAMC 1944.

CUSACK James Joseph Address: Prospect House, Dromolane, Newry, Co. Down. MB, BCh (TCD 1925). Surg. Lt RN (1926).

CUSACK Patrick Bernard Address: 5 Crofton Tce, Dun Laoghaire, Dublin. L.LM (RCPI 1934), MB (1937), L.LM (RCSI 1934). Lt IMS 1st Nov. 1936.

CUSSEN Denis John MB, BCh (TCD 1925). Capt. RAMC.

CUSSEN John MB, BCh (TCD 1925). Surg. Comdr RN. MID.

D

DALES Herbert Calvert Address: Roseville, Lisburn, Co. Armagh. Campbell College. MB, BCh (QUB 1942). Surg. Lt RNVR.

DALTON Hubert William Address: 1 Seaview Tce, Donnybrook, Dublin. MB, BCh (TCD 1931). Maj. RAMC.

DALY George Laurence MB, BCh (TCD 1936), MD. RAMC.

DALY Patrick Joseph MB, BCh (NUI 1938). Lt RAMC 1st May 1938.

DANIELS Henry Aeroux Address: East Grange, Fermoy, Co. Cork. MB, BCh (TCD 1936). Maj. RAMC. MID.

D'ARCY Francis Bertram Address: Etna Lodge, Clones, Co. Monaghan. MB, BCh (TCD 1922) Capt. RAMC (1939).

D'ARCY Thomas Morgan William b. 27th Jan. 1910, Dublin. MB, BCh, BAO (Dublin 1934), DPH (England 1948), MD (NUI 1952). DTM&H (1953). Lt RAMC 23rd Apr. 1936. Capt. 23rd Apr. 1937. PC Capt. 23rd Apr. 1941. A/Maj. 25th Jan. 1942. T/Maj. 25th Apr. 1942. Maj. 23rd Apr. 1946. T/Lt Col. 24th May 1949. Lt Col. 7th Feb. 1951. Lt Col. 16th Apr. 1956. T/Col. 1st Jul. 1956. Col. 29th Jul. 1959. Served Palestine 1936. India 1937–41. E. Africa 1942–44. FARELF 1948–51. OC School of Hygiene Far East 1948–49. ADAH HQ Malaya Dist. 1949–51. AS of Health 1951–53. ADAH HQ W. African Comd 1953–56. ADMS HQ Nigeria Mil. Forces RWAFF 1956. DDAH HQ S. Comd 1956–59. Comdt AS of Health 1959–62. DDAH HQ FARELF 1962–64. CMO HQ UNFICYP Dist. 1965–66. Comdt AS of Health 1966. Medals: GSM (cl. Palestine 1936–39), 1939–45 S., DM, WM, GSM (Malaya cl.), UN Forces in Cyprus Medal, QEII Corn Medal 1953, OStJ 1962. MID 24th Oct. 1950.

D'ARCY Thomas Norman Address: Etna Lodge, Clones, Co. Monaghan. L.LM (1919 RCPI), L.LM (1919 RCSI). Flt Offr RN & RAF 6th Aug. 1942.

DARLING John Singleton Address: Hoophill, Lurgan, Co. Armagh. MB, ChB (QUB 1934), PRCS (England 1940). Lt Col. RAMC.

DAUNT Benjamin James b. 7th Nov. 1892, Ballineen, Co. Cork. s. William Gash (farmer) and Lizzie Daunt, Derrigra, Teadies, Cork. Educ. RCSI. LRCPI (1916), LRCSI, LM (Rot. Hosp.). R. C. of I. T/Lt RAMC SR 22nd Aug. 1916. T/Capt. 22nd Feb. 1917. PC Lt (T/Capt.) 1st Apr. 1919. Capt. 22nd Feb. 1920. Maj. 27th Aug. 1928. A/Lt Col. 11th Aug. 1940. T/Lt Col. 15th Dec.

1940. Lt Col. 17th Apr. 1943. A/Col. 6th Oct. 1941. T/Col. 6th Apr. 1942. Col. 15th Jun. 1947. A/Brig. 19th Jun. 1945. T/Brig. 19th Dec. 1945. r.p. Hon. Brig. 9th Jan. 1956. Served Mesopotamia from 27th Nov. 1916. Salonika Jan.–Feb. 1917. Egypt Feb.–Mar. 1917. India Mar.–Aug. 1917. Mesopotamia 1917–22. BAOR 1923–24. India 1924–30 and 1934–39. Egypt/MEF 1939–43. ADMS HQ British Somaliland Aug.–Sept. 1940. CO 2/3 Cavalry Fd Amb. 1940–41. ADMS HQ 7th Armd Div. 1941–42. ADMS HQ Guards Armd Div. 1943–45. NWE/BAOR 1844–46.: CO 23rd Gen. Hosp. Jan.–Jun. 1945. DDMS HQ 8th Corps. 1945–46. ALFSEA: DDMS HQ Malaya Comd 1946–47. Comdt Depot and Training Estab. RAMC 1947–48. DDMS HQ W. Africa Comd 1948–49. ADMS HQ London Dist. 1950 53. HQ Highland Dist. 1953–55. Medals: OBE (8th Jul. 1941), BWM, VM, GSM (cl. Iraq 1920), 1939–45 S., Africa S., France and Germany S., DM, WM, KGVI Corn Medal 1937, QEII Corn Medal 1953. MID 8th May 1945. d. 12th May 1958, Millbank, London. Commemorated on Roll of Honour RCSI.

DAVEY William Wilkin Address: The Manse, Dunmurray, Co. Antrim. MB, BCh (QUB 1935), MC (QUB 1941). Sq. Ldr (M) RAFVR.

DAVIDSON Thomas Walker b. 10th Nov. 1900 at Clones, Co. Monaghan. Campbell College. MB, BCh, BAO (QUB 1923), LM Rot. Hosp. (1930). PC Lt RAMC 1st Aug. 1923, Capt. 1st Feb. 1927, Maj. 1st May 1934, A/Lt Col. 10th Feb. 1941, T/Lt Col. 10th May 1941, Lt Col. 17th Nov. 1944, A/Col. 13th Feb. 1944, T/Col. 17th May 1944, A/Brig. 8th Sept. 1942, T/Brig. r.p. Hon. Brig. 3rd Apr. 1946. Service Second Sudan Defence Force 1924–31, India 1937–41, Waziristan 1937, Paiforce/MEF 1941–43, CO 32nd Indian Fd Amb. 1941–42, DDMS HQ 21st Indian Corps. 1942, CO 164th Fd Amb. 1945, India 1945. Medals: MID 18th Feb. 1938, OStJ 1950, IGSM with cl. NWF 1937, 1939–45 S., Africa S., Italy S., France and Germany S., DM, WM, KGVI Corn Medal 1937.

DAVIDSON William Mcfarlane Address: 230 Antrim Rd, Belfast. Campbell College. MB, BCh (QUB 1938). Surg. Lt Comdr RN.

DAVIES Henry Rhys Address: Woodlawn, Churchtown Rd, Dundrum, Dublin. Campbell College. MB, BCh (TCD 1933). Maj. RAMC.

DAVIS George Hall. Campbell College. TCD 1918. Maj. RAMC.

DAVIS Walter Samuel Address: Le Sare, Lisburn Rd, Hillsborough, Co. Down. Campbell College. MB, BCh (QUB 1943). Lt RAMC.

DAVISON James Creighton Address: 29 College Gdns, Belfast. MB, BCh (QUB 1925), MD (QUB 1928). Maj. RAMC.

DAVYS Geoffrey Raymond Address: 8 Ailesbury Pk, Ballsbridge, Dublin. MB, BCh (NUI 1942). Flt Lt RAF 14th Feb. 1944.

DAVYS Gerard Irvine MB, BCh (TCD 1901), MD (TCD 1911), DPH, RCPI (1912). IMS. OBE.

DAWSON Donald James Cranston Address: 29 Knock Rd, Belfast. MB, BCh (QUB 1930), MC (QUB 1937). Capt. RAMC.

DAY Charles Lionel MB, BCh (1927 TCD). Younger son of the late Maurice W. Day, Dean of Waterford and husband of Noeline. d. suddenly 30th Jul. 1953, Edinburgh. Lt Col. RAMC.

DEANE Hastings Fitzmaurice TCD 1931. South African Forces. Served in Libya and Greece.

DE BURCA Brian Address: 4 Lower Fitzwilliam St, Dublin. MB, BCh, BAO (UCD 1931). Lt IMS. MBE.

DE COURCY-WHEELER Annesley Eliardo Beresford Address: The Gables, Station Rd, Foxrock, Co. Dublin. MB, BCh (TCD 1936) MD. IMS.

DEENY Patrick Hugh MB, BCh (QUB 1925), DPH (QUB 1931). Maj. RAMC.

DELANEY Patrick Denis Surg. Lt Royal Australian Navy. Only s. Mr & Mrs Denis Delaney, Richmond Avenue, Monkstown, Dublin. Husband of Jocelyn, dt. Mrs Mack and Mr C.W. Mack, Wellington, New Zealand.

DELAP Peter Address: Dangan, Carrickmines, Co. Dublin. MB, BCh (TCD 1936). MD. Capt. RAMC (1940) attd. Commandos. Wounded 1944. MC.

DENNARD Leslie David MB, BCh (TCD 1924). Maj. RAMC.

DENNEHY William Benedict Address: The Square, Listowel, Co. Kerry. MB, BCh (TCD 1940). RAMC.

DEUCHAR Charles Rowland TCD 1941. Flt Offr RAF.

DEVLIN Edward Raymond MB, BCh, BAO (UCD 1926). Flt Offr RAF 25th Jun. 1942.

DEVLIN Henry Richard Tarleton Address: St Owen's Rectory, Ballymore, Co. Westmeath. MB, BCh (TCD 1938). Maj. RAMC. Served in BEF 8th Army, N. Africa and Italy.

DICK James MB, BCh (TCD 1925) FRCS (Edin. 1930). Maj. RAMC.

DICKINSON Richard Frederick O'Toole b. 13th Jan. 1880, Poona, India s. Richard Randall Dickinson. Educ. Blackrock Coll. Dublin and UCD Med Sch. MB (1914), BCh (1914 UCD and London), BAO, MSc, LRCPI (1905), LRCSI, LM (1905), DPH (1909), BCh. Married Ita Mary Pauline dt. Hugh

Macken, Dublin. Lt RAMC 29th Jul. 1907, Capt. 29th Jan. 1911, A/Maj. 7th Aug. 1918, Maj. 29th Jul. 1919, T/Lt Col. 25th Oct. 1931, Lt Col. 1st Nov. 1931. r.p. 13th Jan. 1935. Rempld Maj. 29th Jul. 1940. r.p. Lt Col. 26th Nov. 1946. India 1909–14. France and Belgium 1914–15 invalided. EEF 1916. France and Belgium 1917–19. Germany 1919. Mauritius 1923–27 and 1929–32. War work DAD Hygiene 5th Div. Ire. MO of Unit in 6th Div. 1914–15. Specialist San. Off. Trouville Base and DAD Med. Servs. (sanitation) 1st Brit. A. in the field and later at GHQ Brit. A. of the Rhine. Medals: OBE (3rd Jun. 1919), 1914 S., BWM, VM, DM, WM. MID 10th Jul. 1919. Commemorated on Roll of Honour RCSI.

DICKSON Ronald Ritchie Address: 47 Maryville Pk, Belfast. MB, BCh (QUB 1941). Sq. Ldr (M) RAFVR.

DIMOND William Elliot b. 29th Sept. 1893. L.LM (1915 RCPI), L.LM (1915 RCSI), DPH (RCPSI 1824). s. George Dimond, apothecary and his wife Anna Maude, Dublin St, Queen's County. Married Oonagh Katherine Young (1896–1921) on 22nd October 1919, who died on a voyage to India. Maj. Gen. Indian Medical Service. Served in both World Wars. Twice wounded and MID. Medals: CIE awarded for conspicuous service against cholera, OBE. d. 5th Nov. 1960 aged 67, at Greystones, Co. Wicklow. Buried The Grove Cemetery, Redford.

DIXON Henry Bryan Frost b. 12th Jul. 1891, Kilmainham, Dublin. s. William Henry (Cork merchant and manufacturer) and Henrietta Dixon, 24 James St, Dublin. Educ. TCD BA (1911), MB (1913), BAO, BCh, MD (1934), FRCP London (1938), MB (1926), DTM&H (Eng. 1937). Lt RAMC 5th Aug. 1914. Capt. 1st Apr. 1915. A/Maj. 4th Jan. 1918. PC Capt. 1st May 1919. Maj. 5th Aug. 1926. Lt Col. 28th Apr. 1936. A/Col. 1st Sept. 1939. T/Col. 1st Mar. 1940. Col. 29th Oct. 1941. A/Brig. 4th Apr. 1945. T/ Brig. 4th Oct. 1945. r.p. Hon. Brig. 9th Jun. 1947. Served in Flanders with the London Fd Amb. 1915–19. Mesopotamia 1920–21. India 1921–24. Royal Victoria Hosp. Netley 1926. QA Mil. Hosp. Millbank 1926–28. India 1929–32. EMH Poona. QA Mil. Hosp. 1933–36. Mil. Hosp. Gibraltar 1936–38. Malta CO Mil. Hosp. Amtarfa/90 Gen. Hosp. 1938–42. CO Connaught Hosp. 1942–44. NWE Aug.–Nov. 1944. CO 107 Gen. Hosp. Feb.–Dec. 1944. W. Africa: DDMS GHQ WA Force 1945–46. DDMS HQ London Dist. Jan.–Feb. 1947. Medals: MC (14th Nov. 1916), Bar (26th Jul. 1918), 1915 S., BWM, VM, GSM and cl. Iraq, 1939–45 S., Africa S., France and Germany S., WM, German O. of Cross of Merit 1937. MID 1st Jan. 1916. d. 20th Jan. 1962, Millbank, London.

DIXON Kendal Cartwright MB, BCh (Camb. 1939), TCD (1928). Maj. RAMC. Served in BEF and MEF.

DOBBIN Stafford Address: 46 Grove Pk, Bangor Co. Down. MB, BCh (QUB 1938). Capt. RAMC.

DOCKRELL Thomas Hayes Address: 36 Clarinda Pk East, Dun Laoghaire, Co. Dublin MB, BCh (TCD 1930), FRCS (Ire. 1935). Lt Col. RAMC.

DODDS Robert Leslie MB, BCh (QUB 1920), FRCS (England 1927). Maj. RAMC.

DOHERTY Christopher John Address: Carrantrila, Ballina, Co. Mayo. MB, BCh, BAO (UCG 1938). Lt RAMC.

DOHERTY Francis John MB, BCh (QUB 1931). Lt Col. IMS. DSO.

DOHERTY Reginald Joseph Saunders MB, BCh, BAO (UCC 1932). Lt RAMC.

DOLAN Farrell MB, BCh (QUB 1925). Surg. Comdr RN.

DOMER Robert TCD 1922. Capt. RAMC.

DONAGHY Denis Fitzgerald MB (QUB 1948). NIH (RAC).

DONALDSON George Alexander Address: Rosetta Ave., Belfast. MB, BCh (QUB 1937). Lt Col. RAMC.

DONALDSON Norman Firth Address: 54 Balmoral Ave., Belfast. MB, BCh (QUB 1941). Surg. Lt RNVR.

DONALDSON Raymond Joseph Address: Dundalk Rd, Newtownhamilton, Newry, Co. Down. MB, BCh. DPH (QUB 1943). Capt. RAMC. India and Indo-China.

DONNAN Laurence Frederick Address: 3 Walmer Tce, Holywood, Co. Down. Campbell College. L.M.SSA (London 1931), DPH (QUB 1938). Surgeon RNVR.

DONOVAN John MB, BCh, BAO (UCD 1924). Lt RAMC. First enlisted 5th Jun. 1941.

DONOVAN Timothy Address: 14 St Patrick's Pl., Cork. MB, BCh, BAO (UCC 1922). Lt RAMC.

DOODY William Joseph MB, BCh, BAO (UCD 1924). Surg. Lt RN. First enlisted 4th Aug. 1925.

DOOLIN Walter Michael Address: 2 Fitzwilliam Sq., Dublin. MB, BCh (NUI 1941). Lt IMS 26th Aug. 1941.

DORAN Hugh Joseph Address: 240 Malone Rd, Belfast. MB, BCh (QUB 1937). Maj. RAMC.

DORMAN John Kennedy Addison Address: 102 Somerton Rd, Belfast. MB, BCh (QUB 1940). Maj. RAMC.

DORNAN Frederick Address: 15 Slieve Moyne Pk, Belfast. MB, BCh (QUB 1937). Maj. RAMC.

DORNAN Lloyd Address: 15 Slieve Moyne Pk, Belfast. BDS, MB, BCh (QUB 1931). Capt. RAMC.

DORNAN William Address: Tiralton, Slieve Moyne Pk, Belfast. MB, BCh (QUB 1933). Maj. RAMC.

DOUGALL James Address: 2 Mount Uriel, Belfast. MB, BCh (QUB 1940). Flt Lt RAFVR.

*****DOUGAN** Hampton Atkinson s. Dr George Dougan MD and Mrs Dougan of Portadown, Co. Armagh. Address: 19 Church St, Portadown. Campbell College. MB, BCh (TCD 1938). Maj. RAMC. Lt Col. KIA 20th Oct. 1944 India aged 29. Buried Ranchi War Cemetery, Plot 4.C.10. MC.

DOUGAN John McDonald Address: 19 Church Street, Portadown, Co. Armagh. Campbell College. MB, BCh (TCD 1939). Maj. RAMC. Served MEF. Wounded. MC (for gallant and distinguished service in the Middle East).

DOUGLAS Desmond Joseph Hilliard Address: 135 St Stephen's Green, Dublin. MB, BCh (TCD 1937). Maj. RAMC.

DOUGLAS Gerald Sholto b. 27th Nov. 1891, Dublin City. s. Hugh G. (farmer) and Roberta Douglas, Aughuagurgen, Armahague, Armagh. Educ. RCSI. LRCPI (1914), LRCSI (1914). R. C. of I. Married 1919. T/Lt RAMC 7th May 1915. T/Capt. 7th May 1916. PC Capt. 7th Nov. 1918. Maj. 7th May 1927. Lt Col. 1st Aug. 1941. A/Col. 1st Jul. 1943. T/Col. 23rd Jan. 1944. Col. 28th Nov. 1945. A/Brig. 14th Dec. 1945. T/Brig. 14th Jun. 1946. r.p. Hon Brig. 27th Nov. 1948. Served 1914–18 War. F & F 15th Jun. 1915–14th Aug. 1918. Wounded. Germany 1919. India 1920–24 and 1928–33. Jamaica 1937–42. SMO BEF Dutch W. Indies 1940–42. Specially empld. with Ministry of Info. 1942–43. ADMS HQ 42nd Armoured Div. Jul.–Sept. 1943. ADMS HQ 55th Inf. Div. 1943–44. India/S. East Asia 1944–47: CO BMH Delhi and CMH Ahmednagar 1944. CO 127 IBGH (BT) 1944–45. DDMS HQ 15th Corps. (AFNED) 1945–47. ADMS HQ N. Midland Dist. 1947–48. Medals: 1915 S., BWM, VM. WM, GSM (cl. S.E. Asia 45/46.). d. 1st Nov. 1965 at Innishannon, Co. Cork. Commemorated on Roll of Honour RCSI.

DOWD Denis Address: Ballysheen, Abbeydorney, Co. Kerry. L.LM (RCPI 1938), L.LM (RCSI 1938). Lt RAMC 9th Jan. 1940.

DOWDS Annie Address: 37 Belmont Avenue, Donnybrook, Dublin. MB, BCh (TCD 1940). IMS.

DOWDS John Alexander MB, BCh (TCD 1930). Capt. RAMC. RWAAF (1943). AA Defences, England (1944).

DOWLING Jeremiah Address: Nelson Pl., Co. Tipperary. MB, BCh, BAO (UCD 1927). Lt RAMC 11th Jul. 1942.

DOWLING Kathleen MB, BCh (TCD 1939). Lt RAMC.

DOWSE John Cecil Alexander b. 16th Nov. 1891, Glenageary, Co. Dublin. s. John Clarence (clerk in Holy Orders) and Jane Henrietta Dowse, 5 Seafield Ave., Blackrock, Co. Dublin. Educ. Trent Coll. Derbyshire, TCD. MB (1914), BCh, BAO, LM (Rot Hosp.), MRCOG (1933). R. C. of I. T/Lt (SR) RAMC 5th Aug. 1914. Mobd 28th Aug. 1914. T/ Capt. 1st Apr. 1915. PC Lt 1st Jan. 1917. Capt. 28th Feb. 1918. Maj. 5th Aug. 1926. Lt Col. 15th Apr. 1936. Col. 21st Oct. 1941. Maj. Gen. 28th Nov. 1945. r.p. 26th Dec. 1949. Served 1914–18 War France 11th May 1915–19. India 1919–23. NWF 1919 and 1924–29. Louise Marg. Hosp. Aldershot 1930–32. Gibraltar 1932–36. CO and spec. MFH Tidworth 1937. Louise Marg. Hosp. Aldershot 1937–39. BEF France OC Surg. Div. 7th Gen. Hosp. 1939–40. CO 11th Gen. Hosp. Feb.–May 1940. ADMS HQ 44 Div. 1940–41. Insp. Of Army Med. Services War Office 1941–43. N. Africa/MEF 1943–46. DDMS HQ Med. Services War Office 1941–43. N. Africa/MEF 1943–46. DDMS HQ 15th Army Group Aug.–Sept. 1943. DDMS HQ 57 Base Area 1943–44. DDMS HQ 8th Army Jan.–May 1944. DMS GHQ MEF/MELF 1944–46. DDGAMS War Office 1946–48. KHP 30th Jun. 1946. Comd and D. of studies RAM Coll. 1948–49. Played rugby for Ireland 1913 and 1914. Medals: CBE (1st Jan. 1942), CB (13th Jun. 1946), MC (14th Jan. 1916), bar (11th Jan. 1919), 1915 S., BWM, VM, IGS (1908) cl. NWF (1919), 1939–45 S., DM, WM, Kt Comdr R.O. of the Phoenix (19th Nov. 1948). MID 11th Jan. 1916, 20th Dec. 1940. d. 16th Aug. 1964 Millbank, London. Commemorated on Roll of Honour Sir Patrick Dun's Hosp.

DOYLE Bernard MB, BCh (NUI 1912). George Medal (air raid – saving life public shelter at oil and cake mills, Limehouse, London 19th Mar. 1941 *London Gazette*, 27th Jun. 1941).

DOYLE Eric Edwin Address: Stanley House, Greystones, Co. Wicklow. L.LM (RCPI 1938), L.LM (RCSI 1938). Flt Lt RAF 21st Jan. 1944.

DOYLE Hugh Aidan Daly MB, BCh (NUI 1938). Lt RAMC 13th Jan. 1940. Address: Dunsandle, Wilfield Pk, Ballsbridge, Dublin.

DOYLE William John Address: Drumcora, Cork. MB, BCh, BAO (UCC 1926), DPH (UCC 1928). Lt RAMC.

DRAFFIN David Alexander b. 31st Aug. 1915, s. Alexander and Sarah Ann Draffin, Address: Prospect House, Curnanure, Ballybay, Co. Monaghan. Educ. Clones High School, MB, BCh (QUB 1939). Married Margaret R. Lyle, 1948. Capt. RAMC. BEF. POW Colditz. He invented an apparatus for the operation of tonsillectomy called the Draffin bipod.

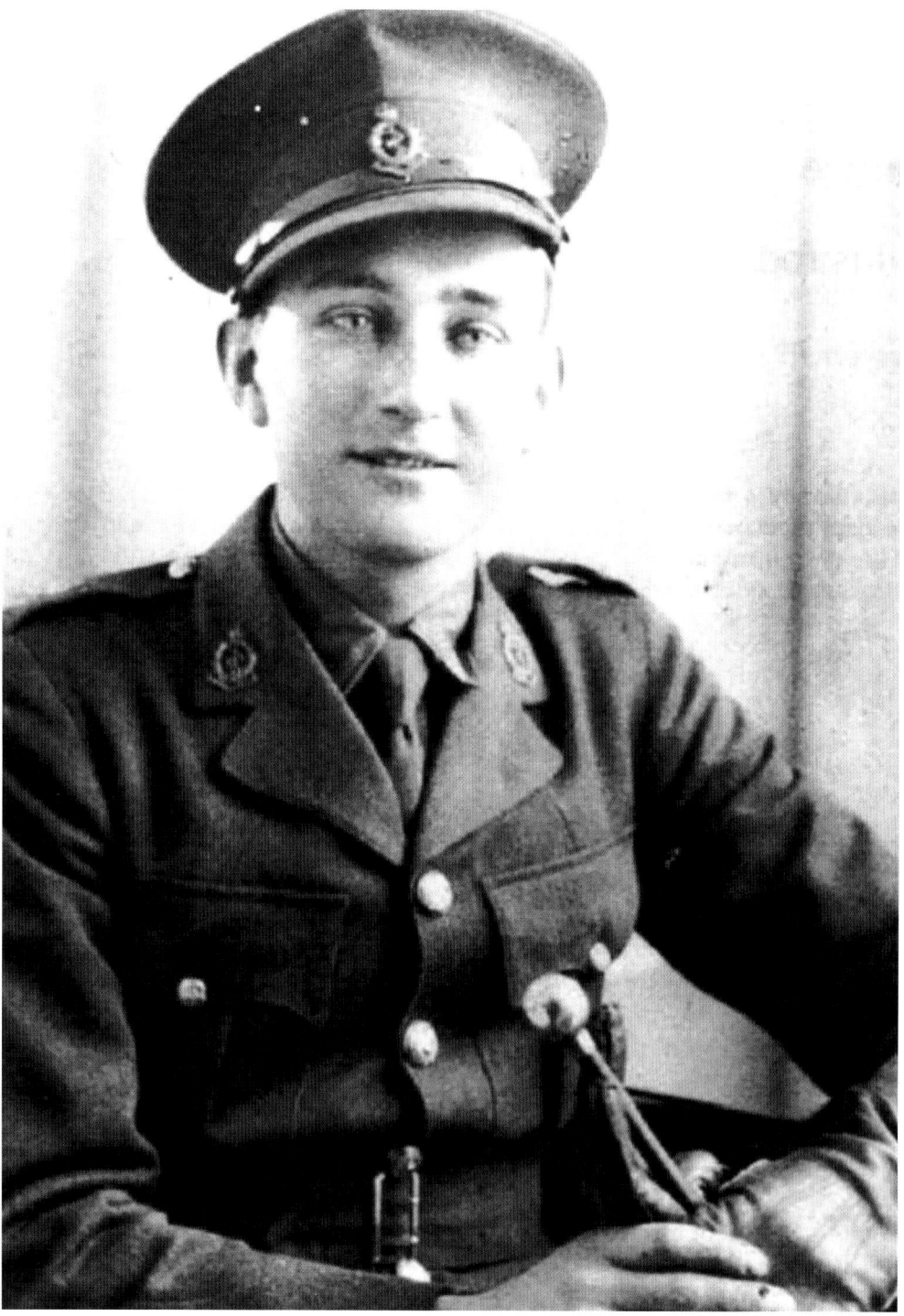

Dr David Alexander Draffin invented an apparatus for the operation of tonsillectomy called the Draffin bipod.

DRAPER Arthur Philip MB, BCh (1912 TCD), MD (TCD 1914). MC.

DRAPER Dare Hastings MB, BCh (TCD 1941). Surg. Lt RNVR (1944).

DRENNAN Alexander James Murray Campbell College. MB, ChB (1938 University of Edinburgh). Maj. RAMC.

DRISCOLL William James Address: 9 Ormiston Dr., Belfast. MB, BCh (QUB 1942). Surg. Lt RNVR.

DRURY Maurice O'Connor MB, BCh (TCD 1939), MD. RAMC.

DUANE William MB, BCh, BAO (UCC 1920). Lt RAMC.

DUFFY James MB, BCh, BAO (1933). Lt IMS.

DUFFY Timothy MB, BCh, BAO (UCD 1926). Lt RAMC 11th Oct. 1939.

***DUGGAN** Dermot Harry Tuthill s. Captain George Grant Duggan, Royal Irish Fusiliers and Dorothy De Courcy Duggan, Foxrock, Co. Dublin. TCD 1933 (MB, BCh). Surgeon Lieutenant RNVR. From Foxrock, Co. Dublin. KIA on HMS *Ardent* Jun. 1940 aged 27 years. Commemorated on Plymouth Naval Memorial, Panel 44, Column 1.

DUGGAN Francis Rupert Address: Ennis, Co. Clare. L.LM (RCPI 1932), L.LM (RCSI 1932). Lt RAMC 22nd Jun. 1940. Captain. MID Italy.

DUNCAN Robert Wilson MB, BCh (TCD 1937). Surg. Lt Comdr RN.

DUNCAN William Linn Address: Waveney Rd, Ballymena, Co. Antrim. Campbell College. L.Med., LS, MB, BCh (TCD 1923). Major. RAMC.

DUNDAS Joseph Address: Lurgandarragh, Enniskillen, Co. Fermanagh. MB, BCh (NUI 1939). Lt RAMC 28th Nov. 1942.

DUNLOP John Boyd Address: Beulah, Dalkey, Co. Dublin. MB, BCh (TCD 1941). Surg. Lt RNVR.

DUNLOP Robert Address: Ardreen, Dreen, Co. Antrim. MB, BCh (QUB 1942). Flt Offr (M) RAFVR. MBE.

DUNN Hugh Wallace McCammon Address: 2 Breda Pk, Belfast. MB, BCh (QUB 1941). Sq. Ldr (M) RAFVR.

DUNN John Hubert MB, BCh (1920), DPH (1922), MD (1924 QUB). Lt Col. RAMC. OBE, TD. MID.

DUNN William James MB, BCh (QUB 1923). Lt RAMC.

DWYER Patrick b. 29th May 1901, Belfast. MB, BCh, BAO (NUI 1926). PB. Lt RAMC 26th Jan. 1928, Capt. 26th Jul. 1931, Maj. 26th Jan. 1938, A/Lt Col. 1st Feb. 1941, T/Lt Col. 1st May 1941, Lt Col. 19th Dec. 1945, r.p. disability 27th Dec. 1949. Served China 1928–29, India 1929–34, Saar 1934–45, India/Burma 1939–44, ADMS HQ L of C area 1942–43, CO BMH Alahabad 1944, NWE: CO 172nd Fd Amb. 1944–45, HQ BAS France 1945, CO Mil. Isolation Hosp. 1946–47, MELF 1947–49: BMH Cyprus 1947–49, CO BMH El Ballah 1949. Medals: 1939–45 S., Burma S., DM, WM.

E

EARLE Brian Vigors MD TCD (1942). RAF.

EARLY Edmund Patrick Noel Mary MB, BCh (TCD 1926). Col. IMS (1928), BEF (Ind. Contingent) 1939–40, ALFSEA (SEAC) 1942–45.

EATON Arthur Hugh McCulloch Address: Camowen Hill, Omagh, Co. Tyrone. MB, BCh (QUB 1922), FRCS (Edinburgh 1927). Lt Col. RAMC. TD.

EDGAR John Herbert Address: 21 Rathmines Rd, Dublin and The Manse, Kerrykeel, Co. Donegal. L.LM (RCPI 1940), L.LM (RCSI 1940). Flt Lt RAF 7th Feb. 1942.

EDMONDSON Lancelot Alistair Stanislaus MB, BCh (TCD 1939). Capt. RAMC.

EDWARDS David Julius (formerly Blumberg) Address: 120 Cliftonville Pk, Belfast. MB, BCh (QUB 1937). Capt. RAMC.

EDWARDS Matthew Dermot Carnalea House, Crawfordsburn, Co. Down. LARCP (Edin. 1938), LRCS (Edin. 1935), LRFPS (Glasgow 1938). Surg. Lt Comdr RNVR.

EDWARDS Sarah Jamison (née Adams) Address: Blackstown House, Ballyligpatrick, Droughane, Ballymena, Co. Antrim. MB, BCh (QUB 1940). Maj. RAMC.

EEDY Bernard Nicholas Address: 9 Belgrave Ave., Lisburn Rd, Belfast. MB, BCh (QUB 1934). Capt. RAMC.

EGAN Eugene MB, BCh, BAO (UCC 1926). Maj. FMS. POW (Singapore).

EGAN John MB, BCh (UCC 1923), DPH RCPS (England 1929). Federal Malaya Services. POW.

EGAN Mary Attracta MB, BCh (NUI 1942). St Bennins Tce, Tuam, Co. Galway. Lt 24th Nov. 1945 RAMC.

EGAN Michael Anthony MB, BCh (NUI 1937). Address: Corohoe, Kiltimagh, Co. Mayo. Lt RAMC. Served in the British Expeditionary Force and was awarded the MC.

ELLIGOT Roger Francis Flt Offr RAF 26th Mar. 1940.

ELLIMAN Hyman MB, BCh (TCD 1936). Capt. RAMC.

ELLIOTT Abraham Hyman MB, BCh (QUB 1920). Capt. RAMC.

ELLIOTT Charles Kennedy Address: Church Sq., Monaghan. MB, BCh (TCD 1942). Capt. RAMC.

ELLIOTT Cyril Mobray L.Med., LCh (TCD 1931). RAMC.

ELLIOTT Elizabeth Address: Olivegrove, Cregagh, Belfast. MB, BCh (QUB 1942). Flt Lt (M) RAFVR.

ELLIOTT James May b. 16th Mar. 1886, Newry, Co. Down. s. Dr J. Elliott, Rathfriland, Co. Down. Educ. St Andrews Coll. Dublin 1st Sept. 1897–31st Oct. 1904. TCD (1909) MB (1910), BCh, BAO, LM (Rot. Hosp). R. Presbyterian. Lt RAMC 28th Jul. 1911. Capt. 28th Jan. 1915. Maj. 28th Jul. 1923. Lt Col. 1st May 1934. r.p. 10th Oct. 1937. Rejoined 1st Sept. 1939. A/Col. 6th May 1943. T/Col. 6th Nov. 1943. r.p. Hon. Col. 1st Oct. 1945. Served India 1913–19 and 1922–27. Spec. Derm. Connaught Hosp. Aldershot 1928–30, Egypt 1930–35, Mil. Hosp. Khartoum 1930–31. Offrs Hosp. Abbassia 1931–33. Spec. Derm. Citadel Mil. Hosp. Cairo 1933–35. Q.A. Mil. Hosp. Millbank 1935–37. BEF France 1939–40. ADMS HQ 2 L of C sub area 1939. Cons. Derm. GHQ BEF 1940. CO 13 CCS Jul.–Sept. 1940. CO 9 CCS 1940–41. CO Mil. Hosp. Colchester 1941–43. West Africa 1943–44 (invalided). CO 68 WA Gen. Hosp. 1943. ADMS HQ 76 Div. Apr. to Sept. 1944. ADMS HQ 47th Inf. Reserve Div. 1944–45. Spec in Derm and VD 1921. BWM, VM, 1939–45 S., DM, WM. d. 6th Jan. 1954.

ELLIOTT Moses Isaac MB, BCh (QUB 1923). Maj. RAMC.

ELLIOTT Robert Andrew George Educ. TCD (1911). MB (1913), BCh, DPH (1923). T/Lt RAMC 5th Nov. 1915. T/Capt. 5th Nov. 1916. Capt. RAF Dec. 1918. Group Capt. (Med) 1st Jul. 1935. Served in 1914–18 War, France from 3rd Dec. 1915. Medals: 1915 S., BWM, VM. Commemorated on Roll of Honour Sir Patrick Dun's Hosp.

ELLIOTT William George TCD 1934. Med. Spec. RAMC. Served in W. Africa. Invalided 1943.

ELMES Euseby Address: New Ross, Co. Wexford. L.LM (RCPI 1935), L.LM (RCSI 1935). Flying O. RAF 18th Feb. 1942.

EMERSON Henry Horace Andrews b. 14th Sept. 1881, Rathmines, Dublin. s. Robert Henry Mulock Emerson, Morehampton Rd, Dublin. Educ. Rathmines Sch. 1891. TCD (1905). BA, BAO (1905), MB, BCh, DPH (Eng. 1914). Lt RAMC 31st Jul. 1905. Capt. 31st Jan. 1909. Maj. 15th Oct. 1915. Bt. Lt Col. 1st Jan. 1928. Maj. Gen. 26th Mar. 1937. r.p. 16th Apr. 1939. Re-employed as Col. 29th Jan. 1941. r.p. Maj. Gen. 17th Jan. 1942. Served in France 25th Sept. 1915, DADMS 1915, CO 44th CCS 1916–19. Dept. Health India 1919–24. OIC Med. Div. in Gen. Hosp 1919. Served in Home Guard. Medals: CB (8th Jun. 1939), DSO (1st Jan. 1917), 1915 S., BWM, VM, KGV Jubilee Medal 1935. MID 15th Jun.

1916, 4th Jan. 1917, 10th Jul. 1919. d. 17th Nov. 1957. Commemorated on Roll of Honour Sir Patrick Dun's Hosp.

EMPEY William Stewart MD, BCh (QUB 1932). Lt Col./Surg. Comdr IMS & RIN. OBE.

ENGLISH Joseph Sandys L.Med., LS, MB, BCh (TCD 1914). POW.

ENTRICAN John Cuthbertson MB, BCh (QUB 1932). Capt. RAMC.

EPPEL Cecil Address: 74 Grosvenor Rd, Rathmines, Dublin. MB, BCh (TCD 1937) RAMC.

EPPEL Isadore Jack. L.LM (EXPI 1936), L.LM (RCSI 1936) RAMC.

ERSKINE Sydney Leslie Wylie Address: Ardshane, Holywood, Co. Down. MB, BCh (1933), DPH (QUB 1936). Sq. Ldr (M) RAFVR.

ESLER William Logan Address: Lisvarna, Broughshane Rd, Ballymena. MB, BCh (QUB 1942). Sq. Ldr (M) RAFVR.

ESMONDE Patrick Address: Drominagh, Borrisokane, Co. Tipperary. L.LM (RCPI 1940), L.LM (RCSI 1940). Lt RAMC 6th Feb. 1941.

EUSTACE John Thomas MB, BCh, BAO (NUI 1926), MC (NUI 1935). Lt RAMC 25th Oct. 1939.

EUSTACE William Desmond Address: Lisconagh, Glasnevin, Co. Dublin. L.LM (RCPI 1936), L.LM (RCSI 1936). Lt RAMC 26th Oct. 1936.

EVANS Robert Address: 32 Cyprus Gdns, Belfast. MB, BCh (QUB 1926), MD (QUB 1929). Maj. RAMC.

EVANS Robert Address: Killorglin, Co. Kerry. MB, BCh, BAO (UCC 1924). Lt RAMC 23rd Jun. 1941.

*EVES Thomas Preston b. 31st Mar. 1884, Donnybrook, Dublin. MB, BCh (TCD 1907), BAO, LM (Rot. Hosp.). Lt RAMC 4th Feb. 1908. Capt. 4th Aug. 1911. T/Maj. 12th–21st Aug. 1916. Maj. 4th Feb. 1920. A/Lt Col. 22nd Aug. 1916–14th Feb. 1919. Lt Col. 13th Feb. 1933. r.p. 1st Mar. 1939. Rejoined 12th Sept. 1939. Served in 1914–18 War. First theatre of war Mesopotamia 17th Mar. 1915. Gallipoli 1915–16. Egypt Jan.–Apr. 1916. France and Belgium 1916–19. CO 36th Fd Amb. 1916–19. Germany 1919 CO 139th Fd Amb Jun.–Oct. Egypt 1921–26 and 1927–31. India 1933–36. CO BMH Calcutta 1934–36. CO Mil. Hosp. Holywood NI 1936–39. CO 6 Hosp. Ship 1939–44. Medals: DSO (1st Jan. 1918), Bar (26th Jul. 1918), 1915 S., BWM, VM, 1939–45 S., Atlantic S., Italy S., WM. MID 13th Jul. 1916, 24th Dec. 1917, 30th Dec. 1918. KIA 24th Jan. 1944, missing at sea when the Hosp. Ship *St David* was sunk by German Aircraft off Anzio. Commemorated on Roll of Honour Sir Patrick Dun's Hosp.

* **EWART** Archibald Robert TCD 1926.
Surg. Comdr RN. d. 13th Jun. 1941.

F

FAHY John MB, BCh (1926 NUI). Lt RAMC 18th Oct. 1939. Resigned due to ill health 11th May 1940.

FALLON Martin Address: 32 Fitzwilliam Sq., Dublin. MB, BCh (TCD 1932), MCh (1936), FRCSI (1934). Lt Col. RAMC. MEF 1940–44. OBE.

FALLON Thaddeus Address: 59 Ranelagh Rd, Dublin. MB, BCh (TCD 1938). Capt. RAMC.

FALLON Walter Martin MB (UCG 1922). Lt RAMC 1940.

FARRELL Henry William MB, BCh, BAO (UCD 1925), DPH (1928), FRCS (Edinburgh 1933). Lt IMS 31st Aug. 1927.

*****FARRELL,** John Andrew (Jack) b. IFS. 2nd s. Mrs T. Farrell, Ardamine, Lower Rathmines Rd, Dublin. Husband of Betty, Lennoxbrook, Kells, Co. Meath. LRCP&S (RCSI 1936). Lt RAMC 1st Feb. 1939. Maj. RAMC East Africa including Abyssinia. KIA 12th Jul. 1945.

FARRELL Michael James Address: 26 Moyne Rd, Ranelagh, Dublin. MB, BCh (UCD 1939). Lt RAMC 8th Feb. 1940.

FARRELL Michael Joseph b. Baganelstown Co. Carlow. Educated in Castleknock College and studied medicine in RCSI (1943). 'Joined the RNVR and saw action in the English Channel as a ship's surgeon on board RVNR Monowai assisting casualties extracted from the Normandy landings in 1944. Posted to Singapore to act as port medical officer following the Japanese surrender. Returning to Ireland after the war he specialised in public health and following appointments in Kilkenny and Kerry he was posted to Leitrim, where he remained for the rest of his life. He died in 1990'.

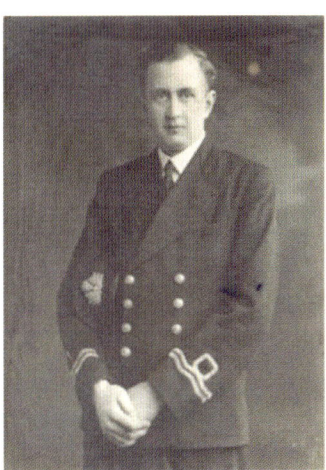

Michael Joseph Farrell. Posted to Singapore to act as port medical officer following the Japanese surrender.

FARRELL Norman George Address: 23 Sandford Rd, Ranelagh, Dublin. MB, BCh (TCD 1935). Flt Lt RAF. MID.

FEARIS Thomas Plunkett MB BCh (QUB 1944). Surg. Lt RNVR.

FEE John Gordon Address: 5 Sicily Pk, Balmoral, Belfast. MB, BCh (QUB 1939). Sq. Ldr (M) RAFVR. MID.

*****FENNELL** P.G. Capt. Died WWII.

FENTON George Irwin Address: Fernayhandrum, Seskinore, Omagh, Co. Tyrone. MB, BCh (QUB 1938). Capt. RAMC.

FERGUSAN George Gordon Address: 65 College Rd, Cork. MB, BCh, BAO (UCC 1942). Lt RAMC.

FERGUSAN Henry Arnott Col. MB, BCh (1926 TCD), DPH (RSPC England 1935). b. 3rd Oct. 1902, Rathmines, Dublin. Youngest s. J.A.O. Fergusan of Dublin. T/Lt 4th Mar. 1927. Capt. 27th Jan. 1931. Major 27th Jul. 1937. A/Lt Col. 27th Jan. 1942. T/Lt Col. 27th Apr. 1942. Lt Col. 29th Oct. 1945. A/Col. 5th Jan. 1944. T/Col. 26th Jun. 1946. Retired Hon. Col. 3rd Nov. 1946. Rempld Major 14th Nov. 1946. d. 27th Dec. 1952 at Basingstoke, Hants. Served India 1928 to 1921, Egypt 1935 to 1936, Burma 1937 to 1940, India 1943, invalided. DDH HQ Eastern Comd 1944. ADMS HQ 80th Division 1944. ADMS Embarkation HQ 1945. Medals: 1939–45 S., France and Germany S., BWM.

FERGUSON Sidney Clement, s. Ion and Annie (née Fisher) Ferguson, Address: Ulster Bank House, Kilcock, Co. Kildare. L.LM (RCSI 1942), L.LM (RCSI 1942). Lt RAMC 5th Aug. 1944.

FERGUSON Thomas Ion Victor, s. Ion and Annie (née Fisher) Ferguson, Address: Ulster Bank House, Ballyconnell, Co. Cavan. L.LM (RCSI 1937), L.LM (RCSI 1937). Joined the RNVR in 1939, HMS *Drake*, but transferred to the RAMC as a result of sea sickness. Was captured when the Germans conquered Athens in 1941 and spent most of the war as a prisoner of war in Colditz Castle.

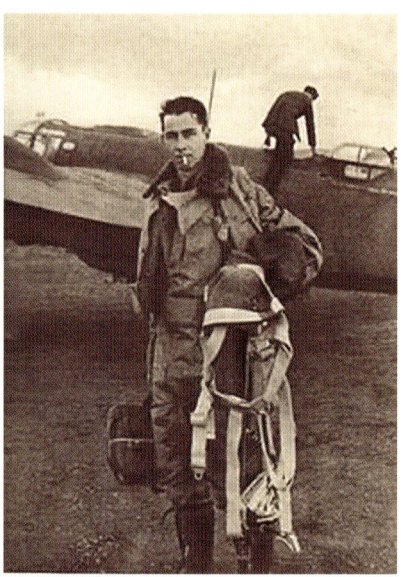

Thomas Ion Victor Ferguson.

FERRIS Robert James Leslie, Address: 4 Windsor Villas, Victoria Rd, Larne, Co. Antrim. MB, BCh (QUB 1939). Sq. Ldr (M) RAFVR. MC.

FETHERSTON Helen Sinclair (née Jackson) MB (QUB 1939). Lt RAMC.

FIELD Claude Marcus Beresford Address: 5 Rosetta Pk, Belfast. MB, BCh (QUB 1942). Surg. Lt RNVR.

FIELD Thomas Eglington b. 24th Sept. 1915, Belfast, Co. Antrim. MB, BCh, BAO (QUB 1939), DTM&H (Eng. 1951), MD (QUB 1963). Lt 12th Apr. 1940. A/Capt. 2nd Oct. 1940. T/Capt. 2nd Jan. 1941. Capt. 12th Par. 1941. A/Maj. 10th May 1942. T/Maj. 10th Aug. 1942. PC Capt. 12th Apr. 1945. Maj. 12th Apr. 1948. A/Lt Col. 6th Jul. 1945. T/Lt Col. 6th Oct. 1945. Lt Col. 4th Sept. 1958. Col. 12th Apr. 1963. r.p. 26th Sept. 1965. BNAF/CMF 1942–47. CO 1st Fd Amb. 1945. CO 14th Fd Amb. 1945 & 1946–47. CO 83rd Gen. Hosp. 1946–47. CO 114th Con. Dep. 1947. Australia 1953. BAOR: ADP and OIC Central Path. Lab. 1955. FARELF 1956–58. ADP E. Comd and OIC E. Comd/London Dist. Lab. 1959–61. CO David Bruce Lab. 1961–64. Prof. Path. RAM Coll. 1964–65. Junior Spec. Path 1952. Senior Spec. 1955. Medals: MBE (28th Jun. 1945), 1939–45 S., Africa S with 1st Army cl., Italy S., DM, WM GSM with cl. Malaya. MID 19th Jul. 1945.

FIELDING Vivian John Address: 20 Leinster Sq., Rathmines, Dublin. L.LM (RCPI 1930), L.LM (RCSI 1930). Flt Offr RAF 5th Nov. 1940. Surg. Comdr RN (1940).

FINN, Josephine Sarah QUB 1932. RAF Feb. 1944.

FINNEGAN Edward Joseph MB, BCh, BAO (UCD 1929). Lt RAMC.

FINNEGAN John Address: 26 Norfolk Dr., Belfast. MB, BCh (QUB 1939). Col. RAMC. MID (2).

FINNY Charles Morgan b. 9th Jul. 1886, Rathdown, Co. Dublin. Educ. TCD. MB (1910), BCh, BAO, DPH (1912), FRCS (Eng.). Lt RAMC 27th Jan. 1911. Capt. 27th Jul. 1914. A/Maj. 2nd Jul–26th Oct. 1919. Maj. 27th Jan. 1923. Lt Col. 1st May 1934. Col. 1st May 1938. T/Brig. 17th Jan. 1941. Maj. Gen. 13th Oct. 1941. r.p. 27th May 1942. Rempld Col. 5th Jun. 1942. r.p. Maj. Gen. 26th Oct. 1946. Served India 1913–19, invalided. NWF 1915 and 1918. Persia and Persian Gulf 1918–19. Surg. Spec. KGV Hosp. Dublin 1921–22. Malta Mil Hosp. Intarfa Surg. Spec. 1922–23. OIC Surg. Div. 1923–27. R. Herbert Hosp. Woolwich 1927–28. Cambridge Hosp. Aldershot 1928–30. India BMH Calcutta, Poona and Rawalpindi 1930–35. Mil Hosp. Catterick 1935–37. Asst Prof. of Mi. Surg. RAM Coll. 1937–38. CO QA Mil. Hosp. Millbank 1938–39. ADMS HQ 3rd Div. 1939–40. DDMS HQ 3rd Corps. 1940–41. DDMS HQ N. Comd 1941–

42. PSMB Scottish Comd 1942–46. Spec. Surg. 1921. Medals: OBE (3rd Jun. 1927), 1915 S., BWM, VM, GSM (cl. Sth Persia), 1939–45 S., DM, WM. MID 3rd Feb. 1920. Commemorated on Roll of Honour Sir Patrick Dun's Hosp.

FISHER Guy Beadon Walmsley MB (QUB 1928), FRCS (Edinburgh 1938). Maj. IMS.

FISHER Leo Henry Grattan MB, BCh, BAO (NUI 1926). Flt Offr RAF 25th Feb. 1942.

FISHER Myer MB, BCh, BAO (UCD 1940). Address: 18 Antrim Rd, Belfast. Capt. RAMC. First employed 14th Feb. 1941.

FISHER Robert Ernest Walmsley Address: Ulster Bank, Connswater, Belfast. MB (QUB 1932). Wing Comdr (M) RAF. MID.

FISHER Robert Lucius Cary MB, BCh (TCD 1922). Wing Comdr RAF.

FITZGERALD Denis Patrick Address: Donewell Rd, Douglas, Co. Cork. MB, BCh, BAO (UCC 1942). Flt Offr RAF.

FITZGERALD Edward Joseph MB, BCh, BAO (UCC 1928). Lt RAMC.

FITZGERALD James Gerard Address: Killanure, Cahir, Co. Tipperary. MB, BCh (NUI 1942). Flt Offr RAF 26th Oct. 1944.

FITZGERALD Michael Joseph MB, BCh, BAO (UCC 1926). Lt RAMC.

FITZGERALD Richard Joseph Address: Dernacaraha, Dunmanway, Co. Cork. MB, BCh, BAO (UCC 1943). Lt RAMC.

FITZGIBBON Henry Address: 9 St James's Tce, Clonskeagh, Dublin. MB, BCh (TCD 1940). Surg. Lt RNVR.

FITZPATRICK John Miles Address: Beulah, Glenageary Hill, Kingstown, Co. Dublin. Youngest s. T.P. Fitzpatrick Captain Royal Irish Fusiliers and Mrs Fitzpatrick, of Glenageary, Kingstown, Co. Dublin. Husband of Eva Diomys 2nd dt. H.G. Travers DFC. L.LM (RCPI 1935), L.LM (RCSI 1935). Flt Offr RAF 28th Nov. 1941.

FITZPATRICK Owen Captain b. Co. Down. Educ. at Clongowes Wood College and Edinburgh University LRCP&S (Edinburgh), LRFPS (Glasgow 1920), MB BCh (Edinburgh 1920). Surg. Sub. Lt RNVR. d. Rathfriland, Co. Down, Feb. 1941.

FITZPATRICK Patrick Ernan Address: 30 Antrim Rd, Lisburn, Co. Antrim. MB, BCh (QUB 1936). Capt. RAMC.

FITPATRICK William Gordon Caulfield Beulah, Glenageary Hill, Kingstown, Co. Dublin. L.LM (1923 RCPI) L.LM (1923 RCSI), LRCP&S. Surg. Comdr RN Jan. 1935.

FLACK George Herbert Address: 1 Hanover Sq., Croagh, Co. Tyrone. MB, BCh (QUB 1940). Flt Lt RAFVR.

FLACK Hugh MB, BCh (QUB 1926). Lt Col. IMS.

FLAHERTY Nicholas Anthony MB, BCh, BAO (UCC 1934). Lt RAMC.

FLANAGAN Michael Brendan Address: 38, High Street, Sligo. MB, BCh (TCD 1942). Surg. Lt RNVR.

FLANIGAN Francis Desmond Address: Aughavanagh, Portadown, Co. Armagh. MB, BCh, BAO (NUI 1943). Lt RAMC 1944.

FLANNERY Alfred Edward Address: Knockbride Rectory, Bailiboro, Co. Cavan. L.LM (RCPI 1929), L.LM (RCSI 1929). Flt Offr RAF 29th Feb. 1942.

FLARIS Thomas Plunkett MB (QUB 1944). Surg. Lt RNVR.

FLEMING Mary Irene Address: Mourne View House, Lurgan, Co. Armagh. MB, BCh (QUB 1942). Capt. RAMC.

FLEMING William MB, BCh, BAO (UCC 1926). Lt IMS.

FLETCHER Evan Address: 52 South Parade, Ormeau Rd, Belfast. MB, BCh (QUB 1939). Maj. IMF.

FLOOD Charles John Stuart Address: 3 Warwick Tce, Leeson Pk, Dublin. Campbell College. MB, BCh (1937 TCD). Captain RAMC.

FLOOD Frederick George b. 5th Mar. 1890, at Omagh, Co. Tyrone. s. Mrs Flood, Glencar, Cowper Downs, Rathmines, Dublin. Educ. St Andrews Coll, Dublin 30th Aug. 1906–30th Jun. 1908. TCD (1912). MB (1914), BCh, BAO, LM (Rot. Hosp.). R. C. of I. Lt RAMC 20th Aug. 1914. Capt. 1st Apr. 1915. A/Maj. 17th May–17th Oct. 1919. Maj. 20th Aug. 1926. Lt Col. 26th Mar. 1937. T/Col. 17th Nov. 1940. Col. 16th Sept. 1942. r.p. 9th Jan. 1948. Served in 1914–18 War France 1915–17. Wounded Sept. 1917. Russia Jan.–Oct. 1919. Served through 1939–45 War RAMC. Medals: OBE (11th Oct. 1945), MC (18th Jun. 1917), Bar (15th Jul. 1919), 1915 S., BWM, VM, GSM Iraq, IGSM Waz. 21–24. MID 1st Jan. 1916 and 20th Dec. 1940. OStStan 3rd class (Jun. 1919), 2nd class (Oct. 1919).

FLOOD Robert Alexander b. 26th Sept. 1885 at Enniskillen, Co. Fermanagh. MB, BCh, BAO TCD (1911) & LM (Rot. 1912). Lt RAMC. 26th Jul. 1912. Capt. 30th Mar. 1915. A/Maj. 4th Jan. 1918. Maj. 26th Jul. 1924. Lt Col. 2nd Aug. 1934. r.p. 8th May 1943. Rempld Maj. 8th May 1943. r.p. Lt Col. 29th Sept. 1946. Served BEF France 1914. POW 1914–15. France, Belgium and Germany 1915–19. Nth Russia 1919. Mesopotamia 1920–21. India 1921–24. China 1927–30. Bermuda 1933–35. India 1938–43. CO BMH Lucknow 1938–42. BMH Nowshera 1942. Medals: MC 16th Sept. 1918, 1914 S., BWM, VM. d. 27th Feb. 1964.

FLOOD James Edward MB, BCh, BAO (UCD 1923). Lt RAMC.

FLYNN Gerald James Address: 29 Belgrave Sq., Monkstown, Dublin. MB, BCh, BAO (UCD 1943). Flt Lt RAF 16th Jan. 1945.

FLYNN William Address: 239 North Circular Rd, Dublin. MB, BCh, BAO (NUI 1936). Flt Lt RAF 15th Aug. 1941.

FOLEY John Joyce Address: Maryville, Athenry, Co. Galway. MB, BCh (NUI 1939). Surg. Lt RNVR 24th Apr. 1941.

FOOT William b. 2nd Dec. 1889, Dublin. Only s. Albert and Eveline Eleanor Foot, 57 Northumberland Rd, Dublin. Educ. Shrewsbury Sch. from 1907. TCD. MB (1914), BCh, BAO, LM (Rot. 1914). T/Lt RAMC 18th Aug. 1914. T/Capt. 18th Aug. 1915. PC Lt 1st Jan. 1917. Capt. 18th Feb. 1918. A/Maj. 9rd Nov. 1918–14th Feb. 1919 and 5th Sept. 1919–23rd Jan. 1920. Maj. 18th Aug. 1926. Lt Col. 2nd Feb. 1937. Col. 4th Jun. 1942. A/Brig. 5th Jan. 1944. T/Brig. 5th Jul. 1944. A/Maj. Gen. 14th May 1946. Maj. Gen. 27th May 1946. r.p. 12th May 1949. Served in France from 27th Aug. 1914. RMO 3rd Coldstream Gds. 1914–16. India 1919–23. Afghanistan 1919. Malta 1926–29. India 1934–39. CO 2nd Armd Div. Fd Amb. 1939–40. BEF France May–Jun. 1940. ADMS HQ 8th Armd Div. 1940–41. Comdt No. 1 Dep. and Training Est. RAMC 1941–43. Paiforce MEF 1943–47. DMS GHQ Paiforce 1945–46. DMS GHQ MEF 1946–47. DDMS HQ E. Comd 1947–49. KHP 1st Jan. 1947. Medals: CB (12th Jun. 1947), MC (1st Jan. 1916), Bar (14th Nov. 1916), 1914 S., BWM, VM, IGS (Afghanistan 1919), 1939–45 S., DM, WM. MID 1st Jan. 1916, 30th Dec. 1918.

FORAN John Edward MB, BCh, BAO (UCC 1925). Flt Lt RAF.

FORBES Robert Alexander Address: 423 Upr Newtownards Rd, Belfast. MB, BCh (QUB 1939). Flt Lt (M) RAFVR.

FORD Richard Alexander Wilson b. 1887, Waterford City. s. Alexander (GP and Surg) and Maria Louisa Ford, 42 Sth Parade, Waterford. Educ. RUI/RCSI L.LM (RCPI 1922), L.LM (RCSI 1911). R.RC. Surg. Lt RN 3rd Aug. 1914. Surg. Capt. Served in 1914–18 War. Flt Offr RAF WWII 14th May 1940. Commemorated on Roll of Honour RCSI.

FORSYTH Robert Lane MB, BCh (TCD 1925). Sq. Ldr RAF.

FORSYTHE Kirk Address: 193 Belmont Rd, Belfast. MB, BCh (QUB 1927), MD (QUB 1931), DPH (QUB 1932). Surg. Comdr RNVR. VD. MID.

FOSTER Peter Alexander Henry McConnell Address: 17 University Sq., Belfast. MB, BCh (QUB 1942). Flt Lt (M) RAFVR.

FOSTER Robert Cowan, Campbell College. MB, BCh (QUB 1925). Surg. Comdr RN.

FOX Edward Gerard Address: 76 Seafield Rd, Clontarf, Dublin. MB, BCh (TCD 1937). Sq. Ldr RAF

FOXE Wilfrid MB, BCh, BAO (UCC 1924). Lt RAMC.

FRASER Ian James Address: 33 Wellington Pk, Belfast. MB, BCh (QUB 1923). Brig. RAMC. DSO, OBE. OStJ.

FRASER Robert Cosbey Address: Bright Rectory, Downpatrick, Co. Down. MB, BCh (QUB 1937). Flt Offr (M) RAFVR.

FREEDMAN Samuel Max Address: 18 Carlisle Street, South Circular Rd, Dublin. L. Med. LCh (1934), MB, BCh (TCD 1939). RAMC.

FREEMAN Michael James (formerly Freedman Max) Address: Ferndale, Howth Rd, Sutton, Co. Dublin and 29 Fitzgibbon Street, Dublin. L.LM (RCPI 1927), L.LM (RCSI 1927). Flt Lt RAF 13th May 1942

FREEMAN Richard George Address: Balscadden House, Kilcock Rd, Howth, Co. Dublin. LRCP&S (RCSI 1925). Flt Lt RAF 14th Nov. 1939.

FREEMAN Thomas Address: 4 Castle Pk, Belfast. MB, BCh (QUB 1942). Maj. RAMC.

FRID JOHN Leslie Address: 120 South Circular Rd, Dublin. L. Med. LCh (TCD 1936). RAF.

FRIEL William Ralph Nicholson MB, BCh (Edin. 1938), TCD 1930. RAMC.

FRIER William b. 20th Jun. 1888, Warringstown, Co. Down. Educ. TCD. MB (1912), BCh, BAO, DPH (QUB 1914). Lt RAMC 27th Aug. 1914. Capt. 27th Aug. 1915. Reg. Army 1st May 1919. Maj. 27th Aug. 1926. Lt Col. 1st Apr. 1937. Col. 25th Mar. 1943. r.p. 20th May 1947. Served in 1914–18 War, France 1914–16, India 1916–18, France 1918–19, India 1920–24. Wazirstan 1920–22. BAOR 1925–26. Shanghai 1928–32. India 1935–44. CO BMH Chakrata 1936–39. BMH Meerut 1939. BMH Ahmed na Gar 1939–44. ADMS HQ N. Highland Dist. 1944–45. PSMB NW. Dist. 1945–47. Medals: 1914 S., BWM, VM, IGS (Waz. 1921–24), DM, WM. MID 19th Sept. 1921, 12th Jun. 1923. Commemorated on Roll of Honour Sir Patrick Dun's Hosp.

FRIZELLE Gordan Macauley MB, BCh (QUB 1926), MD (QUB 1930). Col. RAMC. TD. MID. US Medal of Freedom with silver palm. Gold Medal of Merit Italian Red Cross.

FROST William Arthur b. 30th Mar. 1886, Newmarket on Fergus, Co. Clare. s. Edmond Frost MD, Newmarket on Fergus, Co. Clare. MB, BCh, BAO (RUI 1909), BS. Married Josephine Marion, dt. Col. John Stirling RA, Gargannock,

Stirlingshire, Scotland. Lt RAMC 27th Jan. 1911. Capt. 27th Jul. 1914. Maj. 27th Jan. 1923. Lt Col. 1st May 1934. Col. 26th May 1938. r.p. ill health 27th Sept. 1941. War work served in India, Snr MO Hyderabad, Sind Feb. 1915–Jun. 1919. Invalided. DADH & P Singapore 1921–25. DADP N. Comd 1925–28. DADH and P Malaya Comd 1929–31. DADP Catterick and Northumbrian area 1932–34. China 1934–37. CO Mil. Hosp. Hong Kong 1934–35. DADP Hong Kong 1935–37. ADH and P Scottish Comd 1938. SMO CLRD 1938–39. E. Africa 1939–40. ADMS force HQ Sept.–Dec. 1939. ADMS HQ Central Mid. Area 1940–41. PSMB Scottish Comd 1941. Specialist in Pathology 1921. Medals: OBE (12th Sept. 1919), BWM (only). MID 11th Jun. 1920. d. 2nd Dec. 1953.

***FRY** Humphrey Francis Warren MB (QUB 1944). Flt Lt RAFVR. KIA.

FRY Margaret Fisher Address: 7 Chlorine Gdns, Belfast. MB, BCh (QUB 1942). Flt Lt (M) RAFVR.

FULLERTON Jane Mooney Address: Coolbawn, Dunmurry. Belfast. MB, BCh (QUB 1938). Flt Lt (M) RAF.

FULTON Thomas Terence MB (QUB 1944). Sq. Ldr (M) RAFVR.

FUNSTON William David Dundas b. IFS. s. Margaret Funston of Bundoran, Co. Donegal. Maj. R. Canadian A.M.C. d. 12th Apr. 1945 aged 43. Buried in Hamilton (Woodland) Cemetery, Sec. 24, Lot 167.

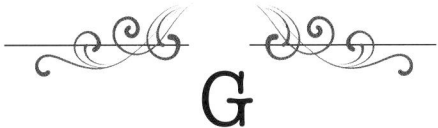

G

GALLAGHER Anna Theresa Address: Joaleen, Hartlands Rd, Cork. MB, BCh (UCC 1941). Lt RAMC.

GALLAGHER Herbert William MB (QUB 1939). Capt. RAMC.

GALLAGHER Mary Bridget Address: Joaleen, Hartlands Rd, Cork. MSc, MB, BCh BAO (UCC 1941). Flt Offr RAF.

GALLAGHER Michael Thomas Address: Hazelwood, Strabane, Co. Tyrone. MB, BCh (NUI 1939). Flt Offr RAF.

GALLAHER Herbert Frederick Llewellyn Address: Ardlui, Myrtlefield Pk, Belfast. MB, BCh (QUB 1934). Capt. RAMC.

*****GAMBLE** Edward Moore b. IFS Capt. RAMC. MB, BCh (TCD 1927). Capt. 246204 RAMC. d. India 26th Dec. 1943. Buried in Kirkee War Cemetery India, Plot 10F6.

*****GANNON** Ciaran Joseph Address: 22 Castlewood Pk, Rathmines, Dublin. MB, BCh, BAO (NUI 1939). b. IFS. s. James J.A. and Bridget Gannon, Rathmines, Dublin. Capt. RAMC. d. Burma 22nd Mar. 1944, aged 29. Commemorated Rangoon Memorial Face 18.

GANNON James Patrick Address: 22 Castlewood Pk, Rathmines, Dublin. MB, BCh (NUI 1941). Lt RAMC 26th Sept. 1942.

GANTLEY William Address: 5 Quay, New Ross, Co. Wexford. MB, BCh (NUI 1940). Lt RAMC 13th Jun. 1942.

GARDINER Robert Address: Carrick House, Ballintra, Co. Donegal. MB, BCh, BAO (UCD 1924). Lt IMS. First enlisted 2nd Apr. 1942.

GARRY James Francis Fitzgerald Address: 12 O'Connell St, Ennis, Co. Clare. L.LM (RCPI 1932), L.LM (RCSI 1932). Lt RAMC 17th Aug. 1940.

GATER Cyril Edward Hammond b. 1888, England. Educ. RCSI. L.LM (RCPI 1915), L.LM (RCSI 1915), DPH (RCPSI 1920). R. C. of I. Capt. RAMC SR. Maj. Served 1914–18 War France from 10th Sept. 1915. Flt Lt RAF 9th Jan. 1940. Medals: 1915 S., BWM, VM. MID. Commemorated on Roll of Honour RCSI.

GAVAGAN Dudley Patrick Address: Rathslevin, Kiltimagh, Co. Mayo. MB, BCh (NUI 1939). Lt RAMC 8th May 1943).

GEANY John Joseph MB, BCh (NUI 1922). Lt RAMC 5th Sept. 1939. Resigned 17th May 1945.

GEOGHEGAN Patrick Joseph MB, BCh, BAO (UCC 1934). Lt RAMC.

GIBBON Edward b. 20th Dec. 1881, Rosslare, Co. Wexford. Educ. TCD. MB (1906), BCh, BAO. Lt RAMC 30th Jul. 1906. Capt. 30th Jan. 1910. Maj. 30th Jul. 1918. Lt Col. 13th Aug. 1930. Col. 1st May 1934. r.p. 1st May 1938. Rempld 1st Sept. 1939. Reverts to Lt Col. 28th Jul. 1940 and Maj. 31st Mar. 1942. r.p. with rank of Col. 1st Sept. 1945. First theatre of war Gallipoli 9th Aug. 1915. attd. Egyptian A. 1908–20. Sudan 1914-16 and 1917–18. EEF 1917. India 1924–30 21st Gen. Hosp. Medals: OBE (3rd Jun. 1918), 1915 S., BWM, VM, DM, WM, GV Jub. 35, O. of the Nile 4th Class (21st Apr. 1917), Sultans Sudan Medal cl. Nyima 1917–18. MID Nov. 1916, Dec. 1919. d. 17th Feb. 1966 at Trillick, Co. Tyrone. Commemorated on Roll of Honour Sir Patrick Dun's Hosp.

GIBBONS Patrick Joseph MB, BCh (NUI 1928). Capt. RAMC 1st Jun. 1939. Resigned 24th Apr. 1940 due to ill health.

GIBSON Clarence Hamilton Address: Killyleagh Street, Crossgar, Belfast. L.LM (RCPI 1940), L.LM (RCSI 1940). Surg. Lt RN 30th Sept. 1938.

GIBSON Eileen McCreary (née Hill) Address: Glengar, Banbridge, Co. Down. MB, BCh (QUB 1928). Capt. RAMC.

GIBSON George Barton Address: 41 Cranmore Gdns, Belfast. Campbell College. MB, BCh (TCD 1941). Lt E. African Forces. Served in Madagascar.

GIBSON John George Address: 32 Wellesley Ave., Malone Rd, Belfast. MB, BCh (QUB 1942). Flt Lt (M) RAFVR.

GIBSON Samuel Address: Loughbaughan, Broughshane, Co. Antrim. MB, BCh (QUB 1938). Sq. Ldr (M) RAFVR.

GIBSON Wilfred Gerard Francis Address: 126 Newlodge Rd, Belfast. MB, BCh (QUB 1938). Sq. Ldr (M) RAFVR.

GILBERT Edward Theodore (formerly Goldblatt) Address: 15 Waterloo Gdns, Belfast. MB, BCh (QUB 1934). Maj. RAMC. DSO, OBE.

GILBERT Jonathan Cordukes Address: Moira Lodge, Bangor, Co. Down. MB, BCh (QUB 1926). Capt. RAMC.

GILL Anthony Mary Joseph Address: Westport, Co. Mayo. MB, BCh (NUI 1940). Flt Offr RAF 22nd Feb. 1944.

GILLESPIE Charles William Address: The Manse, Croagh, Co. Tyrone. Campbell College. MB, BCh, DPH (QUB 1941). Capt. RAMC.

GILLESPIE Frank Sheppard b. 19th Oct. 1889, Killaloe, Co. Clare. Educ. St Columba's Coll., Rathfarnham, Dublin 1904. TCD (1912). BA (1912), MB (1914), BCh, BAO, LM (Rot. Hosp.), MD (1918). T/Lt RAMC 28th Aug. 1914. Mobd 23rd Sept. 1914. T/Capt. 1st Apr. 1915. PC Capt. 1st May 1919. Maj. 28th Aug. 1926. Lt Col. 11th Apr. 1937. T/Col. 23rd Nov. 1940. Col. 16th Apr. 1943. r.p. 21st Oct. 1948. Served in France 1915 and 1916. India 1919–24. BAOR 1924–25. India 1926–30. Malta 1933–37. Egypt 1937–39. CO Mil. Hosp. Holywood Mar.–Sept. 1939. BEF France 1939–40: CO 4th Fd Amb. CO 35 Gen. Hosp. Mar.–May 1940. Iceland ADMS HQ 147 Inf. Brig. May–Jul. 1940. ADMS HQ 5th Div. 1940–42. USA MLO to US Army Washington 1942–46. PSMB Devon and Cornwall area 1947–48. Medals: 1915 S., BWM, VM, IGSM (cl. Afgh. 1919), 1939–45 S., DM, WM. Offr Leg. of M.

GILLESPIE William Alexander Address: 12 Merlyn Pk, Ballsbridge, Dublin. MB, BCh (TCD 1936), DPH (1938), MD (1942). Lt Col. RAMC.

GILMORE John Address: Ballybennox, Macosquin, Coleraine, Co. Derry. MB, BCh (QUB 1938). Lt RAMC.

GILMOUR Anna Elizabeth Address: The Manse, Dromara, Belfast. MB, BCh (QUB 1941). Surg. Lt WRMS.

GILMOUR Dan Kerr Address: 58 Quay Rd, Ballycastle, Co. Antrim. MB, BCh (QUB 1941). Maj. RAMC.

GILMOUR Samuel Joseph George Address: Dunelm, Quay Rd, Ballycastle, Co. Antrim. MB, BCh (QUB 1937). Maj. RAMC. MID.

GILROY John Martin Address: 70 Bishop St, Londonderry. MB, BCh (NUI 1939). Lt RAMC 31st Jan. 1942.

GIRVAN Hugh Lavelle Boyd Address: 19 Hopefield Ave., Antrim Rd, Belfast. MB, BCh (QUB 1940). Sq. Ldr (M) RAFVR.

*****GIVEN** Hugh MacIvor Address: Markstown, Cullybackey, Co. Antrim. MB, BCh (QUB 1940). Flt Lt (M) RAFVR. KIA.

GLASGOW Isobel Little Address: Corbally, Bishopscourt, Downpatrick, Co. Down. MB, BCh (QUB 1923). Capt. RAMC.

GLASGOW William Victor Address: The Mount, Newtownards, Co. Down. MB, BCh (QUB 1941). Flt Lt (M) RAFVR.

GLENDINNING Alan Campbell Address: Glendearg, Dhu Varren, Portrush, Co. Antrim. MB, BCh (QUB 1937). Maj. IMS.

GLENN Robert Address: Ivy Hill, Lisburn, Co. Antrim. MB, BCh (QUB 1933). Maj. RAMC.

GLUCK Bernard MB, BCh (TCD 1922), MCh (1927), FRCS (Edin 1928). Maj. RAMC.

GLYNN Edward John MB, BCh, BAO (UCD 1924). Lt RAMC 8th Oct. 1940.

GLYNN Jarlath Joseph MB, BCh, BAO (UCD 1926). Flt Offr RAF 24th Jun. 1941.

GLYNN Thomas MB, BCh, BAO (UCD 1923). Flt Offr RAF. First enlisted 23rd Jan. 1924.

GOLDING Lesley David Address: Kenilworth Pk, Dublin. L.LM (RCPI 1933), L.LM (RCSI 1933). Lt RAMC 9th Dec. 1944.

GOLDRING Hymon Jack Address: 1 Easton Crescent, Cliftonville Rd, Belfast. MB (QUB 1930). Sq. Ldr (M) RAFVR.

GOLDRING Leslie Address: 9 Sandy St, Newry, Co. Down. MB, BCh (QUB 1942). Flt Lt (M) RAFVER.

GOOD Benjamin Sydney Address: Woodvale, Rineen, Skibbereen, Co. Cork. MB, BCh (TCD 1939). Sq. Ldr RAF.

GOOD Henry William Whately MB, BCh (TCD 1936). Capt. RAMC. Served in Burma. MID.

GOOD Robert Augustine Address: 54 Grand Parade, Cork. MB, BCh, BAO (UCC 1932), DPH (1936). Lt RAMC.

GOODWIN David MB (QUB 1944). Capt. RAMC.

GORDON Charles MB, BCh (TCD 1923), MD (TCD 1930). Capt. RAMC. Invalided out 1943.

*****GORDON** David Shaw s. Robert David and Jeanette Gordon. Husband of Margaret Gordon MB, BCh (QUB 1925). Lt Col. RAMC. d. Active Service 17th Jun. 1947 aged 46. Buried Bulford Cemetery, Yorkshire, Section 2, Row L, Grave 3.

GORDON Ernest Howard Address: 42 Ravenhill Pk, Belfast. MB, BCh (QUB 1940). Sq. Ldr (M) RAFVR.

GORDON Myer Jacob MB, BCh (QUB 1928), MD (QUB 1932), MRCP (London 1933). Sq. Ldr (M) RAF.

GORDON Reginald Edgar MB, BCh, BAO (UCD 1924). Lt RAMC. First enlisted 1st Jan. 1938.

GORE Lionel (Formerly Gorfunkle) MB, BCh (QUB 1932). Capt. RAMC.

GORMAN James Hamilton MB, BCh (QUB 1926), DPH (QUB 1936). Lt Col. IMS, IAMC.

GOULD Reginald Address: 33 Waterloo Pl., Dublin. L.LM (RCPI 1941), L.LM (RCSI 1941). Lt RAMC 29th Aug. 1942.

GRAHAM Francis Malcolm L.LM (RCPI 1940), L.LM (RCSI 1940). Surg. Lt Comdr 19th May 1936.

GRAHAM George Frederick b. 11th Jan. 1885. s. Christopher (assistant insp. to industrial and reformatory schools) and Rachel Graham, 47 Willington Pl., Dublin. Educ. St Andrews Coll. Dublin 31st Aug. 1900–31st Oct. 1902. TCD (1906) MB (1907), BCh, MD (1913), FRCSI (1921). Lt IMS 1st Aug. 1908. Capt. 1st Aug. 1911. Lt Col. Served 1914–18 War IEF Turkish Arabia. Wounded E. Afr. Aug. 1917. Medals: MID 5th Apr. 1916. Commemorated on Roll of Honour Sir Patrick Dun's Hosp.

GRAHAM George Kenneth MB, BCh (TCD 1929). Lt Col. IMS.

GRAHAM John Race Address: 78 Maryville Pk, Belfast. MB, BCh (QUB 1938). Sq. Ldr (M) RAFVR.

*****GRAHAM** M.A. Sub Lt Fleet Air Arm. KIA.

GRAHAM Matthew Joseph MB, BCh (NUI 1915), DPH (Dublin 1920). d. Dun Laoghaire, 15th Feb. 1950.

GRAHAM Roland Harris b. 16th Apr. 1892, Cambridge. s. Christopher (Asst Insp. of industrial and reformatory schools) and Rachel Graham, 47 Wellington Pl., Dublin. Educ. St Andrews Coll. Dublin 31st Aug. 1900–Jun. 1909. TCD (1914), MB, BCh, BAO, LM (Rot. Hosp. 1915), MD. R. C. of I. Lt RAMC SR 12th Aug. 1914. Capt. 1st Apr. 1916. A/Maj. 1918. Maj. 1st Oct. 1927. A/Lt Col. 4th Feb. 1940. T/Lt Col. 4th May 1940–10th Sept. 1941. r.p. Hon. Lt Col. 8th Jan. 1947. Served in 1914–18 War from 11th Jun. 1916. India 1916–18. E. Persia 1918–21. Constantinople 1922–23. India 1925–29 & 1931–35. BEF France 1939–40. CO 2 CCS Feb.–Sept. 1940. Medals: MC (Dec. 1918), BWM, VM, 1939–45 S., DM, WM, IGS Afghan. 1919. MID Jan. 1916.

GRAHAM William MB, BCh (QUB 1923). Col. RAMC. OBE. Mid (2).

GRAHAM William Ewing Address: Tildarg, Ballyclare, Co. Antrim. MB, BCh (QUB 1941). Flt Lt (M) RAFVR.

*****GRAHAM COOK** A.S. Sgt Pilot RAFVR. KIA.

GRANT Alan Proctor Address: Ardmore, Holywood, Co. Down. MB, BCh (QUB 1940). Capt. RAMC. MID (2).

GRANT Frederick George Address: 406 Beersbridge Rd, Belfast. MB, BCh (QUB 1943). Flt Lt (M) RAFVR.

GRAY Edwin Noel Hillman b. 1894, Co. Dublin. s. Thomas Hillman (drapery agent) and Susana Ellen Jane Gray, 1 Fitzwilliam Tce, Dartry, Dublin. Educ. RCSI. L.LM (1915) RCPI, L.LM (1915) RCSI, DPH, RCPSI (1919). R. Methodist. T/Lt RAMC SR. Capt. Flt Lt RAF. Served 1914–18 War BEF France from Sept. 1915. 65th Fd Amb. 21st Div. MO attd. HODS Dover. Surg. Capt. RN 30th Jun. 1934. Medals: 1915 S., BWM, VM. Commemorated on Roll of Honour RCSI.

GRAY George Edward b. 6th Mar. 1906, Belfast, Co. Antrim. MB, BCh, BAO (QUB 1934). Lt 1st Sept. 1939. Capt. 1st Sept. 1940. PC Capt. 1st Sept. 1944. A/Maj. 2nd Aug. 1942. T/Maj. 2nd Nov. 1942. Maj. 1st Sept. 1946. r.p. 7th Aug. 1947. Served BEF France 1940. NWE 1945. Medals: 1939–45 S., France and Germany S., DM, WM.

GRAY James Ernest MB, BCh (QUB 1923). Lt Col. IMS. Officer B. OStJ.

GRAY Muriel Eve Address: Plushayes, Armagh Rd, Portadown, Co. Armagh. MB, BCh (QUB 1941). Capt. RAMC.

GREEN John Harold Address: 23 Myrtlefield Pk, Balmoral, Belfast. Campbell College. MB, BCh (QUB 1933), MD (QUB 1936). Maj. RAMC.

GREEN William Francis Address: 24 Glandore Drive, Antrim Rd, Belfast. MB BCh (QUB 1932), DPH (QUB 1935), MD (1936). Maj. RAMC.

GREENAWAY Mary Isabel (née Allen) MB (QUB 1942). Flt Lt (M) RAF.

GREENE Charles Westland Address: Kilkea Lodge, Mageney, Co. Kildare. MB, BCh (TCD 1936). Col. IMS. Served Eritrea, Italy and Greece. MID (3).

GREENE Elizabeth Margaret (née Rees) Address: Cherry Cottage, Westport, Co. Mayo. MB, BCh (TCD 1938). Capt. RAMC.

GREENE Juan Nassau Address: Kilkea Lodge, Mageney, Co. Kildare. MB, BCh (TCD 1941). Flt Offr RAF.

GREER Charles Olaf MB, BCh (TCD 1934). RAF.

GREEVES Frederick Douglas MB (QUB 1938). Maj. RAMC.

*****GREEVES** Hubert Gough b. Co. Tyrone. Capt. 87080 RAMC. d. at sea 10th. Jul. 1943. 181 Airlanding Fd Amb. Commemorated Cassino Memorial, Italy, Panel 12.

GREGG George Address: Ferndale, Larne Harbour, Co. Down. MB, BCh (QUB 1938). Maj. RAMC. Chev. of the O. of Leopold II with palm, Croix de Guerre with palm. MID.

GREGG Thomas James Myles MB, BCh (TCD 1934). RAF 1935. SMO HQ No. 2 Group 2nd Tactical Air Force B.L.A. Wing Comdr. OBE.

GREMSON Harry Address: 7 Rockboro Rd, Cork. MB, BCh, BAO (UCC 1937). Lt RAMC.

GRIFFIN Charles Robert b. 1919. Address: 9 Dartmouth Sq., Leeson Pk, Ranelagh, Dublin. Educ. Wesley College, Dublin. MB, BCh (TCD 1941). RAMC 1942. Sq. Ldr RAF. Air Vice Marshal. Served in Africa, Egypt, Palestine. Honorary Surgeon to the Queen. Senior Consultant to the RAF. Pioneer of hyperbaric oxygen. d. aged 66 years.

GRIFFIN Patrick Wynne Address: Lindsay Rd, Glasnevin, Dublin. L.LM (RCPI 1939), L.LM (RCSI 1939). Lt RAMC 13th Mar. 1943.

GRIFFIN Thomas Percy Address: Beech Tree House, Curragh, Co. Kildare. MB, BCh (TCD 1938). Surg. Comdr RNVR. Served North Africa. North Atlantic and Italy.

GRIFFIN William Patrick MB, BCh (TCD 1933). Sq. Ldr RAF. Served in Yugoslavia and Greece. MID.

GROVE-WHITE Robert John Address: Rinn na Mara, Blackrock, Co. Dublin. MB, BCh (TCD 1938). Malayan Med. Service. POW Singapore, released 1945.

GROVES James Charles MB (QUB 1936). Sq. Ldr (M) RAF.

GROVES Thomas Alexander MB, BCh (QUB 1936). Maj. RAMC.

GUILBRIDE Arthur Herbert Hamilton Address: 40 Merton Rd, Rathmines, Dublin. MB, BCh (1941 TCD). Lt RAMC 1942. Invalided out 1942.

GUINAN John Stanislaus Address: Millbrook House, Cloghan, Offaly. MB, BCh (NUI 1938). Lt RAMC 19th Jun. 1940.

GUNDERSON Eileen Marguerite (née Logan) Address: 10 Upr Crescent, Belfast. BA, MB, BCh (QUB 1941). Capt. RAMC.

GURD Dudley Plunket MB, BCh (QUB 1932), MC (QUB 1942). Surg. Comdr RN.

GURRIE Norman Solomon (formerly Gurevich) MB, BCh (TCD 1927), MD (TCD 1936). Flt Offr RAF.

GWYNN Arthur Montague Address: Prospect, Templeogue, Co. Dublin. MB, ChB (Aberdeen 1942), TCD 1930. Capt. RAMC. MID.

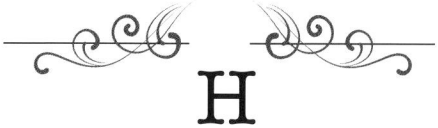

H

HACKETT Edward William Ronald MB, BCh (TCD 1938). Colonial Med. Serv. Interred in Hong Kong 1941–45.

HADDEN George Brownligg b. 16th Feb. 1888 at Arklow, Co. Wicklow. MB, BCh, BAO (1914 TCD). Lt RAMC SR 7th Dec. 1914. Mobd 16th Dec. 1914. Capt. 16th Jun. 1915. PC Lt 1st Jan. 1917. Capt. 16th Jun. 1918. Maj. 7th Dec. 1926. Lt Col. 26th Nov. 1946. r.p. (Hon. Col.) 26th Nov. 1946. Served India 1915–16. Mesopotamia 1916–20. Malta 1920. Constantinople 1922–23. India 1924–28. China 1930–33. Egypt 1935–36. Palestine 1936 and 1938–40. Egypt 1940–43. CO Ind. Fd Amb. 1940. AGMS HQ Alexandria Sub. Area 1940–41. CO 8th Gen. Hosp. 1941–43. Invalided. CO Mil. Hosp. BWLCH 1943–44. and Mil. Hosp. York 1944–46. Medals: 1939–45 S., Africa S., DM, WM.

HADDEN Robert Evans Address: Magharee House, Portadown, Co. Armagh. Campbell College. MB, BCh (TCD 1926), MD (TCD 1932). Capt. RAMC.

HADDICK George MB, BCh (QUB 1920). Capt. RAMC.

HALAHAN Robert Michael MB, BCh (TCD 1940). RAMC.

HALL Ernest Hamilton b. 26th Jan. 1905, Passage West, Co. Cork. MB, BCh, BAO (TCD 1926), DPH (England 1935), RCPS (England 1935). PC Lt RAMC 26th Jan. 1927. Capt. 26th Jul. 1930. Maj. 26th Jan. 1937. A/Lt Col. 23rd Sept. 1941. T/Lt Col. 23rd Dec. 1941. Lt Col. 7th Jul. 1945. A/Col. 17th Apr. 1945. T/Col. 17th Oct. 1945. Col. 7th Nov. 1949. Brig. 8th Jan. 1955. T/Maj. Gen. 1st Apr. 1952. r.p. Hon Maj. Gen. 21st February, 1956. Served Sudan Defence Force 1928–33. India 1938–46. GHQ(I) ADH and P 1941–45. ADP 1945–46. ADP S. Comd 1946–47. CO Emergency Vaccine Lab. 1947–49. AD-GAMS War Office (AMD 1) 1949–52. DDGAMS 1952–54. DMS HQ BAOR 1954–56. Medals: OBE (1st Jan. 1946), DM, WM, OStJ (1952). d. 25th Aug. 1959 at Aldershot, Hants.

HALL Henry Potter b. 21st Apr. 1891. MB, BCh, BAO (QUB 1913), RAMC WWI. Surgical Registrar Royal Victoria Hosp. Asst Prof. of Surgery QUB. Consulting surgeon to the Belfast City Hosp. and the Ulster Volunteer Hosp. In 1922 he submitted a valuable thesis for the Mastership of Surgery, based on his wide experience of the surgery of injuries in peripheral nerves caused by gunshot wounds. During and after WWII he was a member of the Central Medical War Committee. d. 10th Jul. 1962.

HALL Hugh Edwin Address: 23 College Gdns, Belfast. MB, BCh (QUB 1916), MC (QUB 1929). Surg. Comdr RNVR. VD.

HALL Philip Augustus MB, BCh (TCD 1916), MD (TCD 1919), MCh (TCD 1933). RAF.

HALL Robin MB (QUB 1918). Surg. Comdr RNVR. VD.

HALL Thomas Theodore Schoales MB, BCh (QUB 1925), MC (QUB 1929), DPH (QUB 1931). Maj. RAMC. MBE, TD.

HALLEY Walter Address: Kilbarry, Waterford. MB, BCh (NUI 1939). Lt RAMC 7th Feb. 1941.

HALLIDAY John Address: 374 Beersbridge Rd, Belfast. MB, BCh (QUB 1931). Capt. RAMC. MID.

HALLIDAY Robert Address: 2 Cyprus Ave., Belfast. MB, BCh (QUB 1942). Flt Lt (M) RAFVR.

HALLINAN Francis John Address: Castlegrace, Clogheen, Co. Tipperary. MB, BCh (NUI 1938). Flt Lt RAF 15th Aug. 1941.

HAMILL James Norman b. 15th Apr. 1914, Dungannon, Co. Tyrone. MB, BCh, BAO (QUB 1937). Lt 29th Sept. 1939. WS Capt. 29th Sept. 1940. A/Maj. 8th Dec. 1942. PC Capt. 29th Sept. 1944. A/Maj. 18th Aug. 1944. T/Maj. 18th Dec. 1944. WS Maj. 30th Oct. 1945. Maj. 29th Sept. 1947. A/Lt Col. 30th Jul. 1945. T/Lt Col. 30th Oct. 1945. Lt Col. 29th Aug. 1957. Col. 29th Sept. 1962. r.p. disability 6th Apr. 1966. MEF 1941–43. RMO 1st Worcs. 1941–42. India/SEAC 1943–46: CO 14th Indian Fd Amb. 1945–46. Ceylon 1947–48. FARELF 1948–50. PSMB W. Comd 1956. MELF Cyprus: CO 2nd Fd Amb. 1957–59. BAOR 1960–66: CO 29th Fd Amb. 1960–62. Medals: 1939–45 S., Africa S., Burma S., DM, WM, GSM cls Malaya and Cyprus. OStJ (1963). MID 5th Apr. 1945.

HAMILL Mary Address: Swords, Co. Dublin. MB, BCh (NUI 1938). Flt Offr RAF 4th Mar. 1943.

HAMILTON Alexander Drake Monk Address: 25 Cyprus Ave., Bloomfield, Belfast. MB, BCh, DPH (QUB 1941). Capt. RAMC.

HAMILTON John Aloysius MB, BCh (TCD 1935). RAMC.

HAMILTON Robert Stanley Address: Ballymoney, Ballymena, Co. Antrim. Campbell College. MB, BCh (QUB 1942). Sq. Ldr (M) RAFVR.

HAMILTON William Bruce b. Dublin, 23rd Aug. 1905. MB, BCh, BAO (TCD) MD SSC. Lt 25th Apr. 1935. Capt. 25th Apr. 1936. Permanent Capt. 25th Apr. 1940. A/Maj. 24th Dec. 1939. T/Maj. 24th Mar. 1940, Maj. 25th Apr. 1944. A/Lt Col. 17th Dec. 1944. T/Col. 17th Mar.

1945. d. 16th Dec. 1947. Served Egypt 1936–43, M.East 1944–45. Medals: 1939–45 S., Africa S. with 8th Army cl., Defence Medal and Victory Medal.

HAMILTON William Dunlop MB, BCh (QUB 1924). Maj. RAMC.

*****HANLY** Gerard Joseph b. 21st Jul. 1900 at Elphin, Co. Roscommon. Eleventh child of John Hanly, farmer and Winifred Breslin his wife. Educ. Summerhill Coll. Sligo and UCG. MB, BCh, BAO. (NUI 1923). FRCS Edin. 1931. MRCS and FRCS. Dec. 1940. Commissioned RAF Med. Serv. 1924. Flt Lt 1926. Sq. Ldr 1934. Wing Comdr 1938. Group Capt. 1942. Served India, Iraq, Aden, Egypt. Married Miriam Duff 24th Jul. 1937, who survived him with two daughters. d. on active service in the Middle East in Aug. 1942.

HANNA Fredrick Alexander Address: Braemar, Maxwell Rd, Bangor, Co. Down. MB, BCh (TCD 1939). Capt. RAMC. Served in India.

HANNA Frederick Maurice MB, BCh (TCD 1934). Maj. RAMC. MID.

HANNA Hector Ramsay MB TCD (1934). RAMC.

HANNA John Ridgway MB, bcH (TCD 1928). Sgt A/Gnr RAF.

HANNA William Swanston Address: Mayfield, Dunmurry, Co. Down. MB, BCh (QUB 1942). Surg. Lt Comdr RNVR.

HANNAN James MB, BCh (NUI 1925). RAMC 16th Jan. 1940.

HANWAY Aidan Patrick Address: Santry Lodge, Santry, Co. Dublin. MB, BCh, BAO (NUI 1936). Lt RAMC 1944.

HARAN Thomas Kevin Address: 8 Haddon Rd, Clontarf, Dublin. LRCP&S (RCSI 1939). Flt Offr RAF 31st Oct. 1932.

HARBINSON Alfred Forbes Address: Methodist Manse, Omagh. MB, BCh (QUB 1940). Sq. Ldr (M) RAFVR.

HARBINSON David Lowry Address: Glanrye, Newry, Co. Down. MB, BCh (TCD 1940). RAMC.

HARDING Charles Edward Litton b. 20th Sept. 1880, Wellington, New Zealand. Educ. RUI (QCB) MB (1907), BCh, BAO, BS (1907). Lt RAMC 4th Feb. 1908. Capt. 4th Aug. 1911. A/Maj. 22nd Apr. 1919. Maj. 2nd Feb. 1920. Lt Col. 2nd Nov. 1932. r.p. 20th Sept. 1935. Rempld Maj. 20th Jun. 1940. r.p. Lt Col. 7th Dec. 1947. Served in India 1909–14. Aden from 5th Jul. 1915–18. N. Russia Jun–Oct. 1919. Hosp. Ship *Suntemple* 1922–23. India 1924–28. Ceylon 1930–33. SMO RMA Sandhurst 1934–35. Medals: 1915 S., BWM, VM, DM, WM.

HARDY James Denis Address: 39 Kirkliston Dr., Bloomfield, Belfast. MB, BCh (QUB 1933), MD (QUB 1937), MRCP (London 1938). Lt Col. IMS.

HARKIN Thomas Joseph Address: Newtown Villa, Dodder Rd, Rathfarnham, Dublin. L.LM (RCPI 1929), L.LM (RCSI 1929). Flt Lt RAF 23rd Feb. 1934.

HAROLD Charles Gordon MB, BCh, BAO (UCC 1928). Flt Offr RAF.

HAROLD Richard St John Address: 19 Upper Fitzwilliam St, Dublin. L.LM (RCPI 1940), L.LM (RCSI 1940). Med. Officer T. Res. 24th May 1945.

HARPER John Address: 39 Camden St, Belfast. MB, BCh (QUB 1937). Maj. RAMC.

HARPER Thomas Gerald Educ. TCD. MB (1912). Capt. New Z. AMC Apr. 1917. Sq. Ldr New Zealand Med. Servs.

HARRIMAN Denis Gaston Frederick Address: 38 Cranmore Ave., Lisburn Rd, Belfast. MB, BCh (QUB 1943). Capt. RAMC.

HARRIS Cyril Robert MB, BCh (TCD 1928). Maj. RAMC.

HARRIS Derycke Peile Address: Rynnville, Bray, Co. Wicklow. MB, BCh (TCD 1935). Sq. Ldr RAF. Served in Nova Scotia.

HARRIS Frederick b. 21st Jun. 1891, Stewartstown, Co. Tyrone. Educ. TCD MB (1914), BCh, BAO, DPH (Eng. 1928), RCPS (Eng. 1928), LM (Rot. Hosp.). T/Lt RAMC 10th Jan. 1915. Capt. 11th Jan. 1916. PC Capt. 1st Dec. 1918. Maj. 10th Jan. 1927. Bt. Lt Col. 1st Jan. 1939. A/Lt Col. 3rd Sept. 1939. T/Lt Col. 3rd Dec. 1939. Lt Col. 15th Apr. 1940. A/Col. 7th May 1941. T/Col. 7th Nov. 1941. Col. 22nd May 1945. A/Brig. 17th Apr. 1945. T/Brig. 17th Oct. 1945. Brig. 1st Nov. 1947. A/Maj. Gen. 8th Apr. 1947. T/Maj. Gen. 1st Nov. 1947. Maj. Gen. 12th Dec. 1948. T/Lt Gen. 1st Apr. 1952. Lt Gen. 29th Apr. 1952. r.p. 2nd May 1956. Served in the Dardanelles, Egypt 1915–16 and France 1916–17. Gassed and wounded May 1917. RMO 17 Bde.RFA 1915–17. Italy 1918–19. India 1919–24. China 1928–31. DADH Hong Kong Jan.–Jun. 1929 and 1929–30. Shanghai Jun.–Nov. 1929. DADMS/DADH HQ China Comd 1930–31. DADH and P NI Dist. 1932. Hyg. Spec. NI Dist. 1927–28. Asst Prof. of Hyg. RAMC Coll. 1932–36. India 1936–45: NWF 1936–37. DADH Peshawar Dist. 1937–38, ADH and P HQ N. Comd 1938–41. DDH and P/DDH GHQ (I) 1941–45. Burma DDMS HQ 12th Army/Burma Comd 1945–46. ADMS HQ Aldershot and Hants. Dist. 1946–47. DMS GHQ MELF 1947–48. DDGAMS War Office 1948–52. DGAMS War Office 1952–56. KHS 4th Feb. 1946. QHS 1st Apr. 1952. Medals: KBE (1st Jan. 1953), CB (1st Jan. 1949), CBE (1st Jan. 1944), MC (26th Sept. 1917), 1915 S., BWM, VM, IGSM (cl. NW Frontier 36/37), Burma S., DM, WM, QEII Corn Medal 1953. MID 13th Jul. 1916.

HARRIS Gerald Frederik MB, BCh (TCD 1932). Col. IMS. Wounded in Burma. MID.

HARRIS Henry MB, BCh (QUB 1931). Maj. RAMC.

HARRIS Louis MB, BCh (TCD 1923). Maj. RAMC. CMF.

HARRIS St George Eyre Educ. TCD. MB, BCh (1899), MD (1902). LT RAMC Oct. 1915. Capt. 1916. Maj. r.p. 1941. Served in 1914–18 War from 2nd Nov. 1915, Salonika 78th Gen. Hosp. Medals: OBE, 1915 S., BWM, VM.

HARRISON Desmond George Address: 18 Fortfield Pk, Terenure, Dublin. MB, BCh (TCD 1939). Capt. RAMC.

HARRISON Frederick John Address: Shell Hill, Portrush Rd, Coleraine, Co. Derry. MB, BCh (QUB 1941). Capt. RAMC.

HARRISON Thomas James Address: 57 Candahar St, Ormeau Rd, Belfast. MB, BCh (QUB 1942). Flt Lt (M) RAFVR.

HART John Alexander Getty Address: Main St, Ballymoney, Co. Antrim. MB, BCh (QUB 1942). Flt Lt (M) RAFVR.

HARTY Michael Address: Ballinamona, Dungarvan, Co. Waterford. MB, BCh (NUI 1937). Flt Offr RAF 6th Apr. 1944.

HASLETT John Herbert MB, BCh (QUB 1924). Lt Col. RAMC.

HASSAN Bernard Vincent Address: 105 Osborne Pk, Belfast. MB, BCh (QUB 1940). Maj. RAMC.

HASSARD Jason Robert Address: Churchville, Church Avenue, Rathmines, Dublin. MB, BCh (TCD 1941). Surg. Lt RNVR.

HASSETT Cornelius Jeffcott Address: Ard na Greine, Moycullen, Co. Galway. MB, BCh (TCD 1936). Maj IMS. OBE.

HAUGHTON Samuel George Steele Educ. St Columba's Coll. Rathfarnham, Dublin. TCD, BA (1904), MB (1906), MD (1913), MAO (1913), BCh. Occupation A/Professor of Midwifery Lahore Uni. Lt IMS 1905, Capt. 1909. Maj. 1918. Col. Served in 1914–18 War with the Indian Exp. Force. Turkish Arabia 1915. POW Kut el Amara May 1916. Medals: OBE, CIE.

HAWTHORNE Alexander Thomas Address: Fairmount, Burnfoot, Co. Donegal. MB, BCh (QUB 1938). Surg. Lt RNVR.

HAY David Address: The Manse, North Circular Rd, Lisburn, Co. Antrim. MB, BCh (QUB 1942). Surg. Lt RNVR.

HAY Robert Kenneth MB, DPH (QUB 1944). Sq. Ldr (M) RNVR.

HAYDEN Thomas Ernest Address: 100 Cliftonville Rd, Belfast. MB, BCh (QUB 1934), MD (QUB 1937). Capt. RAMC.

HAYES Gerard Thomas Maurice Address: 35 Upr Fitzwilliam St, Dublin. MB, BCh (NUI 1938). Lt IMS 1st Nov. 1938. MC.

HAYES John Marcus Educ. RCSI L.LM (RCPI 1905), L.LM (RCSI 1905). Surg. RN. Surg. Lt Comdr 12th May 1916. Served 1914–18 War. Surg. Lt 16th Jan. 1931. Medals: BWM, VM. Commemorated on Roll of Honour RCSI.

HAYES Patrick MB, BCh, BAO (RUI). b. 20th Mar. 1887 at Rosscarbery, Co. Cork. Lt 27th Jan. 1922, Capt. 27th Jul. 1914, Maj. 27th Jan. 1923, r.p. 27th Jan. 1931. Rejoined 1st Sept. 1939. A/Lt Col. 18th Aug. 1940, T/Lt Col. 18th Nov. 1940. r.p. 1st Apr. 1943. Served India 1912–19, invalided, BAOR 1922–23, India 1927–28, Shanghai Feb. to Oct. 1927. Surg. Spec. Royal Herbert Hospital Woolwich 1929–31. BEF France Surg. Spec. 3 Gen. Hosp. 1939–40, OC Surg. Div. Mil. Hosp. Shaftsbury 1940–41. MEF and India 1941–42. Spec. in Surg. 1922. Medals: BWM, VM, Kaiser-i-hind Medal 1919. d. 12th Aug. 1951

HAYTHORNTWAITE Becher Fitzjames Address: 5 Rathdown Villas, Terenure, Dublin. MB, BCh (TCD 1920). Wing Comdr RAF. No.7 RAF Hosp.

HEADON Patrick Lawrence Address: 12 Haddon Rd, Clontarf, Dublin. MB, BCh, BAO (NUI 1939). Lt RAMC 1940.

HEALY Eugene Address: Main St, Caherciveen, Co. Kerry. L.LM (RCPI 1933), L.LM (RCSI 1933). Lt RAMC 27th Feb. 1940.

HEALY John Rambaut Address: Thormanby, Howth, Co. Dublin. MB, BCh (TCD 1941). RAF Comd.

HEALY Michael Francis Address: 18 Pearse St, Nenagh, Co. Tipperary. MB, BCh (NUI 1941). Lt RAMC 13th May 1944.

HEANY John Ignatius MB, BCh, BAO (UCD 1928), DPH (NUI 1928). Lt RAMC.

HEARD Richard Gerald Patterson Address: 1 Green Pk, Orwell Rd, Rathgar, Dublin. MB, BCh (TCD 1939). Sq. Ldr RAF.

*****HEARNE** James Philip BA, MB, BS, BAO, BCh (TCD 1942). b. IFS. s. Michael James and Teresa Mary Hearne, New Ross, Co. Wexford. Capt. 279095 RAMC Western Europe Campaign 1944/45. KIA 13th Jun. 1944 Normandy, France, aged 27. Buried Bayeux War Cemetery, Plot XIV.

HEATLEY Frederick Charles Address: Seaview House, Glencormac, Bray, Co. Wicklow. MB, BCh (TCD 1937). Maj. RAMC 8th Army.

HEATLEY Seymour Frederick Address: 1 Fitzwilliam Pl., Dublin. MB, BCh (TCD 1926). Lt Col. RAMC. OBE.

HEATON, Samuel Gilbert Address: Hightrees, Athlone, Co. Westmeath. MB, BCh (TCD 1937). Capt. RAMC Indian Comd.

HEDERMAN Joseph Patrick Address: Ballyneale, Ballingary, Co. Limerick. L.LM (RCPI 1925), L.LM (RCSI 1925). Surg. Lt RN 7th Dec. 1932.

HEGY Reginald MB, BCh (TCD 1922), MD (TCD 1934). Capt. SAMC. South Africa and Egypt 1941–45.

HENDERSON Douglas Address: 3 Mount Aboo Pk, Finaghy, Belfast. MB, BCh (QUB 1942). Surg. Lt RNVR.

HENDERSON Edwin MB, BCh (QUB 1933). Maj. RAMC.

HENDERSON Herbert John Reid Address: Northern Bank House, Lisburn, Co. Antrim. Campbell College. MB, BCh (TCD 1938). Capt. RAMC. Served in W. Africa.

HENDERSON John Alexander Holden Address: Glenheather, Garryford, Co. Antrim. MB, BCh (QUB 1937). Capt. RAMC.

HENLEY Wilton Ernest Eldest s. Dr Ernest Albert William Henley. Educ. Wanganui Collegiate and Otago university, New Zealand. Married Wilhelmina Muriel Jean Barnes Graham in 1935. Won a Rhodes Scholarship to London in 1929. MB, ChB (Oxford 1935). Selected for Irish rugby trial. Returned to New Zealand in 1939. Joined the New Zealand Army Medical Corps. Served in Italy and occupation of Japan. MBE for services during the war years.

HENNESSY Alice Patricia Mary Address: 22 Oakley Rd, Ranelagh, Dublin. L.LM (RCPI 1939), L.LM (RCSI 1939). Lt RAMC 12th Dec. 1940.

HENNESSY Edmond Mary b. 1st Aug. 1904, Bombay, India. MB, BCh, BAO (UCC 1928). PC Lt RAMC 30th Jan. 1929, Capt. 9th Nov. 1931, Maj. 9th May 1938, A/Lt Col. 29th Dec. 1941, T/Lt Col. 13th Apr. 1946, Lt Col. 27th May 1946, T/Col. 1st Feb. 1956, Brig. 16th Apr. 1956. r.p. 14th May 1963. Served India 1930–35, China 1937–40, Malaya 1940–42, CO Base Hosp. Tanglin, Singapore 1941–42, POW Far East 1942–45, CO Mil. Hosp. Chepstow 1946–47, BAOR: CO Mil. Hosp. Iserlohn 1947–48, FARELF 1948–51: ADMS /DDMS HQ LF Hong Kong 1948–49, ADMS HQ 40th Div. 1949, CO 33 Gen. Hosp. 1949–51, ADMS HQ N. Midland Dist. 1951–53, BAOR: ADMS & CO BMH Berlin 1952–53, DMS HQ FARELF 1956–57, DDMS HQ Scottish CCMD 1958–60, DMMS HQ MELF/NEARELF 1960–63. Medals: OBE 12th Feb. 1946, MID 12th Sept. 1946, 1939–45 S., Pacific S., DM, WM, GSM and cl. Malaya.

HENNESSY James Noel Address: 22 Richmond Hill, Cork. MB, BCh, BAO (UCC 1936). Lt RAMC.

HENRY Gerald MB, BCh, BAO (NUI 1939). Lt RAMC 1940.

HENRY George Hewitt L Med LS (1927), MB, BCh (TCD 1939). Capt. RAMC. Served in W. Africa.

HENRY James Lawrence Address: Mount Davys, Cullybackey, Co. Antrim. MB, BCh (QUB 1939). Capt. RAMC.

HENRY John Aloysius MB, BCh, BAO (1928). Lt RAMC 1st May 1943.

HENRY Knox Isaac Houston Address: Riverview, Dunman, Cookstown, Co. Tyrone. MB, BCh (QUB 1935). Capt. RAMC.

HENRY Robert Francis Jack Address: 24 Upr Fitzwilliam St, Dublin. MB, BCh (TCD 1924), FRCSI (1927). RAMC.

HEPPLE Robert Alexander b. 13th Mar. 1888, Ballymena, Co. Antrim. s. William Sefton (merchant tailor) and Janet Hepple, 10 Wellington St, Ballymena, Co. Antrim. Educ. Edinburgh Uni. MB (1913), BCh. R. C. of I. Lt RAMC SR 12th Jun. 1912. Mobd 10th Aug. 1914. Capt. 1st Apr. 1915. PC Capt. 1st Jun. 1918. A/Maj. 4th Jan. 1918. Maj. 10th Aug. 1926. Lt Col. 9th Jul. 1936. A/Col. 2nd Sept. 1939. T/Col. 2nd Mar. 1930. Col. 1st Mar. 1942. A/Brig. 24th Oct. 1941. T/Brig. 24th Apr. 1942. r.p. Hon. Brig. 24th Oct. 1947. Served BEF France 21st Aug. 1914–19. India 1919–24. BAOR Path. Spec. Mil. Hosp. Wiesbaden 1926–27. Exp. Stn. Porton 1927–31. India 1931–36: BMH Meerut 1931–35. CIMH Razmak 1935. DADP Baluchistan Dist. 1935–36. ADP S. Comd 1936–39. BEF France: DDP HQ Services (Medical) 1939–40. ADP Aldershot Comd Jul. 1940 and Northern Comd Jul.–Oct. 1940. W. Africa 1940–41. HQ Nigeria Area 1940–41, DDMS HQ Mil. Forces 1941–43. CO 108 Gen. Hosp. 1943–44. BNAF/CMF: DDMS AF HQ 1944–45. ADMS HQ Salisbury Plain Dist. 1945–46. PSNB E. Comd/War Office 1946–47. Medals: CBE (21st Jun. 1945), MC (26th Jul. 1918) Bar (15th Feb. 1919), 1914 S., BWM, VM, IGS cl. Malabar 1921–22, 1939–45 S., Italy S., DM, WM, KStJ. MID 10th Jul. 1919, 22nd Feb. 1945. d. 26th Sept. 1965, Farnham, Surrey.

HEPWORTH Sydney Jacob Address: 332 Antrim Rd, Belfast, MB, BCh (QUB 1939). Maj. RAMC.

*HERBERT Leopold b. Armagh. s. Abraham and Edith Herbert. MD (QUB 1934). Capt. 101137 RAMC. Sicily 186th Fd Amb. KIA 27th Jul. 1943, aged 31. Commemorated on Casino Memorial. MC.

HERMAN Myer Address: 284 Lr Kimmage Rd, Dublin. MB, BCh (TCD 1939). Maj. RAMC. Dunkirk, El Alamein, India.

HERNAN Gerard Charles Address: 97 Bishop Street, Londonderry. MB, BCh (NUI 1939). Lt RAMC 16th Jan. 1940.

HERON Robert James Alexander Address: Greenfield, Katesbridge, Co. Down. MB, BCh (QUB 1939). Capt. RAMC.

HERRON Robert Alexander Crosthwaite MB, BCh (QUB 1932). Surg. Lt Comdr RN.

HETHERINGTON Andrew William Address: Ardkeen, Greenisland, Co. Antrim. MB, BCh (QUB 1941). Surg. Lt RNVR.

HEWITT John Cecil Address: 30 Portmore St, Portadown, Co. Armagh. MB, BCh (QUB 1938). Lt Col. RAMC.

HEWITT Richard Whiteside Address: 169 Malone Rd, Belfast. MB, BCh (QUB 1933). Maj. RAMC.

HICKEY James Finbarr Joseph, Address: 1 College View Tce, Western Rd, Cork. MB, BCh, BAO (UCC 1937). Flt Offr RAF.

HICKEY Michael Patrick Joseph Address: 1 Alexander Tce, O'Connell Ave., Limerick. L.LM (RCPI 1939), L.LM (RCSI 1939). Flt Lt RAF 24th Aug. 1931.

HICKEY Walter Gerard L.LM (RCPI 1935), L.LN (RCSI 1935). Lt RAMC 8th Nov. 1941.

HICKS Denis Ormond Address: Stonehurst, Killiney, Co. Dublin. MB, BCh (TCD 1940). Sq. Ldr RAF.

HICKS Eric Cyril MB, BCh (TCD 1929). Lt Col. IMS.

HIGGINS Robert William MB, BCh, BAO (UCG 1921). Surg. Comdr RN.

HIGSON William James Basil Address: Bangor Rd, Newtownards. MB, BCh (QUB 1943). Surg. Lt RNVR.

HILL Alice Margaret Address: New Court, Bray, Co. Wicklow. L.LM (RCPI 1939), L.LM (RCSI 1939). Flt Offr Canadian Airforce.

HILL Georgina Address: Tirgracey Cottage, Muckamore, Co. Antrim. MB, BCh (QUB 1939), DPH (QUB 1941). Capt. RAMC.

HILL Hannah Erica (née Hinchcliff) Address: 24 Mount Merrion Ave., Blackrock, Co. Dublin. MB, BCh (TCD 1942). Lt RAMC.

*****HILL** Ian b. IFS. Capt. RAMC. West Africa d. 3rd Jul. 1944.

HILL James Roland b. 10th Jul. 1883, Strabane, Co. Tyrone. Educ. Edinburgh Uni. MB (1907), ChB. Lt RAMC 30th Jan. 1909. R of O Jan.

1912. Rejoined 29th Aug. 1914. Capt. 30th Oct. 1914. A/Maj. 12th Mar. 1918. Maj. 19th Oct. 1922. A/Lt Col. 11th Jan. 1919. Lt Col. 1st May 1934. Col. 1st May 1938. r.p. remained employed 10th Jul. 1940. r.p. 28th Sept. 1946. Served Gallipoli Aug.–Oct. 1915. Salonika 1915–19. CO 31st CCS 1918–19 and 40 and 84 Fd Amb. 1919. Russia May–Oct. 1919. India 1923–28. Royal Mil. Hosp. Tidworth and R. Herbert Hosp. Woolwich 1929–31. India Royal BMH Meerut and Chakrata 1931–36. Cambridge Hosp. Aldershot 1936–37. CO Connaught Hosp. Aldershot 1937–38. R. Herbert Hosp. Woolwich 1938–39. ADMS HQ Home Counties area 1939. BEF France. ADMS HQ 1st Div. 1939–40. ADMS Southern area 1940–41. PSMB 1942–46. Specialist in Radiology 1923. Medals: 1915 S., BWM, VM, 1939–45 S., DM, WM, Medal for Mil. Merit 3rd Class Greece (26th Nov. 1919). MID 28th Nov. 1917.

HILL John Patrick Address: Society St, Ballinasloe, Co. Galway. L.LM (RCPI 1936), L.LM (RCSI 1936). Lt Indian Army 11th Jan. 1944.

HILL Samuel Maurice Barklie Address: Ballynure PO, Ballynure, Co. Antrim. MB, BCh (QUB 1939). Ships Surg. MN.

HILL William John Coleman Address: White Staunton, Portrush, Co. Antrim. MB, BCh (TCD 1942). Capt. RAMC. India.

HOBART Edward Guest Address: Currabinny, Crosshaven, Co. Cork. MB, BCh (TCD).

HOFMAN Jacob MB, BCh (TCD 1922). Capt. RAMC 1940.

HOGAN Niall James b. 3rd Jan. 1917. Address: 16 Upr Fitzwilliam St, Dublin. MB, BCh (TCD 1939). Served with the RAMC North Africa and Italy. d. 26th Apr. 1995. Buried in Glasnevin Cemetery Dublin.

HOGG Henry Sydney Address: 17 Eglantine Ave., Belfast. MB, BCh (QUB 1939). Surg. Lt RNVR.

HOLDEN Ernest Edwin b. 28th Jan. 1888. Maryborough, Queen's Co. s. Charles and Caroline Elizabeth Holden, 114 Donore Ave., Sth Circular Rd, Dublin. Educ. St Andrews Coll. Dublin 31st Aug. 1903–31st Mar. 1905. L.LM RCPI (1912), L.LM RCSI (1912), LM and MB. R. C. of I. Lt RAMC 16th Sept. 1914. Capt. 16th Sept. 1915. Reg. Comm. Capt. 1st Jun. 1919. Maj. 16th Sept. 1926. Lt Col. 15th Apr. 1938. A/Col. 1st May 1943. T/Col. 1st Nov. 1943–26th Mar. 1944. r.p. ill health (Hon. Col.) 9th Oct. 1944. Served in 1914–18 War from May 1915 Gallipoli to Sept. 1915. Mesopotamia 30th Nov. 1916–21st Sept. 17. 31st FA 10th Div. India 1920. Invalided 1921–24 and 1928–32. India and Burma 1937–43. ADMS HQ 2AA Gp 1943–44 and 6AA Gp Jan.–Mar. 1944. PSMB W. Comd Jun–Oct. 1944. Medals: 1915 S., BWM, VM, 1939–45 S., Burma S., DM, WMM.

HOLLAND Edward Kennedy Address: 79 Anglesea Rd, Dublin. MB, BCh (TCD 1942). Flt Lt RAF.

HOLLEY William Martin Address: 4 Strand Head, Portstewart, Co. Derry. MB, BCh (QUB 1941). Surg. Lt RNVR.

HOLLINS Frederick Rudolf Theodore Address: Strathearn, Mount Eden Rd, Donnybrook, Dublin. MB, BCh (TCD 1939) RAMC.

HOLMES John Gerard MB, BCh (TCD 1919). Surg. Capt. RN. MID, OBE.

HOLMES John Robert Charles Address: Rose House, Athlunkard, Limerick. MB, BCh (TCD 1941). RNVR.

HOLMES William Edward MB, BCh (TCD 1922). Malaya Medical Service. POW.

HOPKINS William Allen Address: Greenholme, Carrickfergus, Co. Antrim. MB, BCh (QUB 1936). Lt Col. IMS. MID.

HORAN Michael Joseph b. 20th Dec. 1910. MB, BCh (TCD 1933). Married 1938 in the UK. Son John. Address: Locaden, Lee Rd, Cork.

HORAN Victor George MB, BCh (TCD 1926). Surg. Comdr RN.

HORGAN Michael Joseph MB, BCh (UCC 1920), MD (UCC 1925). Lt RAMC.

HOULIHAN John Francis MB, BCh, BAO (NUI 1937). Flt Offr RAF 1940. Flt Lt 30th Apr. 1941.

HOUSTON James MB, BCh (QUB 1935). Cpt. RAMC.

HOUSTON James Montague MD, BSc (QUB 1931). Maj. RAMC.

HOUSTON John Kenneth Address: Northern Bank, Kilrea, Co. Derry. Campbell College. LRCP (Edinburgh 1938), LRCS (Edinburgh 1938), LRFPS (Glasgow 1938), MB, BCh (QUB 1938). Maj. RAMC.

HOWITT Emmanuel MB, BCh (TCD 1933). Capt. RAMC.

HOWLETT Michael Joseph MB, BCh, BAO (UCC 1929). Flt Officer RAF.

HUBBARD Douglas Alan TCD 1936. Capt. RAMC. Served in India.

HUGHES Brian Watson b. 25th Mar. 1914, Dublin. MB, BCh, BAO (Dublin 1928). Lt 19th Sept. 1939. Capt. 19th Sept. 1940. PC Capt. 19th Sept. 1944. A/Maj. 5th Jan. 1945. T/Maj. 5th Apr. 1945. WS Maj. 21st Jun. 1945. Maj. 19th Sept. 1947. A/Lt Col. 12th Feb. 1945. Lt Col. 25th Jul. 1957. Col. 19th Sept. 1962. BEF France 1940. MEF 1941–42. CMF 1943–45. CO 23rd Indian Fd Amb. 1945. W. Africa 1950–53. BAOR: CO BMH Hostert 1956–59. E. Africa 1959–63. CO 24 Brig. Group Med. Coy/24th Fd Amb 1959–61. CO BMH Nairobi 1961–63.

BAOR 31 Fd Amb. 1963–64. ADMS HQ 2nd Div. 1964. Medals: OBE (1st Jan. 1962). 1939–45 S., Africa S., Italy S., DM, WM.

HUGHES Stanley Barton, Campbell College. MB, BCh (QUB 1930). Maj. RAMC.

HUGHES William Dillon b. 23rd Dec. 1900, Ardglass, Co. Down. Campbell College. MB, BCh, BAO (QUB 1923), MD (QUB 1937), MRCPI (1947), DTM&H (Eng. 1947), FRCPI (1953). PC Lt 28th Aug. 1928, Capt. 23rd Feb. 1932, Maj. 28th Aug. 1938, A/Lt Col. 1st Mar. 1941, T/Lt Col. 1st Jun. 1941, Lt Col. 3rd Apr. 1946, T/Col. 23rd Nov. 1950, Col. 9th Jun. 1951, Brig. 25th Jul. 1957, T/Maj. Gen. 1st Apr. 1957, Maj. Gen. 2nd May 1958. R.p. 23rd Dec. 1960. Served China 1929–33, Egypt 1935–36, Palestine 1946–37, Egypt 1937–42, OIC Med. Div. 64 and 105 Gen Hosp. 1944–45, NWE 1944–47, CO 81st Gen Hosp. SMO Belsen Camp 1945, OIC Med. Div. 108th Gen Hosp. 1945–46, 23 Gen Hosp 1946–47, OIC Med. Div. QA Mil. Hosp, Millbank 1947–48, Cambridge Hosp. Aldershot 1948–50.

HUGHES William John MB, BCh (NUI 1926), MD (NUI 1934). MRCP (London 1934). Lt RAMC 8th Jul. 1941.

HUGO Hans Jacob MB, BCh (TCD 1924). Lt Col. S. African Med. Corps.

HUNT Frederick George s. Dr and Mrs Hunt, Coolaney, Co. Sligo. MB, BCh (UCG 1917). Surg. R. Admiral RN. Served China, E. Indies, Mediterranean and Home Fleet. Stationed in hospitals in Hong Kong, Plymouth and Chatham. President of the Admiralty Medical Board, London. Commanding the first hospital ship to operate in forward area with the strike force in the Pacific. After the Japanese surrender, he was one of the first to enter Yokahama Harbour and tend to the thousands of sick POWs. After the war he was in charge of the medical section of the Royal Naval Hospital in Chatham and subsequently the Royal Naval Hospital in Haslar, the largest and most senior of the Royal Hospitals. He was appointed a rear admiral in 1949. Medals: CMG. d. 1975.

*****HURLEY** Cecil Edward BA, MB b. IFS s. Michael and Mary Hurley, Dublin. Lt RAMC France and Belgian Campaign 1939–40 d. 16th Jun. 1940 France aged 43. Buried Escoublac-La-Baule War Cemetery, Plot 1.B.3.

HURLEY Jeremiah Address: Mallowgeton, Bandon, Co. Cork. MB, BCh, BAO (NUI 1936), MCh (NUI 1943). Lt RAMC 1943.

*HURST** Henry b. 6th Feb. 1895, Bantry, Co. Cork. s. Thomas Robert and Mary Hurst. LRCP&S. Married Nan Hurst of Alverstoke, Hampshire. Cmdr Surgeon RN, HMS *Hood*. Joined the *Hood* 16th Aug. 1940. d. 24th May 1941 aged 46 in the sinking of HMS *Hood* by the German battleship *Bismark*. Commemorated Portsmouth Naval Memorial Panel 45, Column 3 and St Brendan's Church, Wolfe Tone Sq., Bantry, Co. Cork.

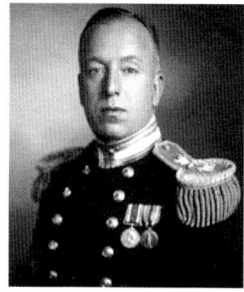

Commander Surgeon Henry Hurst RN.

HUSTON John b. 6th Jul. 1901, Ballykeel, Holywood, Co. Down. MB, BCh, BAO (QUB 1923), FRCS (Edinburgh 1947). PC Lt 30th Jan. 1924, Capt. 30th Jul. 1927, Maj. 1st May 1934, A/Lt Col. 15th Mar. 1940, T/Lt Col. 7th Sept. 1940, Lt Col. 12th Feb. 1946, Col. 12th Dec. 1948, T/Brig. 26th Feb. 1950. r.p. 3rd Dec. 1959. Served India 1925–31 and 1934–39, BEF France 1939–40: CO 1st CCS 1940, CO 196 Fd Amb. 1940–42, Singapore 1941–42, POW Far East 1942–45, OIC Surg. Div. Mil. Hosp. Cowglen 1946–48, E. Africa Adv. Surgery HQ EA Comd 1948–50, Cons. Surg. GHQ MELF 1950–51, Cons. Surg. HQ BAOR 1951–53, D. Surg. Cons. Surg. to the army 1953–59, QHS 1st Jan. 1954. Medals: CBE 12th Jan. 1958, OStJ 1952. MID 4th Mar. 1941, 12th Sept. 1946, 1939–45 S., Pacific S., WM.

HUTCHINSON Henry Tell MB, BCh (TCD 1940). RAMC.

HUTCHINSON James MB, DPH (QUB 1926). Group Capt. (M) RAF.

HUTCHINSON William Edward Address: 69 The Quay, Waterford. MB, BCh (TCD 1923), DPH (1924), MD (1933 TCD). Lt Col. RAMC. POW Singapore 1942–44.

HUTCHINSON William George MB (TCD 1948). RAF.

HUTCHINSON William John MB, BCh (QUB 1923), DPH (QUB 1926). Wing Comdr (M) RAF.

HUTH Mary Clare (née Conlon) MB, BCh (TCD 1938) RAMC.

HYDE Raymond James Garnet MB, BCh (TCD 1925). Lt Col. RAMC. Served BEF, MEF and India.

HYLAND Finbarr Cornelius MB, BCh, BAO (UCC 1934). Lt RAMC.

HYMAN Samuel Address: 37 Lombard St West, Dublin. MB, BCh (TCD 1940). Capt. RAMC. Wounded.

HYNES Thomas Gerard MB, BCh (NUI 1930). Lt RAMC.

I

INGRAM Leslie Lyle MB (QUB 1936). Sq. Ldr (M) RAF. MID. Campbell College. MB, DPH (QUB 1932). Capt. RAMC.

IRVINE Francis Stephen b. 20th Dec. 1873, Belfast. Educ. RUI. MB (QUB 1899), BCh, BAO. Lt RAMC 17th Nov. 1899. Capt. 17th Nov. 1902. Maj. 17th Aug. 1911. T/Lt Col. 4th Oct. 1915. Lt Col. 29th Sept. 1916. Bt. Col. 31st Dec. 1924, Col. 3rd Jun. 1927. r.p. 26th Dec. 1930. Rempld 5th Feb. 1940. Col. 12th Jun. 1940. A/Maj. Gen. 13th Mar–30th Apr. 1946. r.p. 27th Jun. 1946. Served in S. Afr. 1899–1902. India 1902–05. S. Afr. 1906–09. BEF France 16th Aug. 1914–15. POW Aug.–Sept. 1914. Comdt RAMC Sch. Construction and CO D pot RAMC 1915–19. India 1920–24. CO BSH Rawalpindi 1920–22. ADMS AHq (I) 1922–24. VHS CO Camb. Hosp. Aldershot 1926–27. ADMS HQ London Dist. 1927–28. DDMS HQ N. Comd 1928–30. RAM Coll. Assistant Comdt 1940. Comdt 1940–46. Medals: CMG (3rd Jun. 1918), DSO (23rd Jun. 1915), QSA (4 cls), KSA (2 cls), 1914 S., BWM, VM. MID 17th Feb. 1915, 22nd Jun. 1915, 6th Jul. 1918. d. 3rd Jul. 1962, Millbank, London W1.

IRVINE Gilbert Marshal Address: Mountmorris, Co. Armagh. MB, BCh (TCD 1921). Lt Col. IMS.

IRWIN Charles Gibson Address: 29 University Sq., Belfast. Campbell College. MB, BCh (QUB 1941). Capt. RAMC. MID.

IRWIN John Walker Sinclair Address: 29 University Sq., Belfast. Campbell College. MB, BCh (QUB 1937). Capt. RAMC.

IRWIN Samuel Thompson Address: 29 University Sq., Belfast. Campbell College. MB, BCh (QUB 1938). Capt. RAMC.

IRWIN William John b. 16th Jan. 1916, Feenagh, Charleville, Co. Limerick. L.LM (RCPI 1942), L.LM (RCSI 1942). Lt 11th Mar. 1944. Capt. 11th Mar. 1945. T/Maj. 27th May 1950. PC Capt. 13th Jul. 1951. Maj. 11th Mar. 1952. Lt Col. 30th Aug. 1961. Col. 11th Mar. 1967. FARELF Hong Kong 1949–52. Malta 1957–61. BAOR: CO 30th Fd Amb. 1961–65. CO Mil. Hosp. Colchester 1965–67. Medals: WM.

ISAACSON Elliott Address: 7 St Kevin's Rd, South Circular Rd, Dublin. MB, BCh, BAO (NUI 1938). Lt RAMC 1942.

ISAACSON Isidore MB, BCh (TCD 1927), MD (TCD 1935). Maj. UDF.

J

JACKSON Francis Charles MB, BCh (TCD 1931), MD (TCD 1936). Col. IMS. MID.

JACKSON George Boyce s. Mr and Mrs G.B. Jackson, Levitstown House, Mageney, Co. Kildare. MB, BCh (TCD 1936). Married 5th Apr. 1938, Beatrice Wilkinson, dt. Mr and Mrs W.H. Wilkinson, Tyrrelstown, Mulhuddart, Co. Dublin. Col. IMS. MID (4). Served in Burma.

JACKSON Neville Address: 191 Rathgar Rd, Dublin. MB, BCh (TCD 1937). Capt. RAMC. Served W. African Brigade.

JACKSON Norman Address: 33 Lower Baggot St, Dublin. MB, BCh (TCD 1933). Sq. Ldr RAF.

JACOB Samuel Address: 10 St Kevin's Rd, South Circular Rd, Dublin. L.LM (RCPI 1936), L.LM (RCSI 1936). Lt RAMC 11th Dec. 1942.

JAFFE Louis MB, BCh, BAO (UCD 1922). Lt RAMC. First enlisted 3rd Jan. 1941.

JAMES Edwin Francis George Address: Adara, Co. Donegal. MB, BCh (QUB 1937), MD (QUB 1940). Sq. Ldr (M) RAFVR.

JAMES William Bellamy Address: 93 Great Victoria St, Belfast. MB, BCh (QUB 1938). Flt Lt (M) RAFVR.

JAMESON Cecil Edmund BA, Dip.Ed., MB (QUB 1933). Lt Col. RAMC.

JAMESON William Burns MB (QUB 1929). Surg. Lt Comdr RNVR.

JEFFERSON Harold Address: 3 Old Cavehill Rd, Belfast. MB, BCh (QUB 1940). Flt Lt (M) RAFVR.

JENNINGS Charles Blake MB, BCh (NUI 1920). Colonial Medical Service Singapore.

JEWELL, John Hugh Auchinleck MB, BCh (TCD 1936) Surg. Lt Comdr RNVR.

JOHNSON Benjamin b. 19th May 1883, Ballina, Co. Mayo. s. Benjamin (master saddler) and Christina Johnson, 2 Knox St, Ballina, Co. Mayo. Educ. TCD. LM and LCH (1905), L.Med. LS, MB (1913), BCh, BAO. R. C. of I. Lt RAMC 30th Jul. 1906. Capt. 30th Jan. 1910. T/Maj. 3rd Jun. 1917. Bt. Maj. 3rd Jun. 1917. Maj. 30th Jul. 1918. Lt Col. 24th Sept. 1930. Col. 10th Jul. 1934. r.p. 10th Jul. 1938. Rempld 28th Nov. 1939. r.p. 22nd Jul. 1940. Rempld May 13th Nov. 1941. r.p. Col. 8th Oct. 1942. Served in France from 17th Oct. 1914 attd. 16th LCRS. POW Oct. 1914–Jun. 1915.

Salonika 1915. France and Belgium 1915–16. Salonika 1916–19. CO 18th FA. BAOR 1924. Medals: DSO (3rd Jun. 1918), 1914 S., BWM, VM. 1939–45 S., WM. MID 21st Jul. 1917, 28th Nov. 1917. 11th Jun. 1918. d. 20th Nov. 1952 at Tavistock, Devon.

*JOHNSON Reginald b. 13th Sept. 1888, at Kew, Surrey. s. Prof. Thomas Johnson (Prof. Botany) and Bessie Stratton, 13 Palmerston Pk, Rathmines, Dublin. Educ. Archbishop Holgates Grammar School, York. TCD, MB (1912), BCh, BAO, MD (1915). R. Presbyterian. Married Agnes dt. Thomas McHugh, Kings Co. T/Lt RAMC 10th Jan. 1916. Capt. 10th Jan. 1917. RAC Capt. 1st Sept. 1920. Maj. 10th Jan. 1918. T/Lt Col. 27th Jun. 1940. Served in 1914–18 War France 1916–17. Gassed Sept. 1917. India 1921–26. Medals: MBE (10th Oct. 1918), BWM, VM, IGS cl. Waziristan, WM. d. 4th Feb. 1941 at Kings Lynn, Norfolk.

JOHNSTON Hugh Clyde Armstrong MB, BCh (QUB 1933). Surg. Comdr RNVR.

JOHNSTON James Cleland Address: 10 Wellington Pk, Belfast. MB, BCh, DPH (QUB 1939). Maj. RAMC.

JOHNSTON John MB, BCh (TCD 1926). Surg. Comdr RN.

JOHNSTON Robert Stewart MB, BCh (QUB 1925), DPH (London 1933). Lt Col. RAMC.

JOHNSTON William Rankin Address: Ingledene, Lodge Rd, Coleraine. MB, BCh (QUB 1938). Maj. RAMC.

JOHNSTON William Samuel Address: 45 Mayville Pk, Belfast. MB, BCh (QUB 1940). Surg. Lt RNVR.

JOHNSTON Wilson MB, BCh (QUB 1929). Maj. RAMC.

JONES Arthur Edward Booth b. 29th May 1879, St John's, Sligo. Educ. TCD MB (1901), BCh, BAO, MD (1902). R. Methodist. Civil Surg. In S. African War 1902. Lt RAMC 29th Jul. 1907. Capt. 29th Jan. 1911. A/Maj. 19th Dec. 1918. Maj. 29th Jul. 1919. Lt Col. 1st Feb. 1932. r.p. 29th May 1934. Rempld 2nd Sept. 1939. r.p. 1st Feb. 1941. Rempld (Maj.) 1st Dec. 1943. r.p. Lt Col. 3rd Oct. 1946. 1914–18 War served in France and Belgium 1914–16, India 1916–18, Egypt 1918. OC 328th and 340th home Fd Amb. 1918–19. China 1923–26. OC Mil Hosp. Hong Kong 1923. Mil Hosp. Peking 1923–25. Malta 1929. Palestine 1929–30. Malta 1931–32. SMO Dover 1932–34 and 1939–40. Medals: QSA 4 cls, 1914 S., BWM, VM.

JONES Edward Warburton TCD 1935. Lt Col. Allied Land Forces.

JONES, George James b. 24th Nov. 1876, Warrenpoint, Northern Ireland. Educ. MB, BS (1904 RUI), MD (QUB 1918). From the former RUI 1904 MD (1918), QUB. RAMC 1915. Served in France. Invalided 1918. During WWII was in charge of a First Aid post. d. 8th Mar. 1953 at Smethwick.

JONES William Address: Austinleigh, Western Rd, Cork. MB, BCh (TCD 1939). RNVR.

JORDAN John MB, BCh, BAO (UCD 1934). Surg. Lt RN. HMS Bideford DSO awarded for Dunkirk.

JOYCE Eric Austin Address: 2 Belgrave Villas, Rathmines, Dublin. L.LM (RCPI 1933), L.LM (RCSI 1933). Lt RAMC 1940.

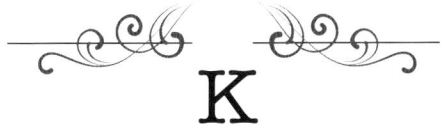

K

KANE Frank Address: Moyargel, Ballycastle, Co. Antrim. MB, BCh, BAO (UCD 1922). Lt RAMC. First enlisted 11th Sept. 1941.

KANE George Alfred Address: Anesfield, Broughshane St, Ballymena, Co. Antrim. MB, BCh, DPH (QUB 1931). Lt Col. RAMC.

KAVANAGH Edward Address: St John's Manor, Enniscorthy, Co. Wexford. L.LM (RCPI 1938), L.LM (RCSI 1938). Surg. Lt Comdr RNVR.

KEANE Patrick Joseph Address: The Square, Lisdoonvarna, Co. Clare. MB, BCh (TCD 1943). Maj. RAMC. SMO hospital ships and troop ships.

KEANE Percival Maurice L.LM (RCPI 1907), L.LM (RCSI 1907), DPH (RCFS England 1913). Served in WWI Surg. RN. Flt Offr and RN 1941.

KEANE William Giles MB TCD (1942). Capt. RAMC. East Africa.

KEATING Claude L.LM (RCPI 1924), L.LM (RCSI 1924). Lt RAMC 1940.

KEATING Michael Joseph, Address: 19 Sheare's Street, Cork. MB, BCh (NUI 1940). Lt RAMC 19th Sept. 1942.

KEATING Stephen Richard MB, BCh (NUI 1942). Lt RAMC 25th Sept. 1943.

KEATING Victor James b. 24th May 1913, Dublin. MB, BCh, BAO (NUI 1937), DA (England 1938). Lt 1st Feb. 1939. Capt. 1st Feb. 1940. PC Capt. 1st Feb. 1944. A/Maj. 26th Mar. 1940. T/Maj. 26th Jun. 1940. Maj. 1st Jul. 1946. A/Lt Col. 31st May 1945. T/Lt Col. 31st Aug. 1945. r.p. Hon Col. 29th Feb. 1952. BEF France 1939–40. Gibraltar 1940–42. ADMS HQ Beach Bde. 1945. India 1945–46. Singapore AFNEI: CO 75th Indian Fd Amb. 1946. ALFSEA: CO 6th Fd Amb. 1946–47. Burma 1947. Hong Kon 1947–49. CO BMH 1949. Medals: 1939–45 S., WM, GSM with cl. SE Asia, MID 26th Jun. 1947.

KEATINGE Alan Francis Heber b. 13th Jul. 1911, Dublin. MB, BCh, BAO (TCD 1934), DPH (England 1948). Lt RAMC 23rd Oct. 1936. Capt. 1st Jan. 1938. A/Maj. 1st Sept. 1939. T/Maj. 1st Dec. 1939. PC Capt. 1st Jan. 1942. T/Maj. 15th Feb. 1943. Maj. 1st Jan. 1946. A/Lt Col. 20th Oct. 1943. T/Lt Col. 20th Jan. 1944. Lt Col. 24th May 1950. T/Col. 8th Nov. 1954. Col. 27th Jan. 1959. T/Brig. 31st Jul. 1966. Brig. 5th Mar. 1967. Served Malta 1937–38 and 1939–42. Palestine 1938–39. MEF 1942–44. CO RAMC Base Depot MEF 1943–44. CO 221 Fd Amb. 1944–45. NWE 1945–46.

ADMS HQ 6 L of C 21 Army Group and 7 Base sub area 1945. CO 130 Fd Amb. 1945–46 and 156 Fd Amb. 1946. MELF Cyprus 1950–52. BAOR 1953–54. DDAH HQ Eastern Comd 1954–58. BAOR: ADMS HQ and CO BMH Berlin 1958–60. FARELF 1962–65. CO BMH Singapore 1962–63. ADMS HQ Singapore Base 1963–65. CO Camb. Hosp. Aldershot 1965–66. DDMS HQ Scottish Comd 1966. Medals: MC (14th Feb. 1939), GSM (with cl. Palestine 1936–39), 1939–45 S., Africa France and Germany S., DM, WM.

KEATINGE Lesley Reginald Heber b. 17th Jul. 1901, Dublin. Educ. at Ellesmere Coll. MB, BCh, BAO (TCD 1928). PC Lt 27th Jul. 1928. Capt. 27th Jan. 1932. Maj. 27th Jul. 1938. A/Lt Col. 19th Jun. 1941. T/Lt Col. 19th Sept. 1941. Lt Col. 29th Mar. 1946. A. Col. 7th Sept. 1944. T/Col. 7th Mar. 1945. Col. 13th Apr. 1951. T/Brig. 9th Jun. 1956. Brig. 29th Apr. 1957. r.p. Hon. Maj. Gen. 16th Sept. 1960. Served Sudan Defence Force 1929–31. India 1932–38, BEF France 1939–40 evacuated from Dunkirk. CO 8th Fd Amb. 1941–42. ADMS HQ 2nd Army 1943–44. NWE 1944–45. ADMS HQ 7th Armoured Div. 1944–45. India 1945–47: CO 17th Gen. Hosp. 1945. CO 21st Gen. Hosp 1945–46. ADH HQ Northern Comd 1946–47. DDH HQ S. Comd 1947–49. DDAH GHQ FARELF 1949–52. ADMS HQ Singapore Base Dist. 1952. DDAH HQ S. Comd 1952–56. BAOR: DDMS HQ 1st Br. Corps. 1956–57. DMS HQ FARELF 1957–60. Medals: CBE (11th Jun. 1960), OBE (1st Feb. 1945), IGSM (with cl. NWF 1936–37), 1939–45 S., France and Germany S., DM, WM, GSM (Malaya), QEII Corn Medal 1953.

KELLEHER Daniel Mortimer Address: West St, Tallow, Co. Waterford. b. Macroom in 1908, the eleventh of thirteen children. Educated at Castleknock College and studied medicine in Cork. MB, BCh, BAO (UCC 1936). Joined the RAMC, 1936, and sent to Palestine. He served in Palestine, Egypt, Germany, Korea and Kuala Lumpur. Promoted to colonel, 1955, on his posting to MELF in Cyprus as consulting physician. Later to the military hospital in Catterick as physician in charge before transferring to the GHQ Far East and subsequently HQ BAOR. Promoted to brigadier. Awarded the OBE in 1959 and appointed Physician to the Queen in 1966. Retired in 1968 to Surrey where he died in 2006 at the age of 98.

KELLEHER Francis Stephen Address: Athdara, Lee Rd, Cork. MB, BCh, BAO (UCC 1933). Flt Offr RAF.

KELLEHER James Stephen Address: Athdara, Lee Rd, Cork. Husband of Patricia. MB, BCh, BAO (UCC 1933). Lt RAMC.

KELLETT John Robert b. 25th Jul. 1913, Syracuse, New York. Address: Hibernian Marine School, Clontarf, Dublin. Married Marjory Sweetman, Monkstown Parish Church, 21st Apr.

1948. MB, BCh, BAO (TCD 1935), DOMS (England 1937). Lt RAMC 24th Oct. 1935. Capt. 24th Oct. 1937. A/Maj. 1st Sept. 1939. T/Maj. 1st Dec. 1939. PC Capt. 24th Oct. 1941. T/Maj. 3rd May 1943. Maj. 24th Oct. 1945. Lt Col. 7th Feb. 1950. Col. 15th Nov. 1958. r.p. 26th Jul. 1959. Served Malaya 1937–42. Ceylon 1942–44. NWE 1945–46. BTA 1949. BAOR 1949–51. USA: MLO British Joint Services Commission 1951–52. BCFK 1953–54. FARELF 1954–56. Medals: MBE (4th May 1953), 1939–45 S., Pacific S., France and Germany S., DM, WM, UNSM and cl. Korea.

KELLS Robert Address: Grange Lower, Annaghmore, Portadown, Co. Armagh. MB, BCh (QUB 1939). Capt. RAMC.

KELLY Cornelius Ignatius Address: Portumna, Co. Galway. MB, BCh (NUI 1942). Flt Lt RAF 7th Dec. 1944.

KELLY Daniel MB, BCh, BAO (UCC 1927). Lt RAMC.

KELLY Daniel Howard Address: 22 Clooney Tce, Londonderry. MB, BCh, BAO (UCD 1924). Lt RAMC 17th Sept. 1939.

KELLY Geoffrey Edward Patrick MB, BCh (TCD 1939). Sq. Cmdr RAF.

KELLY Gerard Joseph Address: Dunlo Hill, Ballinasloe, Co. Galway. L.LM (RCPI 1934), L.LM (RCSI 1934). Lt RAMC 1941.

KELLY Harry Beatty b. 24th Oct. 1879, Rangoon, Burma. s. W.B. Kelly (Ins. Gen. Jails, Burma). Educ. MB, BCh, BAO (TCD 1902) LM (Rot.). Husband of H.M. Filby Kelly. Lt RAMC 31st Jan. 1904. Capt. 31st Jul. 1906. Maj. 31st Oct. 1914. T/Lt Col. 1st Sept. 1915–27th May 1918. Lt Col. 1st Nov. 1925. Col. 15th Sept. 1930. r.p. 15th Sept. 1934. Rempld 11th Oct. 1939. r.p. 11th Aug. 1940. Served in India 1904–09 and in 1914–18 War from 21st Aug. 1914 with the 14th FA and was CO of the 99th FA. POW Sept. 1914–Jul. 1915. Rotterdam 1918–19. India 1919–24. Army Med. Service Home Guard. Medals: DSO (1st Jan. 1917), bar (28th Jul. 1918), 1914 S., BWM, VM. MID 4th Jan. 1917, 24th Dec. 1917, 30th Dec. 1918. d. 20th Dec. 1953 at Swanage, Dorset.

KELLY James Patrick Address: 20 Fitzwilliam Ave., Ormeau, Belfast. MB, BCh DPH (QUB 1934). Sq. Ldr (N) RAFVR.

KELLY John Address: 81 Howth Rd, Dublin. MB, BCh (NUI 1940). Lt RAMC 24th Oct. 1942.

KELLY John Address: 28 St Patrick's Hill, Cork. MB, BCh, BAO (UCC 1926), FRCS (London 1931). Lt RAMC.

KELLY Mary Brielen MB, BCh (TCD 1943). RAMC.

KELLY Matthew Clement MB, BCh (QUB 1935). Lt Col. RAMC.

KELLY Patrick Joseph MB, BCh (NUI 1939). Flt Lt RAF 27th Aug. 1941.

KELLY Thomas MB (NUI 1942). Lt RAMC 22nd Aug. 1942.

*****KELLY** Thomas Anthony b. IFS. s. Jack and Anne Kelly. Husband of Pauline M. Kelly of Cork. MB, BCh, BAO (UCC 1932). Capt. 157851 RAMC. Died 7th Dec. 1942 at sea aged 35. Commemorated at Brookwood 1939–45, Surrey. Memorial Panel 18, Column 1.

KELLY Thomas Bernard b. 1870. LRCP (Edin. 1891), L (1891), F (1895), RCS (Edin.), LFPS (Glasgow 1891). With the MN and helped evacuation of Dunkirk. DSO.

KELLY Thomas James b. 18th Apr. 1890, Killarney, Co. Kerry. Educ. Clongowes Wood Coll. TCD. MB (1913), BCh, BAO, LRCPI, LRCSI, MD (1929), MA (1929). Lt RAMC SR 26th May 1913. Mobd 6th Aug. 1914. Capt. 1st Apr. 1915. PC Lt RAMC (T/Capt.) 1st Jan. 1917. Capt. 6th Feb. 1918. A/Maj. 25th Feb.–30th Sept. 1918. RAF MS 25th May 1920. WWII Air Vice Marshal Bomber Comd. Served with BEF France Sept.–Oct. 1914, 1915–17, 1918–20. Wounded Nov. 1917 and Oct. 1918. DADMS. Went on to serve in Bomber Comd RAF 1941–42. Medals: CBE, MC (1st Jan. 1917), 1914 S., BWM, VM, Russian OStStan 3rd Class (14th Jan. 1918), L. of Merit (US). MID 30th May 1918 and three times for WWII.

KELLY Thomas Leary Address: The Rectory, Dungiven, Co. Derry. MB, BCh (TCD 1941). Capt. RAMC.

KELLY Veronica Mary Address: Portumna, Co. Galway. MB, BCh (NUI 1942). Lt RAMC 7th Oct. 1944.

KELLY William MB, BCh, BAO (1926). Lt RAMC 14th Nov. 1938.

KELLY William MB, BCh, BAO (UCD 1933). Capt. RAMC.

KENNEDY Alan Francis b. 23rd Sept. 1903 at Belgaun in India. MB, BCh, BAO (TCD 1929), MD (Dublin 1946), MRCPI (1947), FRCPI (1951). PC Lt RAMC 12th Feb. 1930. Capt. 13th Feb. 1933. Retired 8th Jul. 1936. Rejoined 1st Sept. 1939. A/Maj. 12th Jan. 1940. T/Maj. 12th Apr. 1940. A/Lt Col. 1st Mar. 1941. T/Lt Col. 1st Jun. 1941. A/Col. 16th Jul. 1945. Hon. Lt Col. 15th Nov. 1945. Served India 1931–36. BEF France 1940. CO 180 Fd Amb. 1941–43 and 210 Fd Amb. 1943–44. NWE 1944–45.: CO 8th Gen. Hosp. 1944. 10 CCS 1944–45. ADMS HQ Netherlands Dist. 1945. CO 105 Gen. Hosp. 1945. Medals: OBE (19th Mar. 1045), 1939–45 S., France and Germany S., DM, WM, Netherlands O. of Orange Nassau with Swords (Offrs) 16th Jan. 1948. d. 20th Mar. 1959.

KENNEDY Charles Denis MB, BCh, BAO (1927). Flt Offr RAF 7th Jan. 1943.

KENNEDY David McMaster Address: Irish Hill House, Ballynure, Co. Antrim. MB, BCh (QUB 1942). Capt. RAMC.

KENNEDY, Dermot Patrick Address: Hollywood, Carrickmines, Co. Dublin. MB BCh (NUI 1932), FRCSI (1936). Volunteered for the RAMC in 1942. Served in Tunisia, Sicily and Italy (Monte Casino) EMS Hosps. Algeria with 1st Army (Op. Torch Nov. 1942), 31st Fd Surgical Hosp.

KENNEDY Harold Address: 463 Upr Newtownards Rd, Belfast. MB, BCh (QUB 1937). Capt. RAMC. MBE.

KENNEDY Kenneth Rodney Address: 332 Ormeau Rd, Belfast. MB, BCh (QUB 1939). Surg. Lt Comdr RN.

KENNEDY Robert Hunter Address: Clements Hill, Ballyclare, Co. Antrim. MB, BCh (QUB 1939). Surg. Lt RNVR.

KENNEDY Thomas Fuller b. 12th Jun. 1892, Dublin. s. James S. (bank manager) and Martha Kennedy, Donnybrook, Dublin. Educ. RUI, MB (1914), BCh, BAO, DPH (London), RCSP (1922). R. C. of I. Lt SR 22nd Oct. 1914. Mobd RAMC 31st Oct. 1914. Capt. 30th Apr. 1915. PC Lt (T/Capt.) 1st Jan. 1917. Capt. 30th Apr. 1918. A/Maj. 29th May 1918–28th May 19. T/Maj. 13th Mar. 1922–9th Dec 24. Maj. 22nd Oct. 1926. Lt Col. 20th Apr. 1939. A/Col. 10th Dec. 1941. T/Col. 10th Jun. 1942. Col. 5th Dec. 1944. A/Brig. 6th Jun. 1944–4th Jul. 46. r.p. Hon. Brig. 26th Feb. 1949. Served in 1914–18 War. EEF Aug. 1915. Gallipoli, Serbia, Macedonia. Palestine 1919. Egypt 1919–20. India 1924–29. China 1933–36: DADH China Comd 1934–36. ADH HQ Aldershot Comd 1936–39. Palestine 1939–40: SMO 18th Inf. Brig. May–Jun. 1939. CO Mil. Hosp. Haifa 1939–40. HQ Scottish Comd ADH 1940–41. DDH 1941–43. Prof. Hyg. RAM Coll. 1943–44 and 1946–48. NWE/BAOR 1944–46. Dep. of Public Health CA Div. SHAEF 1944–45, PMO Public Health Branch CCG 1945–46. Medals: OBE (1st Jan. 1919), 1915 S., BWM, VM, 1939–45 France and Germany S., DM, WM, Kt Comdr O. of Orange Nassau with Swords. MID 22nd Jan. 1918.

KENNEDY Walter Alexander Address: 463 Upr Newtownards Rd, Knock, Belfast. MB, BCh (QUB 1942). Flt Lt (M) RAFVR.

KENNY Michael Martin Augustine MB (NUI 1944). Flt Offr RNVR 29th Nov. 1945.

KENNY William Thomas Address: Strathdoon, Marlboro Rd, Glenageary, Dublin. MB, BCh (TCD 1938), FRCSI (1943). Sq. Ldr RAF.

KENT Pierce Address: 13 Rostrevor Tce, Rathgar, Dublin. MB, BCh (NUI 1938). Lt IMS 1st May 1939.

KERLEY Peter James MB, BCh (UCD 1923), MC (NUI 1932), FRCP (London 1943). Lt RAMC. First enlisted 18th Dec.1939.

KERNOHAN David Herbert Address: Springhill, Cullybackey, Co. Antrim. MB, BCh (QUB 1921). Surg. Comdr RNVR.

KERNOHAN Robert Alexander MB, BCh (QUB 1923). Maj. RAMC.

KERNOHAN Robert James Address: 57 Knutsford Dr., Belfast. MB, BCh (QUB 1941). Capt. RAMC.

KERR Arthur Ian Keith Address: Garvagh, Co. Derry. MB, BCh (QUB 1942). Capt. RAMC.

KERR Cecil Hugh MB, BCh, MC (QUB 1923). Col. RAMC. DSO. MID.

KERR Eric David Address: 2 Anglesea Rd, Ballsbridge, Dublin. MB, BCh (TCD 1941). Capt. RAMC. Served in Burma.

KERRIGAN Henry Address: Westlands, Glen Rd, Belfast. MB, BCh (QUB 1942). Capt. RAMC.

KERRIGAN Thomas Address: Westlands, Glen Rd, MB, BCh (QUB 1940). Maj. RAMC.

KIDD Cecil William Address: 1 Hampton Tce, 180, Lisburn Rd, Belfast. MB, BCh (QUB 1925), MD (QUB 1933). Wing Comdr (M) Royal Australian Air Force. OBE. MID.

KILLEEN Oscar Henry TCD 1939. MB (1946). Royal Marine Commandos. Wounded three times.

KILLIAN Patrick Aloysius MB, BCh, BAO (1926). Flt Offr RAF 19th Dec. 1941.

KILPATRICK James MacConnell b. Belfast, 1st Mar. 1902. Educ. Royal Belfast Academical Institution and MB (QUB), BCh, BAO (1924). RAF 1925. Princess Mary's R. Airforce Hosp. Halton 1927. Served in Iraq and W. Africa. Spent the year 1936 at the RAF Institute of Pathology and Tropical Medicine Halton. 1937–39 at the Chemical Defence Experimental Estab. Porton. OC RAF Hosp. Church Village, Raucbey and Northallerton. Director of Hygiene and Research 1947. Deputy Director General 1950. Appointed Director General of Medical Services 1951. Dean of the London School of Hygiene and Tropical Medicine. Director General of RAF Medical Services 1957. Medals: Knighted 1953. CB (1952), OBE (1946). Awarded Arnott Memorial Gold Medal by the Irish Medical Schools and Graduates Association for work at Halton during an outbreak of cerebrospinal meningitis. d. Suddenly in London on 4th Apr. 1960.

KING Cecil b. 11th Aug. 1903, Castlepollard, Co. Westmeath. MB, BCh, BAO (TCD 1929). PC Lt RAMC 28th Apr. 1933. Capt. 1st May 1934. A/Maj. 29th Jul. 1940. T. Maj. 29th Oct. 1940. Maj. 28th Apr. 1943. A/Lt Col. 17th Jun. 1942. T/Lt Col. 17th Sept. 1942. h.p. (disability) 18th Mar. 1945. f.p. 10th May 1945. Retired Hon. Lt Col. 21st Jun. 1955. Served India 1934–30. BEF France 1940.

India/SEAC 1941–44 (invalided). CO 62nd Indian Fd Amb. 1942–43. CMF 1946–49. CO 48 Gen. Hosp. 1946–47. 70th Gen. Hosp. 1947–49. 31 Gen. Hosp./BMH Klagenfurt 1948–49. Mil. Hosp. Waringfield 1950–52. BAOR 1952–54. CO 31 Fd Amb. 1952. Medals: IGSM and cl. NWF (1935), 1939–45 S., Burma S., DM, WM.

KING Francis b. 15th Jun. 1906, Castlepollard, Co. Westmeath. MB, BCh, BAO (TCD 1932), MA (Dublin 1935). PC Lt RAMC 24th Jan. 1923. Capt. 1st May 1934. A/Maj. 5th Jan. 1940. T/Maj. 5th Apr.–30th Jun. 1940. Maj. 24th Jan. 1943. A/Lt Col. 6th Feb. 1947. T/Lt Col. 8th May 1947. Lt Col. 21st Feb. 1948. r.p. 21st Sept. 1954. Served India 1934–39. BEF France 1939–40. MEF/CMF 1942–46. ADMS HQ BAS France 1947. W. Africa: CO 44 (Kaduna) Mil. Hosp. 1947–49. ADMS HQ W. Comd 1949–51. CO 5th Fd Amb. 1951–53: MELF 1951–53 (invalided). CO Mil. Hosp. Waringfield 1953–54 and Mil. Hosp. Shorncliffe 1954. Medals: 1939–45 S., Africa S (with 8th Army cl.), Italy S., DM, WM.

KING Martin Edward Matthew Address: 3 Eaton Sq., Monkstown, Co. Dublin. L.LM (RCPI 1933), L.LM (RCSI 1933). Lt RAMC 1941.

*****KING** Maurice Baylis b. 15th Mar. 1890, Dublin. Educ. TCD. MB (1915), BCh. Lt RAMC SR 9th Aug. 1914. Mobd 1st Oct. 1915. Capt. 1st Apr. 1919. A/Maj. 25th Feb. 1918–23rd Feb. 19. Maj. 1st Oct. 1927. A/Lt Col. 5th Mar. 1940, T/Lt Col. 5th Jun. 1940–22nd Feb. 42. Lt Col. 13th Apr. 1942. A/Col. 8th Jun. 1942. T/Col. 8th Dec. 1942–4th Mar. 43 and 15th Sept. 1943–9th Feb. 45. Served in 1914–18 War. Egypt 1915–16. France 1916–19. Egypt 1919–21 (invalided). Constantinople Sept.–Oct. 1922. India 1922–25. BAOR 1926. India 1928–36 and 1937–40. BEF France Apr.–May 1940. N. Africa 1942–43. MEF 1943. CMF 1943–45. HQ Allied Control Comm. Italy to 1945. Medals: OBE, MC (1st Jan. 1917), bar (16th Sept. 1917), BWM, VM. MID 10th Jul. 1919. d. 9th Feb. 1945, Italy. KIA.

KINNEAR Nigel Alexander b. 3rd Apr. 1907. s. James and Margaret (née Robinson) Kinnear, Palmerstown, Glenageary, Co. Dublin. MB, BCh (TCD 1930), FRCSI (1934). President RCSI 1961–63. RAMC Belsen Concentration Camp.

KINSELLA John Address: Coolgreany, Edenderry, Co. Offaly. L.LM (RCPI 1938), L.LM (RCSI 1938). Lt RAMC 1941.

KIRK Christopher Address: 56 Rugby Rd, Belfast. MB, BCh (QUB 1930). Maj. RAMC.

KIRK Hector Howard Address: Dromore St, Ballynahinch, Co. Down. LRCP (Edinburgh 1940), LRCS (Edinburgh 1940), LRFPS (Glasgow 1940). Surg. Lt RNVR.

*KIRKPATRICK** Ross McFaul Address: 30 Rosetta Pk, Ormeau Rd, Belfast. MB, BCh (QUB 1940). Surg. Lt RNVR. DSC. KIA.

KIRWAN Michael Edward L.LM, LS (1929), MB, BCh (1931), DPH (TCD 1932). Maj. IMS.

KNIGHT William Alexander Young MB, BCh (TCD 1929). Col. RAMC. Served in Malta, France and N. Africa.

KNOTT Harold Edwin MB, BCh (TCD 1928), MD (TCD 1935), DPH RCPS (England 1936). Col. RAMC. Served India. OBE.

KNOX Harold Joseph Address: 41 Cliftonville Rd, Belfast. MB, BCh (QUB 1935). Flt Lt (M) RAFVR.

KNOX William Alexander Address: Knowehead, Ballymoney, Co. Antrim. MB, BCh, DPH (QUB 1941). Capt. RAMC.

KYLE James Taylor MB, BCh (QUB 1912), FRCS (Edinburgh 1920). Lt Col. RAMC.

KYLE John Bruce Address: 109 Malone Rd, Belfast. MB, BCh (QUB 1939). Capt. RAMC.

KYLE Samuel Wasson b. 8th Mar. 1884, Ballymena, Co. Antrim. s. James (farmer) and Lizzie Kyle, Galgorm Parks, Galgorm, Co. Antrim. Educ. RUI Belfast and Dublin. MB (QUB 1906), BCh, BAO. R. Presbyterian. Lt RAMC 1st Aug. 1908. Capt. 1st Feb. 1912. Bt. Maj. 3rd Jun. 1918. A/Maj. 8th Nov. 1918. Maj. 1st Aug. 1920. Bt. Col. 1st Jul. 1932. Lt Col. 13th Oct. 1933. T/Col. 10th Jan. 1936. Col. 11th Apr. 1937. r.p. remained employed 8th Mar. 1941. A/Maj. Gen. 26th Mar. 1941. T/Maj. Gen. 26th Mar. 1942. r.p. Hon. Maj. Gen. 12th Jan. 1945. Served India 1911–15. Mesopotamia from 6th Dec. 1915–19. Invalided in India Oct.–Dec. 1919. BAOR 1922–24. India 1924–25. Egypt 1932–36. SMO and CO Mil. Hosp. Ras-el-Tin 1934–35. ADMS HQ 5th Div. 1936. ADMS HQ BF in Palestine 1936–37. ADGAMS War Office 1937–41. DDMS HQ E. Comd 1941–45. Medals: 1915 S., BWM, VM, DM, WM. MID 19th Oct. 1916, 27th Aug. 1918.

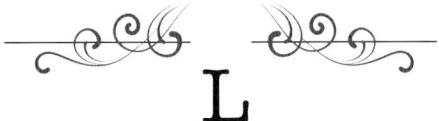

L

LAHIFF Michael James L.LM (RCPI 1932), L.LM (RCSI 1932). Lt RAMC 1939.

LAIRD Robert Marshal Address: 11 Hampton Pk, Ormeau, Belfast. MB, BCh (QUB 1942). Flt Lt (M) RAFVR.

LAIRD William Herbert Address: 48 Myrtlefield Pk, Belfast. MB, BCh (QUB 1941). Sq. Ldr (M) RAFVR.

LALOR Thomas Francis MB, BCh (NUI 1938). Lt RAMC 18th May 1939. Capt. 1st Sept. 1940.

LAMB Henry Harold Brian Address: Lisnadill Rectory, Armagh. MB, BCh (TCD 1942). RNVR.

LAMBKIN Ernest Charles b. 9th Aug. 1884, Donnybrook, Dublin. s. Charles (wine merchant) and Sophia Lambkin, 4, Avoca Tce, Blackrock, Co. Dublin. Educ. MB (TCD 1908), BCh, BAO, LM (Rot. Hosp.). R. RC. Lt RAMC 30th Jan. 1909. Capt. 30th Jul. 1912. A/Maj. 6th Jun. 1918–15th Dec. 1919. Maj. 30th Jan. 1921. A/Lt Col. 5th Jul. 1917. r.p. with rank of Lt Col. 20th Sept. 1931. Rempld 2nd Sept. 1939. A/Col. 15th Feb. 1944. T/Col. 15th Aug. 1944. r.p. 21st Aug. 1945. Served in Hong Kong 1911–15. EEF 2nd Jun. 1915–19. CO 147th Fd Amb. 1917–18. India 1928–31. CO Mil. Hosp. Holywood NI 1939–44. CO Mil. Hosp. Bangor 1944–45. Spec. in Dermatology and VD. Medals: DSO (11th Apr. 1918), 1915 S., BWM. VM. MID Aug. 1915, 21st Jun. 1916, 7th Oct. 1918. d. 4th Dec. 1958 at Liskilleen, Shankill, Co. Dublin.

LAMBKIN John Charles b. 21st Nov. 1912, Hong Kong. Address: Liskillen, Shankill, Co. Dublin. MB, BCh, BAO (TCD 1937). Lt RAMC 22nd Oct. 1937. Capt. 1st Jan. 1939. PC Capt. 1st Jan. 1945. A/Maj. 25th Jun. 1941. T/Maj. 25th Sept. 1941. Maj. 1st Jul. 1946. A/Lt Col. 21st Sept. 1943. T/Lt Col. 21st Dec. 1943. Lt Col. 14th Nov. 1952. A/Brig. 28th Jan. 1960. r.p. 21st Nov. 1962. Served Palestine 1938–39. Sudan/MEF 1939–42: RMO 1st Worcs. 1938–41. India 1942–44. CO 189th Fd Amb. 1943–44. NWE/BAOR 1945–46. CO 146th Fd Amb. 1945–46. MELF 1947–48. CO 132nd Fd Amb. 1947. CO Mil. Hosp. Gaza 1947–48. CO Mil Hosp. Haifa 1948. FARELF 1948–51. CO 1st Fd Amb. 1948–49. BMH Kowloon 1949–50. SMO Br. Gurkhas India 1950–51. BAOR: CO 29th Fd Amb. 1952–53. CO Mil. Hosp. Wheatley, Oxford 1953–54. E. Africa CO Mil. Hosp. Nairobi 1954–57. ADMS HQ Scottish Comd 1958–60. CO Mil. Hosp. Cowglen 1960–62. Medals: OBE (28th Aug. 1956), GSM (cl. Palestine 1936–39),

1939–45 S., Africa S., WM, GSM (cl. Palestine 1947–48, cl. Malaya, AGSM (cl. Kenya).

LANDAU Ernest Myer MB, BCh (TCD 1923). Capt. UDF.

LANE Jeremiah Patrick Address: 3 Maymount, Friars Walk, Cork. MB, BCh, BAO (UCC 1937). Lt RAMC.

LANE Wilfred Francis b. 20th Oct. 1924 at Dharmsala, India. MB, BCh, BAO (TCD 1927), DPH (England 1936), MSc (TCD 1939). PC Lt RAMC 27th Jul. 1927. Capt. 27th Jan. 1931. Maj. 27th Jul. 1937. A/Lt Col. 1st Jan. 1942. T/Lt Col. 1st Apr. 1942. Lt Col. 1st Mar. 1946. A/Col. 14th Feb. 1946. T/Col. 14th Mar. 1947. r.p. Hon. Col. 21st Jun. 1948. Served India 1929–34. Burma 1939–41. ADP HQ Army 1942. India 1942–44. ADP GHQ (I) 1943–44. ADP S. Army 1944. ADP Western Comd 1946. DDP GHQ MELF 1946–48. Medals: 1939–45 S., Burma S., WM. MID 28th Oct. 1941.

***LANG** William Hunter b. Belfast. s. Douglas H. Lang and Agnes M. Lang of Glasgow. MB, ChB. Capt. 23912 RAMC. d. Italy 17th Dec. 1943 aged 24. Buried in Sango River War Cemetery, Plot IXA42. MC.

LANGFORD Cyril Coplen MB BCh (TCD 1933). RNVR.

LANIGAN-O'KEEFE Francis Martin TCD 1940. Flt Lt RAF. Served in India.

LANTIN Harold Address: 15 Cliftonpark Ave., Belfast. MB, BCh (QUB 1942). Capt. RAMC.

LAPEDUS Bethel Address: 38 Bloomfield Ave., South Circular Rd, Dublin. MB, BCh (TCD 1936). Maj. RAMC. Served India, Western Desert and Tunisia. Wounded.

LAPPIN William Parsons MB, BCh, BAO (UCD 1928). Lt IMS. 4th Feb. 1929. 1945 Lt Col. OBE 14th Jun.1945.

LARGE Stanley Dermott b. 21st Oct. 1889, Larne, Co. Antrim. s. W.H. Large. Educ. R. High Sch. Edinburgh, Coll. Surgs Edin. LDS (Edin. 1911), LRCP&S (Edin.), LRFPS (Glasgow 1912). Married Violet Muriel Elise, dt. D. Cowan. Lt RAMC 24th Jan. 1913. Capt. 30th Mar. 1915. A/Maj. 25th Feb. 1918. A/Lt Col. 3rd Sept. 1918. r.p. Lt Col. 6th Jan. 1923. Rempld 2nd Sept. 1939. A/Col. 1st Aug. 1944. T/Col. 1st Feb. 1945. r.p. Hon Col. 7th Sept. 1945. Served BEF France and Belgium from 18th Aug. 1914–19. CO 76th Fd Amb. 1918–19. RMO 1st Scots Guards 1920–21. India 1921–22. BEF France 1939–40. CO 113 Con. Dep. 1940–42 and 102 Con. Dep. 1942–45. Medals: DSO (1st Jan. 1918), MC (14th Jan. 1916), 1914 S., BWM, VM, 1939–45 S. MID 1st Jan. 1916, 24th Dec. 1917. d. 2nd Apr. 1965, Lochgoilhead, Argyll.

LAVELLE John MB, BCh, BAO (NUI 1940). RAMC Lt 14th Nov. 1939.

LAVELLE Kenneth Norman Address: 15 Chichester Ave., Antrim Rd, Belfast. MB, BCh, DPH (QUB 1928). Capt. RAMC.

LAVELLE Ronald Featherston Address: 15 Chichester Ave., Antrim Rd, Belfast. MB, BCh, LDS (QUB 1932). Surg. Lt RNVR.

LAWLESS Desmond James s. John and Mrs B. Lawless (née Mullen). b. Monaghan. Address: 550 North Circular Rd, Dublin. MB, BCh, BAO (UCD 1934). Col. RAMC. Served in Burma. d. aged 60, leaving a wife and three daughters. OBE.

LAWLESS John Robert Address: North Circular Rd, Dublin. L.LM (RCPI 1938), L.LM (RCSI 1938). Lt RAMC 1939.

LEAHY James Daly MB, BCh (TCD 1921). Air Commodore RAF. MC.

LEANE Michael Gerard MB, BCh (TCD 1931). IMS.

LEASK Norman Hogarth MD. MB, BCh (TCD 1931). Maj. RAMC.

LEE George Angus McLean Address: 8 Iona Crescent, Glasnevin, Dublin. MB, BCh (TCD 1942). Surg. Lt RNVR.

LEE Percy Alexander MB, BCh (TCD 1942). Wing Comdr (M) RAFVR.

LEE William Patrick Address: Croaghter Pk, Glasheen Rd, Cork. MB, BCh (NUI 1940). Lt RAMC 27th Feb. 1943.

LEHANE Dermot Address: Rock Fern, Carrigrohane, Co. Cork. MB, BCh, BAO (UCC 1940). Lt RAMC.

LENNON Robert Wilson Address: Waverley House, Knock, Belfast. Campbell College. L.LM (RCPI 1937), L.LM (RCSI 1937). Capt. RAMC.

LENNON William Address: Crescent House, Belfast. MB, BCh (QUB 1922), MD (QUB 1925), MRCP (London 1933). Surg. Lt Comdr RNVR.

LENNOX Thomas Madill Address: 58 Eglantine Ave., Belfast. Campbell College. MB, BCh, DPH (QUB 1939). Capt. 114982 RAMC. MID 20th Dec. 1939. Married Veronica in Belfast 1947. d. 1986 Belfast.

LENTIN Michael MB, BCh, BAO (UCC 1937). Sq. Comdr RAF.

LESSELBAUM Harvey Phillips MB, BCh (TCD 1941). RNVR.

L'ESTRANGE Francis Albert b. 9th Oct. 1889, Co. Dublin. s. Lt Col. Albert H. L'Estrange (AMS) and Martha E. L'Estrange, 10 Eglington Rd, Donnybrook, Dublin. Educ. TCD. BA (1913), MB (1915), BCh, BAO, LM (Rot. Hosp.). R. C. of I. Lt RAMC 24th Mar. 1915. Capt. 24th Mar. 1916. Pc. Capt. 1st Jun. 1919. Maj. 28th Mar. 1927.

A/Lt Col. 2nd Apr. 1940. T/Lt Col. 2nd to 4th Jul. 1940. r.p. ill health 28th Oct. 1940. Served in France from 6th Apr. 1915–16 and 1917–18. Egypt 1918–19. India 1920. Mesopotamia 1920–23. W. Africa 1934–35 & 1926–27. BAOR 1928–09. India 1930–34. Malaya 1936–40. CO 196th Fd Amb. Apr.–Jul. 1940. MID 12th Jan. 1920. Medals: 1915 S., BWM, VM, GSM cls Iraq and Kurdistan, MID Jun.1918.

LEVIS Richard Desmond TCD 1942. Surg. Lt RNVR.

LEWIS Joseph Tegart Address: 25 College Gdns, Belfast. Campbell College. MB, BCh (QUB 1921), MD (QUB 1924), LRCP (London 1927). Lt Col. RAMC. MID.

LIGGETT Samuel Wilberforce Address: Tullyhue House, Tandragee, Co. Armagh. MB, BCh (QUB 1935). Sq. Ldr (M) RAFVR.

LIGHTBODY John Address: 21 Hamilton Rd, Bangor, Co. Down. MB, BCh (QUB 1937). Lt Col. IMS.

LILLIE John MB, BCh (QUB 1939). Flt Lt (M) RAFVR.

LINEHAN Richard Stephen Address: 42 Earlswood Rd, Belfast. MB, BCh (QUB 1940). Sq. Ldr (M) RAFVR.

LINTON Robert MB, BCh (QUB 1923). Lt Col. IMS.

LISTON James Campbell Address: 4 Victoria Tce, Larne, Co. Antrim. MB, BCh (QUB 1922). RAMC. Deceased.

LITTLE Gerald William Address: 22 Mountjoy Sq., Dublin. MB, BCh (TCD 1940). Surg. Lt RNVR.

LLOYD Coote William Address: 15 Ailesbury Rd, Dublin. MB, BCh (TCD 1942). Flt Lt RAF.

LOANE Robert Cecil Ronald Address: 50 Rugby Rd, Belfast. MB, BCh (QUB 1941). Sq. Ldr (M) RAFVR.

LOFTUS John Michael BSc (1920), MB, BCh (1921), DPH (1923), DPM (1931), MD (1932 NUI). RMO 23rd London Bn. Home Guard during WWII. Did Trojan work during the Blitz. d. 18th Sept. 1961 at the Mater General Hospital.

LOGAN Joan Beatty Thomasina Address: Knocknagulla, Whitehead, Co. Antrim. MB, BCh (QUB 1941). Sq. Ldr (M) RAF.

LOGAN John Stephen Address: Knocknagulla, Whitehead, Co. Antrim. MB, BCh (QUB 1939). Lt Col. RAMC.

LOGAN Mary Sinclair Thompson (née Irwin) Address: Bovally, Limavady, Co. Londonderry. MB, BCh (QUB 1940). Flt Lt (M) RAFVR.

LOGAN Robert Francis Leslie Address: 101 Bryansburn Rd, Bangor, Co. Down. MB, BCh (QUB 1940). Troop Ship MO Royal Netherlands Marine Service.

LONGMORE Louis Heaton Valentine MB, BCh (QUB 1940). Maj. NZAMS.

LORD John Graham MB, BCh (QUB 1930). Capt. RAMC. From Mullingar, Co. Westmeath. MC. On May 29th, 1940, when one of our anti-tank guns was in action near his aid post, engaging advancing enemy tanks, Lieutenant Lord displayed courage and devotion to duty of a very high order. In the ensuing actions, while fighting at a very close range, the anti-tank gun was gradually overcome by superior numbers and all the gun crew hit. Lieutenant Lord attended to each casualty at the gun position as it occurred, under heavy fire, treated them at this aid post and eventually got the wounded away in his truck under heavy machine-gun fire. MC.

LOUGHRIDGE David Address: 100 Upr Newtownards Rd, Belfast. MB, BCh (QUB 1921). Maj. RAMC.

LUDLOW Charles Malachi Address: 41 St Laurence Rd, Clontarf, Dublin. MB, BCh (TCD 1939). RAMC.

*****LUSK** George Ian Wilson s. John Brown Lusk and Margaret Dewar Lusk. Address: c/o Dr Samuel Finlay, Lusk, Loughbrickland, Co. Down. MB, BCh (QUB 1940). Capt. RAMC. KIA 30th Apr. 1943, aged 27 years.

LYBURN Rex St John b. 9th May 1906 in Dublin. MA, MB, BCh, BAO (TCD 1929), DPH (1932), MD (Dublin 1935), MRCPI (1935), DObst. RCOG (1947), RCPI (TCD 1954). PC Lt RAMC 22nd Feb. 1932. Resigned 5th Aug. 1933. Rejoined Lt 8th Mar. 1934. Capt. 1st May 1934. A/Maj. 2nd Sept. 1939. T/Maj. 2nd Dec. 1939. Maj. 25th Sept. 1942. A/Lt Col. 9th Feb. 1943. T/Lt Col. 9th May 1943. Lt Col. 22nd Nov. 1947. T/Col. 24th Dec. 1953. Col. 16th Apr. 1956. T/Brig. 10th May 1963. Brig. 29th Oct. 1963. r.p. 9th May 1966. Served India 1933. Egypt 1934–39. BEF France 1939–40. W. Africa 1940–41. Paiforce/MELF 1944–47: ADH HQ Paiforce 1944–45. HQ Palestine 1945–46. GHQ MELF 1946–47. Gibraltar 1949–53: CO Mil Hosp. 1949–52. ADMS FHQ 1952–53. FARELF: CO 33 Gen Hosp. 1953–55. CO QA Mil. Hosp. Millbank 1955–59. Gibraltar ADMS FHQ and CO Mil. Hosp. 1959–63. FARELF: DDMS HQ 17 Burkha Div./OCLF/Malaya area 1963–64. DDMS HQ W.Comd 1964–66. Medals: 1939–45 S., DM, WM, GSM and cl. Palestine 1946, QEII Corn Medal 1953.

LYDON Francis Leo MB, BCh (NUI 1924). Lt RAMC 6th Nov. 1939.

LYLE John Scott MB, BCh (QUB 1922). Maj. RAMC.

LYLE Thomas Address: The Topp, Ballymoney, Co. Andrim. LRCP (Edinburgh 1941), LRCS (Edinburgh 1941), LRFPS (Glasgow 1941). Flt Offr RAF Sept. 1941.

LYNAGH Thomas Bernard MB, BCh (QUB 1926). RAMC.

***LYNCH** Edward George William s. Michael Edward and Grace Penelope (née Kennedy) Lynch. MB, BCh (TCD 1940). Lt IMS 1940. KIA 14th Mar. 1942 aged 26. Buried in Madras War Cemetery, Chennai, Plot 1F4.

LYNCH Patrick Thomas Desmond Address: Eyre Sq., Galway. MB, BCh (NUI 1936). Flt Lt RAFVR 21st Jul. 1944.

LYNCH Philip Vincent Address: 9 Fernside Villas, Summerhill, Cork. MB, BCh, BAO (UCC 1942). Lt RAMC 25th Nov. 1943.

LYNCH Thomas Joseph MB, BCh, BAO (UCD 1923). Lt RAMC. First enlisted 6th Jun. 1940.

LYND William John Address: 24 Alexandra Gdns, Somerton Rd, Belfast. MB, BCh (QUB 1939). Sq. Ldr (M) RAFVR. MID.

LYNHAM John Michael Address: 27 Londonbridge Rd, Sandymount, Dublin. MB, BCh (NUI 1938). Lt RAMC 13th Apr. 1940.

LYONS Arnold Richard Address: 11 Glencoe Pk, Antrim Rd, Belfast. MB, BCh (QUB 1940). Flt Lt (M) RAFVR.

LYONS Clare Frances, Trinity St, Drogheda, Co. Louth. L.LM (RCPI 1938), L.LM (RCSI 1938). Lt RAMC 1940.

LYONS Frederick Maxwell MB, BCh (TCD 1930) RAMC.

LYONS James Francis Louis b. 18th Jun. 1918, Melrose, Sundays Well, Cork. MB, BCh, BAO (NUI 1942). Lt 3rd Jun. 1944. Capt. 3rd Jun. 1945. T/Maj. 30th Dec. 1947. PC Capt. 22nd Jul. 1949. Maj. 3rd Jun. 1952. r.p. disability 11th Feb. 1961. CMF 1945–46. Malta 1946–47. MELF 1947–48. Physn. Mil. Hosp. Chester 1948–49. Mil. Hosp. Catterick 1949–50. W. Africa Mil. Hosp. Accra 1952–55. Lecturer in Trop. Med. RAM Coll. 1955–57. Mil Hosp. Colchester 1957–60. Medals: WM.

LYONS Reginald Francis George Address: Tyrconnel, Perrott Ave., Cork. MB, BCh (TCD 1940). RNVR.

LYTLE Samuel Norman Campbell College. MB, BCh (QUB 1927). Lt Col. RAMC. Polish O. Merit in gold.

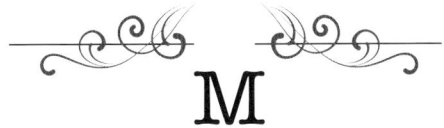

M

McALEER Gerard Ward MB, BCh, BAO (UCD 1926). Flt Offr RAF 1st Jun. 1927.

MacARTHUR Albert Charles Address: 156 Pembroke Rd, Dublin. MB, BCh (TCD 1941). Capt. RAMC 1942.

MacARTHUR Sir William Porter b. 11th Mar. 1884, Belfast. s. John Porter MacArthur (tea merchant), 6 Raglan Rd, Bangor, Co. Down. Educ. RUI (QUB), MB (1908), BCh, BAO, MD (1911), MRCPI (1911), F (1913), MRCSI, DPH (Oxford 1910), DTM&H (Camb.), Hon. DSc (Belfast 1935), FRCP (London 1937). R. Presbyterian. Married Eugenie Therese, dt. Dr L.F. Antelme. Lt RAMC 30th Jan. 1909. Capt. 30th Jul. 1912. Maj. 30th Jan. 1921. A/Lt Col. 24th Oct. 1918. Bt. Lt Col. 9th Feb. 1921. Lt Col. 26th Mar. 1929. T/Col. 26th Dec. 1929. Bt. Col. 29th Sept. 1930. Col. 1st May 1934. Maj. Gen. 16th Sept. 1925. Lt Gen. 1st Mar. 1938. r.p. 1st Aug. 1941. Served Mauritius 1911–14. France and Flanders 1915–16. CO and Chief Instructor AS of Hyg. 1918–21. Prof. Tropical Med. RAM Coll. 1922–29. Shanghai May–Dec. 1927. Aden Sept.–Nov. 1927. Consultant Physn. to Army 1929–32. KHP 29th Sept. 1930. Prof. Trop. Med and Cons. Physician RAM Coll. 1932–34. DDG AMS War Office 1938–41. Col. Comdt RAMC 1946–51. Medals: KCB (8th Jun. 1939), CB (1st Jan. 1938), DSO (14th Jan. 1916), OBE (12th Dec. 1919), 1915 S., BWM, VM, KGV Silver Jub. Medal 1935. MID 1st Jan. 1916. d. 30th Jul. 1964, London.

MacAULEY Henry Treaton, qualified as a doctor in Dublin L.LM (RCPI 1920), L.LM (RCSI 1920) and was practising as a GP in Broadstairs. He volunteered for the RAF in 1940 where he became a squadron leader. He was awarded the OBE for rescuing airmen from a burning aircraft. Medals: OBE. MID.

McAULEY Patrick Matthew Address: Kircubbin, Co. Down. MB, BCh (QUB 1939). Surg. Lt RNVR.

McAULEY William Fergus Address: Kircubbin, Co. Down. MB, BCh (QUB 1942). Surg. Lt RNVR.

McBRIDE William Scott Address: Dromara, Co. Down. MB, BCh (TCD 1930). Maj. RAMC.

McCABE Harold Francis Patrick Address: 26 Rathgar Rd, Dublin. L.LM (RCPI 1941), L.LM (RCSI 1941).

McCABE James MB, BCh (QUB 1938). Capt. RAMC.

McCABE John Knox MB, BCh (QUB 1938). Flt Lt (M) RAFVR. MID.

McCAFFREY Hugh Albert Address: Brownlow Arms Hotel, Lurgan, Co. Armagh. MB, BCh (QUB 1938). Capt. RAMC.

McCANN Henry James b. 26th Aug. 1914, Dublin. MB, BCh, BAO (NUI 1938). Lt 1st May 1939. Capt. 1st May 1940. PC Capt. 1st May 1944. A/Maj. 16th Oct. 1943. T/Maj. 16th Jan. 1944. Maj. 1st May 1947. BEF France 1939–40. MEF 1940–43. BNAF/CMP 1943–44. NWE/BAOR 1945–47. MELF Egypt, Greece 1948–50. Medals: 1939–45 S., Africa S with 8th Army cl., Italy S., France and Germany S., DM, WM. d. 23rd Apr. 1951 at Aldershot, Hants.

McCANN Henry Joseph MB, BCh, BAO (UCD 1926). Surg. Lt RN 19th Jun. 1928.

MacCARTHY Charles Borromeo Address: 74 Old Pk Rd, Belfast. MB, BCh (QUB 1928). Capt. RAMC.

MacCARTHY Joseph Aidan b. 19th Mar. 1913. Address: The Square, Castletownbere, Co. Cork. s. Denis Florence McCarthy (publican and businessman) and Julia MacCarthy (née Murphy). Educ. Dominican Convent and Clongowes Wood College. MB, BCh, BAO (UCC 1939). Flt Lt RAF. Posted to Hastings and then France. Evacuated from Dunkirk. In May 1941 he rescued men from a bomber which had crashed into a bomb store while returning to base. He entered the burning plane with another officer and rescued two men. He received burns to his hands and face and for his bravery he was awarded the George Cross in November 1941. He was ordered to Singapore when the Japanese attacked and was captured in Sumatra. While being transported to Japan with other POWs his ship was sunk by an American submarine. The prisoners were rescued by a Japanese destroyer, but then thrown back into the sea. MacCarthy was picked up by a Japanese fishing boat and endured terrible conditions in a Japanese concentration camp. He was in a working party in Nagasaki when the atomic bomb was dropped on 9th Aug. 1945 and witnessed the explosion. He was the senior Allied Service man when the Japanese surrendered. He was awarded the OBE and retired in 1971 with the rank of Air Commodore. d. 11th Oct. 1995 at Northwood, London.

McCARTHY Charles Thomas MB, BCh (TCD 1923). Malayan Medical Service. POW.

***McCARTHY** Daniel Waldron BA, MB, BCh, BAO (TCD 1937). s. Daniel R. and Claire McCarthy, Fairview, Skibbereen, Co. Cork. Capt. RAMC. KIA. d. Egypt 27th Oct. 1942, aged 26. Buried in El Alamein War Cemetery, Plot XVII.D.5.

McCARTHY Denis Francis Address: Hill Farm, Innishannon, Co. Cork. MB, BCh (UCC 1926), DPH (NUI 1929). Lt IMS.

McCARTHY John Joseph Address: Corlbee, Listowel, Co. Kerry. MB, BCh, BAO (UCC 1936). Lt RAMC.

McCARTHY Thomas Gerald MB, BS, BAO (UCD 1931). Lt RAMC.

McCARTHY Timothy Address: Abbeyside, Dungarvan, Co. Waterford. L.LM (RCPI 1939), L.LM (RCSI 1941).

MacCARTNEY Donald William Address: 9 St Jude's Ave., Ormeau Rd, Belfast. MB, BCh (QUB 1931), MD (QUB 1935), DPH (QUB 1936). Lt Col. RAMC.

MacCARTNEY James Norman MB, BCh (QUB 1935) DPH (QUB 1938), MD (QUB 1940). Lt Col. RAMC. MBE. MID.

McCARTNEY Ernest Thom Address: Lincluden, Lodge Rd, Coleraine, Co. Derry. MB, BCh (TCD 1936). Capt. RAMC. POW Middle East 1943. Released by RN 1943. MC.

McCAUL Kevin L.LM (RCPI 1937), L.LM (RCSI 1937).

McCAULLY Desmond George MB, BCh TCD 1930. Lt Col. RAMC & IMS. Invalided out 1944.

McCAULLY Douglas Robert Address: Ardlynn, Harbour Rd, Bray, Co. Wicklow. MB, BCh (TCD 1941) RAMC.

McCAULLY Menzies Llwelyn 4th s. Mr and Mrs James Mc Caully, Clogbeg. Educ. Clongowes College. MB, BCh (TCD 1926). British Colonial Service, Fiji. d. 8th Aug. 1952.

McCAW David Address: 23 St Ives Gdns, Stranmillis Rd, Belfast. MB, BCh (QUB 1940). Flt Lt (M) RAFVR.

McCAW John William Address: Harbour Rd, Dalkey, Co. Dublin. MB, BCh (TCD 1946). AC/2 RAF 1944.

McCLATCHEY Samuel Jones Address: Dunroman, Old Stranmillis Rd, Belfast. MB, BCh (QUB 1939), DPH (QUB 1941). Sq. Ldr (M) RAFVR.

McCLAY Andrew Oswald Address: 29 Cliftonville Rd, Belfast. MB, BCh (QUB 1941). Maj. RAMC.

McCLEARY Cecil Allen Address: 64 Victoria St, Lurgan, Co. Armagh. MB, BCh DPH (QUB 1939). Capt. RAMC.

McCLELLAND John Alexander Harold Address: 45 Lisburn Rd, Belfast. MB, BCh (QUB 1937). Capt. RAMC.

McCLELLAND John Dunlop Address: Rosebank, Gracehill, Ballymena, Co. Antrim. L.LM (RCPI 1932), L.LM (RCSI 1932). Lt RAMC 1941.

McCLELLAND Robert Sherrard Address: 33 Charlotte St, Ballymoney, Co. Antrim. MB, BCh (QUB 1941). Maj. RAMC.

McCLINTOCK Joseph Address: Cooneen, Fivemiletown, Co. Tyrone. MB, BCh (QUB 1939). Surg. Lt RNVR.

*****McCLOGHRY** Charles Edward b. 11th Nov. 1912, Rusheen. 2nd s. James Palmer and Matilda McCloghry of Ballincar, Rosses Point, Co. Sligo. MB, BCh, BAO (QUB 1930–36). Lt RAMC 23rd Apr. 1937. Capt. 23rd Apr. 1938. Served Palestine, invalided 16th October. MO 1st R. East Kent Regt. MO 1st W. York Regt. OC 3rd Cav. Fd Amb. Indian Div. Attd Rifle Brig. 5th Gen. Hosp. Discharged permanently unfit 3rd Jul. 1940. Medals: GSM Palestine, Africa S., DM. d. Renislow Hosp. Durban, South Africa 18th Mar. 1941, aged 28. Buried in Durban (Stellawood) Cemetery, Block F, Grave 14. Commemorated QUB War Memorial.

McCLURKIN Thomas MB, BCh (QUB 1915), DPH (RCPS England 1923). Air Commodore (M) RAF.

McCOLLUM David Hugh Address: Islandeffrick, Coleraine, Co. Derry. MB, BCh (QUB 1940). Capt. RAMC. MC.

McCOLLUM James Kinloch Address: 2 University Sq., Belfast. MB, BCh (QUB 1929), MC (QUB 1937), MRCPI (1939). Col. RAMC.

McCOLLUM John Kinloch Address: Drumcroon House, Coleraine, Co. Derry, MB, BCh (QUB 1933). Lt Col. RAMC.

McCOLLUM William Kinloch MB, BCh (QUB 1930). Capt. RAMC.

McCOMBE John Smith b. 9th Apr. 1885, Edinburgh. Educ. RUI. MB (QUB 1907), BCh, BAO, BS (1907). Lt RAMC 4th Feb. 1908. Capt. 4th Aug. 1911. Maj. 4th Feb. 1920. Lt Col. 4th Jun. 1933. Col. 1st Mar. 1937. r.p. Remained employed 1st Mar. 1941. A/Brig. 6th May 1943. T/Brig. 6th Nov. 1943. r.p. Hon. Brig. 1st Dec. 1944. India 1909–14. Served in 1914–18 War Mesopotamia 25th Nov. 1914–21st Apr. 1917. India 1917–19 and 1920–25. Egypt 1925–30. ADMS HQ S. Comd 1932–34. India 1934–36. CO BMH Mhow 1934–35. BMH Calcutta 1936. Invalided. DDMS HQ Malta Comd 1937–42. ADMS HQ NI Dist. 1942–43. DDMS HQ NI Comd 1943–44. Medals: DSO for bravery in the field (25th Aug. 1917), 1915 S., BWM, VM. MID 15th Aug. 1917. Holder of the ancient Memorial Medal and 2 Royal Humane Society medals. Twice married, to Mrs Doris Leach who died in 1946 and secondly, in 1951, to Joyce, widow of the 6th Baron Talbot of Malahide. He had a lifelong interest in the RAMC and purchased the Hale VC and other medals and presented them to the Headquarters Mess of the Corp at Millbank. d. 19th Oct. 1959, Dublin. Buried St Patrick's C. of I, Enniskerry, Co. Wicklow.

McCONKEY George Sydney b. 21st Apr. 1890, Dublin. s. George McConkey (RIC Staff Offr) 4 Mount Temple Tce, Dartry Rd, Dublin. Educ. St Andrews Coll. Dublin 28th Aug. 1900–30th Jun. 1901. TCD (1912) MB (1914), BCh, BAO, MD (1923). R. C. of I. Lt SR RAMC 28th Aug. 1914. Capt. 1st Apr.1915. PC. Capt. 1st Apr. 1919. Maj. 28th Aug. 1926. Lt Col. 6th Jun. 1937. A/Col. 26th Feb. 1940. T/Col. 26th Aug. 1940–3rd Apr. 1941 and 18th Jun. 1941–14th Jun. 1943. Col. 15th Jun. 1943. T/Brig. 19th Mar–1st Oct. 1945 and 14th Jun. 1946 to 10th Sept. 1947. r.p. Hon Brig. 8th Jul. 1948. Served in 1914–18 War France 11th May 1915–19. India 1919–23. Afghanistan 1919. Waziristan 1919–20. India 1919–23. Bermuda 1929–32. Egypt 1935–36. BEF France: OIC Med. Div. Gen. Hosp. 1939–40. CO 32 Gen. Hosp. 1940–41. MEF 1940–43: CO 9 Gen. Hosp. Jun.–Sept. 1941. DDMS HQ Alexandria area 1941–43. DDMS HQ 13 Corp Jan. 1943. ADMS HQ E. Riding and Lincs. Dist. May–Jul. 1943. ADMS HQ E. Kent Dist. 1943–44. Syria and Palestine DDMS 1944–45. DDMS HQ BT Palestine and Trans-Jordan 1946–47. Medals: OBE (9th Sept. 1942), 1915 S., BWM, VM, IGS Medal with cl. Afghan. 1919 and Waz. 1919–21 and Mahsud. 1919–20. 1939–45 S., Africa S. with 8th Army cl., DM. WM. MID 26th Jul. 1940, 30th Dec. 1941. d. 26th Jul. 1960, Millbank, London.

McCONKEY John Travers b. 30th May 1890. LRCPSI LM (Dub). T/C Lt 12th Apr. 1915. Capt. 12th Apr. 1916. PC Capt. 1st Apr. 1919. Maj. 12th Apr. 1927. A/Lt Col. 25th Oct. 1939. T/Lt Col. 24th Mar. 1940. Lt Col. 1st Mar. 1941. A/Col. 1st Aug. 1941. T/Col. 1st Feb. 1942. A/Brig. 14th Jan. 1945. T/Brig. 14th Jul. 1945. r.p. Hon. Brig. 20th Nov. 1948. Served France Sept.–Nov. 1915. Salonika 1915–18 (invalided). N. Russia Mar.–Oct. 1919. Mesopotamia 1920–23. W. Africa 1924–25 and 1916–27. India 1929–34. NWF 1931. Egypt 1934–39. Palestine Sept.–Oct. 1936. CO 197 Fd Amb. 1940–41. ADMS HQ 11th Armoured Div. 1941–44. NWE Jun.–Aug. 1944 (invalided). NWE Oct. 1944–Nov. 1945: DDMS HQ 1 Corp/Dist. Jan.–Oct. 1945. MELF Apr.–Jul. 1946 (invalided). ADMS Apr.–May 1946. PSMB London Dist. and Southern Comd 1946–48. Medals: CBE 11th Oct. 1945, IGSM (cl. NWF 1931), GSM and Palestine with 1936/1939 cl., 1939–45 S., France and Germany S., DM, WM. d. 26th Oct. 1958 at Bishopsteignton.

McCONNELL Albert Arthur McGowan Address: 548 Upr Newtownards Rd, Belfast. MB, BCh (QUB 1942). Surg. Lt RNVR.

McCONNELL Alexander Address: 19 Clifton Dr., Belfast. MB, BCh (QUB 1940). Capt. RAMC.

McCONNELL Brian Edmund Address: 35 Stormount Pk, Belfast. Campbell College. MB, BCh (QUB 1939). Capt. RAMC.

McCONVELL Dermot James Redmond b. 9th Feb. 1913, Twickenham, Middx. Address: 3 Auna Ville, Western Rd, Cork. MB, BCh, BAO (NUI 1938), DPM RCPSI (1948). Lt 10th Dec. 1939. Capt. 10th Dec. 1940. PC Capt. 10th Dec. 1944. A/Maj. 30th Aug. 1943. T/Maj. 30th Nov. 1943. Maj. 10th Dec. 1947. T/Lt Col. 4th May 1953. Lt Col. 4th Sept. 1958. E. Africa 1941–44. Burma 1944–45. FARELF 1950–53. Comd Psych. W. Comd and Mil. Hosp. Wheatley 1953–60. A/ADMS Mid-West Dist. 1960. BAOR 1960–62. Graded Spec. Psych. Medals: 1939–45 S., Africa S., Burma S., DM, WM, GSM with cl. Malaya. d. 7th Dec. 1962 at Wegberg, West Germany.

McCORMACK Thomas Henry Address: Omeath, Co. Louth. MB, BCh, BAO (UCD 1937). Flt Offr RAF.

McCOY John Henry Address: High St, Ballymoney, Co. Antrim. MB, BCh, DPH (QUB 1941). Sq. Ldr (M) RAFVR. MID.

McCREA Alexander Hope Address: Edgehill, Lennoxvale, Belfast. MB, BCh (QUB 1941). Surg. Lt RNVR.

McCRORY Lawrence Address: Ballygelly, Broughshane, Ballymena, Co. Antrim. MB, BCh (QUB 1938). Capt. RAMC.

McCULLAGH Graham Patterson. b. Belfast 1904 s. a Belfast medical practitioner. Scholarship to Campbell Coll. MB, BCh, BAO (Hons.) QUB 1927. BSc (Hons) 1928. MD 1931. DPH 1932. Lecturer in Pathology QUB. Demonstrator in Pathology Cambridge 1935. Fellowship of Queens' Coll. 1937. Tutor of Queens' Coll. 1938. R. Naval Volunteer Reserve 1930. Surg. Comdr 1941. Spec. Pathologist to Naval Hosps. during the war. Principal Med. Officer for the Suez Canal. Returned to admin. duties at Cambridge after the war. Awarded the Volunteer Reserve Decoration in 1945.

McCULLAGH Lewis Patrick Address: Eyre Sq., Galway. MB, BCh, BAO (UCG 1923). Flt Offr RAF.

McCULLAGH William McKim Herbert BA, MB, BCh (QUB 1913), FRCS (England 1922). Col. Late RAMC. DSO, MC.

*****McCULLOUGH** William Errol Charles MB, BCh (QUB 1939). Ships Surg. MN. Lost at sea.

McCURDY John L.LM (1930 RCPI), L.LM (1930 RCSI). Lt RAMC Oct. 1939.

McCURRY Arthur Llewellyn MB, BCh (QUB 1922). Wing Comdr (M) RAFVR.

McCUTCHEON James Educ. TCD 1898. BA, MB (1903), BCh. Surg. RN 23rd May 1904. Staff Surg. RN 23rd May 1912. Surg. Comdr 1916. Surg. Rear Adm. Served in 1914–18 War. MID Apr. 1918.

McDERMOTT Francis Joseph MB, BCh, BAO, DPH (UCD). Lt RAMC. First enlisted 7th Sept. 1939.

McDERMOTT John Francis Address: Galdonagh, Manorcunningham, Co. Donegal. MB, BCh, BAO (NUI 1941). Lt RAMC 13th May 1944.

MacDOWEL Francis Lewis Hartwell L.LM (RCPI 1917), L.LM (RCSI 1917). RN.

McDOWELL Leslie Alexander Address: 35 Marlborough Pk North, Belfast. MB, BCh, DPH (QUB 1936). Lt Col. RAMC.

McDOWELL James Gillespie MB, BCh (TCD 1926), MD (TCD 1937). Maj. RAMC. France and N. Africa. Wounded.

McDOWELL Robert Wyatt Address: 1 Kensington Pk, Bangor, Co. Down. MB, BCh (QUB 1940). Flt Lt (M) RAFVR. MBE.

McELDERRY Robert Knox Address: 34 Sans Souci Pk, Belfast. MB, BCh (QUB 1939). Flt Lt (M) RAFVR.

McELLIGOTT H.F. Only s. the late Francis (Major RAMC). Married Marie Therese Monica, eldest dt. Denis O'Driscoll of Carrick on Shannon, Co. Leitrim, 3rd Mar. 1948.

McELMEY W.H. Surg. Pilot RAFVR.

McELROY John Richard Address: 26 Claremont Rd, Dublin SE5. MB, BCh (TCD 1935). Capt. RAMC. Served in East Africa.

McENERY Jeremiah Joseph MB, BCh, BAO (UCC 1926). Lt RAMC.

McERVAL Thomas b. 9th Jun. 1912, at Belfast, Co. Antrim. Campbell College. MB, BCh, BAO BSc (QUB 1937), DA (England 1949), FFA RCS (England 1954). Lt 1st May 1938. Capt. 11th Mar. 1940. PC Capt. 11th Mar. 1944. A/Maj. 18th Dec. 1941. T/Maj. 18th Mar. 1942. Maj. 1st Jul. 1946. A/Lt Col. 10th Nov. 1944. T/Lt Col. 10th Feb. 1945. Lt Col. 14th Sept. 1953. A/Col. 17th Apr. 1946. r.p. 11th Mar. 1954. Rejoined 10th Sept. 1956. India 1930–40 MEF 1940–44. CMF/MEF 1944–46. CO 31st Indian Fd Amb. 1944–45. CO 26th Indian Fd Amb. 1945. ADMS HQ Brit. Mil. Mission Greece 1945–46. CO 78 Gen. Hosp. 1946. FARELF 1950–53. CO MBH Kluang 1952–53. Cyprus 1956. Medals: 1939–45 S., Africa S with 8th Army cl., Italy S., WM, GSM with Malaya cl.

McEVOY Fergus Bryan MB, BCh, BAO (UCD 1924). Lt RAMC 1st May 1943.

McFADDEN John b. 6th Jun. 1889, Badoney House, Newtownstewart, Co. Tyrone. MB, BCh, BAO (QUB 1913). PC Lt RAMC 3rd Oct. 1914, Capt. 3rd Oct. 1915, Maj. 3rd Oct. 1926, Lt Col. 27th Aug. 1938, A/Col. 31st May 1940, T/Col. 4th Apr. 1941, Hon. Col. 28th Sept. 1946. Served Serbia Feb.–Apr. 1915, Salonica 1916–17, Italy 1917–18, Mesopotamia 1920–22, Egypt 1922, invalided, and 1922–24, Palestine 1924–25, Malaya 1928–31, India 1934–39:

CO BMH Jullundur 1938–39, CO 18 CS Jan.–May 1940, CO 36 Gen. Hosp. May–Jul. 1940, CO 37 Gen. Hosp. 1940–41, W. Africa 1941–42. Medals: DM, WM.

McFARLAND William Douglas Haig Address: Gortin, Omagh, Co. Tyrone. MB, BCh (QUB 1941). Flt Lt (M) RAFVR.

MacFARLANE Gordon Nelson MB, BCh (TCD 1937). Capt. RAMC. Wounded. POW Singapore 1942–45.

MacFARLANE Lenox Ross Selby MB, BCh (TCD 1927), DPH (QUB 1935). Lt Col. RAMC. OBE.

MacFETRIDGE Herbert Fitzroy Townsend (TCD 1936). Lt Col. RAMC.

McFETRIDGE Margaret Elizabeth (née McClelland) Address: The Manse, Drumcroom, Coleraine, Co. Derry. MB, BCh (TCD 1940). RAFVR.

McGLADE John MB, BCh, BAO (UCD 1934). Lt RAMC.

McGORRY Henry Desmond Address: The Diamond, Clones, Co. Monaghan. MB, BCh (TCD 1934), DPH (TCD 1936). Surg. Lt RNVR.

McGOVERN John MB, BCh, BAO (UCC 1930). Flt Offr RAF.

*****McGRATH** Cornelius b. IFS. Educ. MB, BCh, BAO (UCC 1936). Lt Col. RAMC. Address: Ballymaw, Waterfall, Co. Cork. s. Patrick and Margaret McGrath of Waterfall, Co. Cork. Husband of Margaret Mary McGrath née Long, 5 Moretimo Tce, Blackrock, Dublin who died 22nd Jan. 1948. d. 18th May 1942 Burma. Buried Imphal War Cemetery, Plot 4.B.S.

McGRATH Daniel Desmond MB (TCD 1942). RAF.

McGRATH John Joseph b. 17th Feb. 1915, Cork. Address: 4 Abbey Sq., North Mall, Cork. MB, BCh, BAO (NUI 1939). Lt RAMC TA 1st May 1939. Capt. 1st May 1940. PC Capt. 1st May 1944. A/Maj. 29th Jun. 1944. T/Maj. 29th Sept. 1944. Maj. 1st May 1947. A/Lt Col. 19th May 1945. T/Lt Col. 29th Aug. 1952. Lt Col. 17th Oct. 1955. BEF France 1939–40. India 1941–45: ADMS GHQ (I) 1945. BAOR 1948–50. Comd Psych. N. Comd and Mil. Hosp. York, 1952–53. BCFK 1953–55. CO 26th Fd Amb. 1953. HQ FARELF & BMH Singapore 1955–56. Comd Psych. N. Comd and Mil. Hosp. York. and Catterick 1956–60. Comd Psych. E. Comd and QA Mil. Hosp. Millbank 1960–61. Comd Psych. HQ W. Comd 1962. Medals: 1939–45 S., Burma S., DM, WM, UN SM and cl. Korea, GSM and cl. Malaya.

*****McGRATH** Liam Henry Address: Wesley Lodge, Dublin Rd, Omagh, Co. Tyrone. MB, BCh (QUB 1939). Wing Comdr 63389 (M) RAFVR. Accidently shot 28th Jan. 1947, buried Omagh (Dublin Rd) Cemetery, Special section 33–39.

McGRATH William Wilson Address: Ruabon, Portrush, Co. Antrim. MB, BCh (TCD 1938). Wing Comdr RAF 1940.

MacHALE James J. Address: Woodville, The Hill, Monkstown, Co. Dublin. MB, BCh (NUI 1936), DPH (NUI 1939). Lt RAMC 15th Aug. 1940.

MacILRATH John Hamilton Address: Windcroft, Knock, Belfast. MB, BCh (QUB 1939). Sq. Ldr (M) RAFVR.

MacILRATH William Acton Address: Windcroft, Knock, Belfast. MB, BCh (QUB 1928). Capt. RAMC.

McILVEEN James Alexander MB, BCh (TCD 1934). Maj. RAMC. BEF 1939.

***MacILWAINE** Alexander Gillilan Johnston CSIE LRCP&SI (QUB). Lt Col. 50557 RAMC. Died 3rd Mar. 1942 aged 55. CIE.

McINTYRE William Percival Edwin MB, BCh (1925), MD (TCD 1929). Surg. Comdr RN. HMS Southampton and Hospital Ship Oxfordshire.

McKAY Alexander Taylor LAH (Dublin 1924) MB, BCh (1926). MD (1935 NUI), MRCPI (1936). Address: 64 South Circular Rd, Dublin. OStJ 21st Jun. 1938.

McKEAN William Thomas Sinclair Address: 4 Shandon Pk, Knock, Belfast. MB, BCh (QUB 1940). Sq. Ldr (M) RAFVR.

McKEE Clifford Wilson Address: 9 Ascot Pk, Knock Rd, Belfast. MB, BCh (QUB 1943). Capt. RAMC.

McKEE John Francis Scott Address: 24 Mount St, Donaghadee, Co. Down. MB, BCh (QUB 1940). Flt Lt (M) RAFVR.

McKENNA Anne Carmel Address: Church Pl., Carrickmacross, Co. Monaghan. L.LM (RCPI 1940), L.LM (RCSI 1940).

McKENNA Francis Hector MB, BCh (TCD 1925). Capt. RAMC. Served in W. Africa.

McKENZIE Kenneth QUB. Flying Officer RAF. DFC.

McKEOWN Robert Adams Address: Church St, Ballymoney, Co. Antrim. MB, BCh (QUB 1943). Surg. Lt RNVR.

McKERNAN Percy Edward MB, BCh, BAO (NUI 1925). Lt RAMC 16th May 1942.

McKERR William Cecil Address: 71 Maryville Pk, Belfast. MB, BCh (QUB 1942). Capt. RAMC.

McKIBBIN Frederick b. 20th Jan. 1892, Belfast. s. John Scott (telegraph clerk) and Margaret McKibbin, 3 Eglantine Ave., Antrim. Educ. QUB MB (1915), BCh, DPH (Camb. 1924). R. Presbyterian. Lt RAMC SR 5th Feb. 1914. Mobd 25th Mar. 1915. Capt. 25th Sept. 1915. PC Capt. 1st Mar. 1921. Maj. 25th Mar.

1927. Lt Col. 8th Dec. 1940. A/Col. 10th Dec. 1941. T/Col. 10th Jun. 1942. Col. 21st Oct. 1945. r.p. 30th Jun. 1949. Rempld Maj. 1st Jul. 1949–30th Nov. 1951. Served France 23rd Apr. 1915–16. Egypt 1917–21. India 1924–29. Ceylon 1932–36. Medals: OBE (1st Jan. 1943), 1915 S., BWM, VM, DM, WM, O. of El Nahda 4th Class (30th Sept. 1920). d. 12th Sept. 1952.

McKINLAY Robert b. 17th Jun. 1892, Castlefinn, Co. Donegal. s. Robert (farmer and asst land commr), Sessiagh, Castlefinn, Co. Donegal. Educ. Campbell Coll. Sept. 1907–Apr. 1908. Edinburgh Uni and QUB. MB (Edin. 1915), ChB, DPH (QUB 1926). R. Presbyterian. Lt RAMC SR 17th Aug. 1914. Mobd 14th Apr. 1915. Capt. 14th Oct. 1915. A/Maj. 4th Jan. 1918. PC Capt. 1st Apr. 1919. Maj. 14th Apr. 1927. A/Lt Col. 18th Jul. 1940. T/Lt Col. 18th Oct. 1940. Lt Col. 26th Mar. 1941. A/Col. 7th Aug. 1942. T/Col. 7th Feb. 1943. Col. 29th Oct. 1945. r.p. 21st May 1948. Served in 1914–18 War. Black Sea 1916–23. India 1929–36. Palestine/MEF 1938–43: OIC Med. Div. 62 Gen. Hosp. Jul–Sept. 1940. ADH HQ BTE 1940–43. Foreign Office 1943–45. DDH HQ N Comd 1946. DDH HQ E. Comd 1946–48. Medals: OBE (6th Jan. 1944). 'This officer has served as the chief adviser to the Deputy Director of Medical Supplies in Egypt, in hygiene and preventive medicine since September 14th 1940; he was mentioned in despatches October 27th 1941. Throughout this long period he has shown remarkable devotion to duty, and a large portion of the credit for the exceptionally low sick rate of the troops who have been in his area either in transit or permanently stationed there is apportioned to his efforts and those of the special staff under his direction, and his sound knowledge and judgement have been invaluable. The results obtained speak for themselves.' BWM, VM, 1939–45 S., Africa S., DM, WM. MID 30th Jan. 1919, 30th Dec. 1941, 30th Jun. 1942.

McKNIGHT Arthur Anderson TCD 1903. Col. S. Rhodesian Med. Corps.

McKNIGHT Edward MB (QUB 1940). Sq. Ldr (M) RAFVR.

MacLAINE Albert Address: Red House Hotel, Portballintrae, Co. Antrim. MB, DPH (QUB 1938). Sq. Ldr (M) RAFVR.

MacLAINE Edmund Address: Red House Hotel, Portballintrae, Co. Antrim. MB, BCh (QUB 1940). Maj. RAMC. OBE. MID.

MacLAINE Francis Victor Address: Portballintrae, Co. Antrim. MB, BCh (QUB 1933). Wing Comdr (N) RAF.

MacLAUGHLIN Francis Alexander Address: 32 Wellington Pk, Belfast. MB, BCh (QUB 1921). Surg. Comdr RNVR. VD.

McLAUGHLIN Francis Leo MB, BCh, BAO (NUI 1922), MD (NUI 1930). Lt RAMC. First enlisted 3rd Jun. 1939.

MacLAUGHLIN John Herbert Address: Lisburn Rd, Finaghy, Belfast. MB, BCh, DPH (QUB 1936). Maj. RAMC.

McMAHON John Ernest MB, BCh (TCD 1928). Served Malaya. POW.

MacMAHON William John Alexander MB, BCh (TCD 1925). Capt. RAMC.

McMANUS Patrick Joseph MB, BCh, BAO (UCD 1930). Lt RAMC.

McMANUS William Address: Ardnanure, Bealnamulla, Athlone, Co. Westmeath. MB, BCh, BAO (NUI 1937). Lt RAMC 27th Dec. 1940.

McMECHAN Eric Wilson Address: Thomastown House, Portaferry, Co. Down. MB, BCh (QUB 1933). Lt Col. RAMC.

McMURRAY James Address: Lauraville, Lisburn Rd, Finaghy, Belfast. MB, BCh (QUB 1937), MD (QUB 1940). Maj. RAMC.

McMURRAY Susan Doris Dickson Lauraville, Balmoral, Belfast. MB, BCh (1941 QUB). Lt RAMC Nov. 1942.

McMURRAY Thomas Address: Co. Down. Campbell College. LRCP (Edinburgh 1941), LRCS (Edinburgh 1941), LRFPS (Glasgow). Captain RAMC.

MacNAMARA Charles Vere b. 21st Oct. 1895, Kilmallock, Co. Limerick. s. Patrick Joseph (MD FRCSI) and Barbara Marian MacNamara, Kilmallock Town, Limerick. Educ. NUI MB, BCh (1918), BAO, DPH (Eng. 1931), RCPS (England 1931). R. RC. T/Lt RAMC 27th Jun. 1918. PC Lt 1st Apr. 1919. T/Capt. 27th Jun. 1919. Capt. 27th Dec. 1921. Maj. 27th Jun. 1930. Lt Col. 11th May 1944. A/Col. 14th Jan. 1943. T/Col. 14th Jul. 1943. Col. 13th May 1948. A/Brig. 14th Jan. 1946. r.p. 21st Nov. 1955. Served Salonika 6th Aug. 1918–19. Serbia Feb–Jun. 1919. Turkey 1919–23. India 1924–29 and 1932–37. Gibraltar 1940–42. DDH HQ Scottish Comd 1943–45. India 1945–47. DDH HQ Eastern Comd 1945–46. Dir. Food Inspection GHQ (I) 1946–47. DDAH HQ Eastern Comd 1948–49. DDAH HQ ABOR 1949–53. DDAH HQ Western Comd 1953–55. Medals: BWM, VM, DM, WM. Awarded the Alexander Memorial Prize for 1937 consisting of a gold medal and a sum of £40. The prize is awarded annually to an officer of the RAMC for professional work of outstanding merit.

MacNAMARA Charles Wesley Lewis MB, BCh (TCD 1937). Sq. Ldr RAF.

*McNAMARA James Michael s. John McNamara, Roscommon. MB, BCh, BAO (NUI 1923). Surg. Comdr RN. First enlisted 19th Dec. 1928. KIA Apr. 1942, HMS *Hermes* aged 42.

MacNAMARA John Philip b. 24th May 1893, Dublin. Educ. TCD (1911). MB (1916), BCh, BAO, LM (Coombe). Lt RAMC 9th Aug. 1914. Mobd 1st Jan. 1917. Capt. 1st Jul. 1917. PC 1st Apr. 1919). LT (T/Capt). Capt. 1st Jul. 1920.

Maj. 1st Jan. 1929. Lt Col. 1st Aug. 1943. Col. 13th Aug. 1947. A/Brig. 20th Feb. 1945. r.p. Brig. 20th Dec. 1950. Served in India 1917–20. Mesopotamia 1920–22. BAOR 1925–27. India 1927–32 & 1936–39. CO 187 Fd Amb. 1940–42. Iceland 1940–41. CO Mil. Hosp. Bracebridge May–Jul. 1942. ADMS HQ 47 Div. 1942–43. W. African ADMS HQ Gold Coast area 1943–44. SEAC/Burma 1944–46. ADMS HQ 81 (WA) Div. 1944–45. DDMS HQ 505 Dist. Feb.–Oct. 1945. ADMS HQ N. Burma area 1945–46. CO Mil. Hosp. Chepstow Feb.–May 1947. MELF: ADMS HQ Canal Central and North Dists 1947–49. DDMS HQ E. African Comd 1949–50. Medals: BWM, VM, IGS cl. NWF (1919) and WAZ (1919–20) and NWF (1930–31), GSM cl. Iraq. WM. MID 27th Sept. 1945, 19th Sept. 1946. d. 1st Aug. 1962, Co. Kildare.

MacNAMARA Patrick Joseph Address: Rhine, Mullagh, Co. Clare. L.LM (RCPI 1936). L.LM (RCSI 1936). Lt T/Surg. Lt RNVR 1941.

***McNAMARA** Robert William Address: Railway St, Ballinahinch, Co. Down. MB, BCh (QUB 1935). Capt. RAMC. KIA.

McNEILLY James Craig Address: Connor Manse, Kells, Co. Antrim. MB, BCh (TCD 1938). Capt. RAMC. POW Singapore. Released 1945.

McNEILLY Robert MB, BCh (TCD 1933). Maj. RAMC.

McPARTLAND John Joseph Address: Cloonone, Drumkeeran, Co. Leitrim. MB, BCh, BAO (UCD 1936). Lt RAMC.

McQUAID Thomas Mayne Address: 108 Sandford Rd, Dublin. L.LM (RCPI 1938), L.LM (RCSI 1938). Lt RAMC 1940.

McQUEEN Campbell b. 29th Jul. 1885, Queenstown, Co. Cork. Address: 3 Anna Ville, Western Rd, Cork. Educ. RCSI LRCPI, LRCSI (1907). Lt RAMC 4th Feb. 1908. Capt. 4th Aug. 1911. A/Maj. 4th Jan. 1918. Maj. 4th Feb. 1920. A/Lt Col. 4th–17th Dec. 1917 and 24th–26th Dec. 1917. Lt Col. 22nd Jul. 1933. r.p. remained employed 29th Jul. 1940. Maj. 7th Aug. 1942. r.p. disability Lt Col. 10th Nov. 1946. Served S. Afr. 1909–13. BEF France 18th Aug. 1914–15. Salonika 1916. Egypt and Palestine 1920–21. Spec. Gynae. MFH Shorncliffe 1922–24. India 1925–27. Iraq Jan.–May 1926. OC MFH Devonport 1928–30. India 1930–36. BMH Rawalpindi and Murree 1931–33. CO BMH Bareilly 1933–36. CO BMH Colaba 1939–41. 2 POW Camp Hosp. 1941–42. Invalided. Medals: MC (14th Jan. 1916), 1914 S., BWM, VM, DM. WM. MID 17th Feb. 1915, 1st Jan. 1916. d. 27th Jan. 1959, Rushbrook, Co. Cork.

MacQUILLAN Bernard Leo MB, BCh (QUB 1929), DPH (QUB 1931). Maj. RAMC. TD.

McQUILLAN John b. 25th Apr. 1911, Dublin. Address: 2 Fitzwilliam Tce, Bray, Co. Wicklow. TCD (1934). MB, BCh, BAO (Dublin 1937), DPM (1948). Lt 23rd Nov. 1939. Capt. 23rd Nov. 1940. PC Capt. 23rd Nov. 1944. Maj. 23rd Nov. 1947. T/Lt Col. 1st Dec. 1950. Lt Col. 4th Sept. 1958. r.p. 18th Mar. 1961. Singapore 1939–42, RMO 2nd Gordons 1940–41, POW Far East 1942–45, BAOR 1947, Psych. N. Comd and Mil. Hosp York 1950–52 and 1955–56. Adv. in Psych. FARELF and BMH Singapore 1952–55. OIC Psych. Wing, Royal Victoria Hosp. Netley 1956–57. Comd Psych. E. Comd and QA Mil. Hosp. Millbank 1957–58. Asst Prof. Army Psych. RAM Coll. 1958–60. Spec. Psych. Cambridge Hosp. Aldershot 1960–61. Graded Psych. 1957. Spec. Psych. 1949. Medals: 1939–45 S., Pacific S. DM, WM, GSM with cl. Malaya. MID 12th Sept. 1946

McQUISTON Andrew Address: Nyora Fitzwilliam Ave., Belfast. MB, BCh (QUB 1933), DPH (QUB 1936). Maj. RAMC.

McROBERT John Address: 61 Wellington Pk, Belfast. MB, BCh (QUB 1942). Sq. Ldr (M) RAFVR.

McSHARRY Noel Address: 35 Rathgar Rd, Dublin. MB, BCh, L Med., LCh (TCD 1939). RAF.

McSORLEY John MB, BCh, BAO (UCD 1934). Lt RAMC.

McSWEENEY Terence Address: Rosalea, Wilton Rd, Cork. MB, BCh, BAO (UCC 1943). Flt Offr RAF.

McSWINEY Myles Joseph Address: Rathpeacon, Cork. MB, BCh, BAO (UCC 1941). Lt RAMC.

McSWINEY Patrick Michael MB, BCh, BAO (UCC 1932). Surg. RN.

McVICKER Rowland Alexander Melville Address: 32 College Gdns, Belfast. MB, BCh (QUB 1939). Capt. RAMC.

*****McWHIRTER** James Russell MB (QUB 1934). Sq. Ldr (M)RAFVR. KIA 31st Aug. 1941. Commemorated on the Ismailia War Memorial.

McWILLIAMS Lionel Francis Address: 37 Princetown Rd, Bangor, Co. Down. MB, BCh (QUB 1938). Capt. RAMC. MC. MID.

MACKENZIE Derek St Clair b. 10th Jun. 1902. MB, BCh (TCD 1926). Served as a captain in the RAMC throughout WWII. d. 17th Dec. 1960 at Kew Gardens, Surrey.

MADILL, Thomas MB, BCh (TCD 1919). Surg. Rear Admiral RN. CB. OBE.

MAGILL Henry George Address: 204 Duncairn Gdns, Belfast. MB, BCh (QUB 1935). Sq. Ldr (M) RAFVR.

MAGNER Jeremiah John b. 26th Jun. 1891, Cork. Educ. NUI. MB (1914), BCh, BAO, DMR (London 1936). Lt RAMC SR 22nd Sept. 1914. Mobd 7th Oct. 1914. Capt. 7th Apr. 1915. PC Capt. 1st Apr. 1919. Maj. 22nd Sept. 1926. Bt. Lt Col. 1st Jan. 1938. Lt Col. 1st May 1938. A/Col. 20th Jun. 1941. T/Col. 20th Dec. 1941. Col. 23rd May 1944. A/Brig. 4th Feb. 1944. T/Brig. 4th Aug. 1944. A/Maj. Gen. 1st May 1947. T/Maj. Gen. 1st Nov. 1947. Maj. Gen. 1st Mar. 1948. r.p. 24th Jul. 1951. Served BEF France 14th Aug. 1914–15 and 1917–19. Salonika 1915–16. N. Russia May–Oct. 1919. Black Sea 1920–23. Seconded to Egyptian Army 1923–25. India 1929–34. Malta 1938–39. Comdt 11 Depot and Trg. Estab. RAMC 1940–31. Chief Instructor 1929–40. ADMS HQ 56 Div. 1941–44. Paiforce 1942–43. MEF 1943–44. DDMS GHQ. MEF 1943–44: DDMS GHQ. MEF Feb.–May 1944. Palestine: DDMS HQ 1944–46. DDMS HQ NI Dist. 1946–47. DDMS HQ Scottish Comd 1947–48. DDMS HQ N. Comd 1948–51. KHP 9th Jul. 1948. Medals: CB (4th Jun. 1948), MC (3rd Feb. 1920), 1914 S., BWM, VM, 1939–45 S., Africa S., Italy S., DM, WM, GSM 1 cl. Palestine. MID 1st Jan. 1916, 5th Aug. 1943, 11th Dec. 1945.

MAGNER John William MB, BCh, BAO (UCC 1925), MC (NUI 1934). Flt Lt RAF.

MAGNER Raymond George Address: 8 Pembroke Rd, Ballsbridge, Dublin. MB, BCh (NUI 1942). Flt Lt RAF 18th Mar. 1944.

MAGOWAN William MB, BCh (TCD 1926). Maj. RAMC. 1940.

MAGUIRE John George MB, BCh (TCD 1925). Surg. Comd RN.

MAGUIRE Joseph Ballantyne Address: Ardeevin, Highfield Rd, Rathgar, Dublin. MB, BCh (TCD 1920). Surg Merchant Marine. SS *Queen Elizabeth*.

MAGURRAN Gordon Fullerton MB, BCh (QUB 1930). Flt Lt (M) RAFVR.

MAHER John Vincent Address: Hughenden, Albany Rd, Ranelagh, Dublin. L.LM (RCPI 1937), L.LM (RCSI 1937). Surg. Comdr RNVR 1937.

MAHON James Raymond Address: Greenlands, Rosses Point, Co. Sligo. MB, BCh (TCD 1938). RAMC.

MAJURY Arthur Stuart Address: The Manse, Greystone Rd, Co. Antrim. MB, BCh (QUB 1941). Wing Comdr (M) RAFVR.

MALLEN Colm Brendan MB, BCh, BAO (NUI 1935). Lt RAMC 1942.

MALLOY Thomas Robert Address: St Abbs, Jordanstown, Co. Antrim. MB, BCh (QUB 1941). Sq. Ldr (M) RAFVR.

MALONE Albert Edward MB, BCh (TCD 1911). Surg. Rear Admiral RN. Served in WWII. CB for distinguished service.

MALONE Evan Kenneth MB, BCh (TCD 1929). Capt. Sudan Defence Force. Served in Kaimakam.

MALONY John George MB, BCh, BAO (NUI 1925). Flt Offr RAF 1st Jan. 1940.

MANNING John Charles MB, BCh, BAO (UCD 1926). Lt RAMC 24th Apr. 1940.

MANSFIELD Michael Matthew MB, BCh, BAO (UCC 1926). Lt IMS.

MANWELL William Address: Flowerfield, Lisburn, Co. Antrim. MB, BCh (QUB 1930). Maj. RAMC.

MARCUS Basil Address: 18 Dufferin Avenue, South Circular Rd, Dublin. MB, BCh (TCD 1942). Surg. Lt RNVR. 1944.

MARK James Allison Address: Dunboe Manse, Castlerock, Co. Derry. MB, BCh, DPH (QUB 1938). Capt. RAMC. MID.

MARK John Frederick Address: Dunboe Manse, Castlerock, Co. Derry. MB, BCh (QUB 1942). Maj. RAMC. MID.

*****MARKS** Hugh Only s. the late Hugh and Mrs A.E. Marks of Randalstown, Co. Antrim. Educ. Portora Royal School, Enniskillen, and Queen's College Belfast. LRCPI (1939 QUB). Surg. Lt RNVR. He was posted to a ship in the east and sailed from England as a passenger in a convoy to take up his position. The convoy was attacked by an armed raider and the boat on which he was a passenger was sunk. After two days on a raft he died from exposure (Mar. 1941).

MARREN John Patrick MB, BCh, BAO (UCD 1927). Lt RAMC 19th Dec. 1939.

*****MARSHAL** Robert William Address: 9 College Gdns, Belfast. MB, BCh (QUB 1940). Sq. Ldr (M) RAFVR. KIA.

MARTIN David Stanley b. 1st Jun. 1889, Newry, Co. Down. s. Samuel Edgar (MD) and Eliza Martin, 1, Downshire Rd, Newry, Co. Down. Educ. MB (TCD 1914), BCh, BAO, LM (Rot. Hosp). R. Presbyterian. Lt RAMC SR 17th Aug. 1914. Mobd 10th Dec. 1914. Capt. 16th Jun. 1915. A/Maj. 14th Jan. 1917. Maj. 16th Dec. 1926. Lt Col. 2nd Mar. 1940. A/Col. 10th Sept. 1940. T/Col. 10th Sept. 1945. r.p. Hon. Col. 5th Jun. 1948. Served in Balkans from 24th Oct. 1915. Egypt 1916. Salonika 1916–17. Palestine 1917–18. India 1918–21 and 1924–29. Medals: 1915 S., BWM, VM, Africa S. (with 1st Army cl.), DM, WM.

MARTIN John Leslie b. 25th Oct. 1905, Durban, South Africa. MB, BCh, BAO (TCD 1931), LM Rot. TCD (1938). PC Lt RAMC 26th Jul. 1932. Capt. 1st May 1934. A/Maj. 7th Aug. 1940. T/Maj. 7th Nov. 1940. Maj. 12th Jan. 1942. A/Lt Col. 6th Aug. 1943. T/Lt Col. 6th Nov. 1943. Served India 1933–38. MEF 1940–41. POW Western Front 1941–43. CO 88th Gen.

Hosp. 1943. SMO 135th Inf. Bde. 1945. ADMS HQ W. African Comd 1945–46. BAOR 1946–47. Medals: 1939–45 S., Africa S., DM, WM. d. 8th Mar. 1947, Oxford.

MARTIN John Robert Aylner Address: Castleview, Rushbrooke, Co. Cork. MB, BCh (TCD 1940). Lt Col. RAMC. POW Italy 1942. Escaped 1943.

MARTIN John Stuart Address: Ballyronan, Magherafelt, Co. Derry. MB, BCh (QUB 1939). Capt. RAMC. b. Robinstown, Co. Meath. MC. On August 9th, 1943, the battery was in action south of Bronte and Captain Martin was with the battery. During the evening the road between the battery position and Bronte was very heavily and accurately shelled and mortared. This road was very congested with stationary guns and vehicles and Captain Martin, realising that there were likely to be casualties, immediately proceeded to the place which was being most heavily shelled. A vehicle had been hit and there were a number of casualties, making it very dangerous to remain in the open. Captain Martin was quite undaunted by this heavy shellfire and attended to the wounded men without regard to his personal safety. By his brave action he undoubtedly saved some lives and his example had a steadying effect on all around him. Lt Col. MC.

MARTIN Justin Francis Address: Ballisodare, Co. Sligo. MB, BCh, BAO (NUI 1936), DPH (Bermingham 1939). Flt Offr RAF 1941.

MARTIN Miles Patrick Campbell College. MRCS (England 1940), LRCP (London 1940). b. Dun Laoghaire, Co. Dublin, T/Surg. Lt. DSO for gallantry, daring and skill in the combined attack on Dieppe in August 1942.

*****MARTIN** Noel s. Bertie Martin (founder of the firm of R. Martin & Sons, Insurance Brokers, Belfast). Educ. Coleraine Academical Institution, Campbell College and QUB. FRCS (England). Qualified in 1937. Served with the Royal Navy during the war. Demobilised with the rank of Surg. Comdr Killed in a car collision on the Antrim Road 2 miles outside Belfast City together with his half-sister Margaret Young, aged 22 years and his mother was seriously injured. He was 34 years of age.

MARTIN Norman Samuel Address: The Manse, Keady, Co. Armagh. Campbell College. MB, BCh (QUB 1935). Maj. RAMC. MBE.

MARTIN Robert McKee Address: Croft, Holywood, Co. Down. MB, BCh (QUB 1937). Capt. RAMC.

MARTIN Robert Noel Address: Mountsandel, Coleraine, Co. Derry. Campbell College. MB, BCh (QUB 1937). Surg. Lt Comdr RNVR. MID.

*****MARTIN** Thomas Gerald MB, BCh, BAO (UCD 1931), DPH. s. Patrick Phelan and Margaret Mary Martin, Macroom, Co. Cork. Maj. RAMC. d. 26th Jul. 1942 Eritrea, aged 36. Buried Asmara War Cemetery, Plot 2.E.10.

MARTIN Thomas Joseph MB, BCh, BAO (UCD 1931). Lt RAMC.

MARTIN Victor Alexander Faris Address: Thornhill, Lisburn. MB, BCh (QUB 1936). Wing Comdr RAFVR.

MARTIN Wilfred Bruce Address: 25 Brighton Rd, Rathgar, Dublin. MB, BCh (TCD 1942). Surg. Lt RNVR.

MARTIN William Desmond Address: Mount Oriel, Whitehead, Co. Antrim. MB, BCh (QUB 1941). Capt. RAMC.

MASON Henry Seacombe MB, BCh (TCD 1932) Flt Lt RAF 1941.

MASON Maureen Nancy Stewart Address: Imaal, Butterfield Ave., Templeogue, Dublin. MB, BCh (TCD 1937). RAMC.

MATHER Norman James MB, BCh (TCD 1927). Younger son of Mrs Mather, Mount Merrion Dublin and the late Robert Mather, Rathdown Road, Dublin. Husband of Doris (née Oliphant). Lt Col. RAMC and IMS. Served in Burma. d. 7th Nov. 1948 at his residence Bryn, Meddyg, Llanaelhaearn, Wales.

MATHERS Henry MB, BCh (QUB 1924). Maj. RAMC.

MATHEWS James Wallace Address: Ballinaloob, Dunloy, Co. Antrim. MB, BCh (QUB 1942). Surg. Lt RNVR.

MATHEWS Samuel Brown Address: Ballinaloob, Dunloy, Co. Antrim. MB, BCh (QUB 1940). Capt. RAMC.

MATHEWS William Address: Ballinaloob, Dunloy, Co. Antrim. MB, BCh (QUB 1940). Maj. RAMC 1901, 4th Jul. 1916, 18th May 1920. d. 16th Jul. 1953 at Nottingham.

MAXWELL Ian Lowry Address: Kilcrubbin, Co. Down. MB, BCh (QUB 1941). Surg. Lt RNVR.

MAXWELL Joseph Archibald MB, BCh (TCD 1912), FRCS (Edinburgh 1926). Surg. Rear Admiral RN. Served on the hospital ship *Oxfordshire*. CB, CBE, OBE, CVO.

*****MAXWELL** Robert Montgomery s. James and Catherine Maxwell. Husband of Bridget Mary Maxwell, Carrickmacross, Co. Monaghan. Capt. 90156 RAMC. d. 27th May 1940, France, aged 30. Buried Dunkirk Town Cemetery, Plot 1, Row 1, Joint Grave 37.

MAY Peter Joseph b. Dun Laoghaire, Co. Dublin. MB, BCh (NUI 1923). Major RAMC 24th Jul. 1945. OBE. 'As Officer Commanding a motor ambulance convoy, Major May has been responsible for the care and welfare of thousands of casualties from forward casualty clearing station to railroad or hospital ship port. It was due to his unbound enthusiasm that, although the distance involved was far greater than could have been anticipated, there was at no time any hitch and an even flow of casualties along the line of evacuation was always ensured. Major May's willing and intelligent co-operation with all concerned has earned the highest praise. A very all-round standard was set by the unit, and by ensuring efficient and skilful maintenance it was at all times possible to call on 100 per cent of his ambulance cars for the evacuation. This is no small achievement when it is realised that these vehicles travelled over 190,000 miles in under two months.'

MAYBIN Robert Patrick Address: Clady House, Dunadry, Co. Antrim. MB, BCh (QUB 1938). Capt. RAMC. MID.

MAYNE Brian Address: Hillside, Killiney, Co. Dublin. MB, BCh (TCD 1938). Capt. RAMC. POW Singapore. Released 1945.

MEARES Denis Edmund Address: Woodview, Stillorgan Rd, Dublin. MB, BCh (TCD 1938). RNVR.

MEARNES Charles Wilson Address: Gas Works House, Newry, Co. Down. MB, BCh (QUB 1938). Maj. RAMC. MID.

MEENAN John Francis William MB, BCh, DPH (QUB 1916). Lt Col. RAMC.

MEGARRY Benjamin Vincent MB, BCh (QUB 1935). Capt. RAMC.

MEGAW John McIlroy Address: 50 Martinez Ave., Belfast. MB, BCh (QUB 1938). Maj. RAMC.

MEHARG William Address: Castlerock, Co. Derry. MB, BCh (QUB 1941). Sq. Ldr (M) RAFVR.

*****MELLETT** Michael Kevin Address: Swinford, Co. Mayo. s. Joseph and Margaret Mellett, Swinford. MB, BCh, BAO, DPH (UCD 1935). Captain 78563 RAMC. d. 26th May 1945 aged 24. Remembered Kilconduff Graveyard.

MEREDITH James Florence MB, BCh, BAO (UCD 1931). Lt RAMC.

*****MILES** William Daniel MB (QUB 1935). s. Henry and Mary Miles of Newtownstewart, Co. Tyrone. Captain 125329 RAMC. KIA 25th Mar. 1943, aged 30 years in Tunisia. Buried in Sfax War Cemetery, Plot XIIIC.23.

MILLAR Bruce Andrew MB, BCh (QUB 1941). Maj. RAMC.

*****MILLAR** Edward Cecil Jackson MB, BCh (TCD 1940). Address: 73 Lower Drumcondra Rd, Dublin. Only s. Ernest and Grace Millar. Captain RAMC. d. 10th Apr. 1948.

MILLAR Edward Graham Address: 13 Anglesea Rd, Ballsbridge, Co. Dublin. MB, BCh (TCD 1939). Capt. RAMC.

MILLAR Frederick Graham Address: 13 Anglesea Rd, Ballsbridge, Dublin. MB, BCh (TCD 1938). Capt. RAMC. Served India. MID.

MILLAR Ian Brown Address: Knocklayd, Knockbreda Rd, Belfast. MB, BCh (QUB 1939). Sq. Ldr (M) RAFVR.

MILLAR John Harold Dundee Address: 95 Princetown Rd, Bangor, Co. Down. Campbell College. MB, BCh (QUB 1940). Surg. Lt RNVR.

MILLAR Stanley MB, BCh (QUB 1936). Capt. RAMC.

MILLEN James Hastings Address: Auburn, Adelaide Ave., Coleraine, Co. Derry. MB, BCh (QUB 1941). Sq. Ldr (M) RAFVR.

MILLEN John Llewlyn Edgar Address: 1 Downshire Rd, Bangor, Co. Down. MB, BCh (QUB 1935). Capt. IMS.

MILLER Anthony Alexander McCutcheon Address: Straidarran House, Straidarran, Co. Derry. MB, BCh (QUB 1942). Surg. Lt RNVR. MBE.

MILLER Geoffrey Arthur Chambers Address: Straidarran House, Straidarran, Co. Derry. L.LM (RCPI 1938), L.LM (RCSI 1938). Flt Offr RAFVR 1943.

MILLER Raymond Address: Briarwood, Urney Rd, Strabane. MB, BCh, DPH (QUB 1943). Surg. Lt RNVR.

MILLIGAN James Redvers MB, BCh (QUB 1924). Capt. RAMC.

MILLIKEN Thomas George Address: 35 Queen St, Ballymena, Co. Antrim. MB, BCh (QUB 1940), MC (QUB 1943). Ship's Surg. MN.

MILLS Elizabeth Mary MB, BCh (QUB 1940). Capt. RAMC.

MILNE James Edward Address: Tynet, Lower Mounttown Rd, Kingstown, Co. Dublin. MB, BCh (TCD 1938). Capt. RAMC.

MINFORD Hugh Jackson Address: 180 Grosvenor Rd, Belfast. MB, BCh (QUB 1934). Lt Col. RAMC. MC.

MITCHELL Duncan b. Glendaruel, Marino, Co. Down. MB, BCh (1939 QUB). Capt. RAMC 6th Medium RA. Medals: MC, Burma S., Defence Medal, BWM. Citation 'During the period January, to April, when 6th Medium Regiment was in 7th Indian Division East Amyu Arakan, this officer performed all duties expected from him in an exemplary manner. Particularly during the period 6th February to the 23rd March in the admin box was this devotion of duty marked. He established his regimental aid post within the perimeter of the east Nyak Pass Garrison on the evening of the 6th February, 1944. He showed consistently – throughout the period during which the garrison was in close contact with the enemy – the highest sense of duty and a noble example of gallantry. His regimental aid post was consistently sniped, shelled and bombed and Captain Mitchell attended to his duties with the upmost zeal, going about on occasions to visit the wounded who could not really be brought to him during periods of enemy attack. His example has endeared him to all ranks in contact with him and he has proved himself a man of great courage and a stout-hearted officer worthy of his calling.'

MITCHELL, John Howard MB, BCh (TCD 1931). Surg. Comdr RN.

MITCHELL John Myles Campbell College. MB, BCh (QUB 1926). Lt RAMC.

MITCHELL William Rowan Donovan Address: Brook House, Holywood Rd, Belfast. Educ. Campbell College. MB, BCh (QUB 1934), FRCS (Edinburgh 1937). Lt Col. RAMC.

MOCKLER Edmond Joseph MB, BCh, BAO (UCC 1924), DPH (NUI 1931). Flt Lt RAF.

*****MOCKLER** John s. John and Margaret Mockler Address: The Square, Thurles, Co. Tipperary. MB, BCh (UCC 1940). Capt. M/775 IMS attached RAPWI. KIA 5th Nov. 1945, aged 29, Indonesia. Buried in Jakarta War Cemetery, Plot 3.K.18.

MOFFETT Eveline 24 Malone Pk, Belfast. MB, BCh (QUB 1941). Capt. RAMC.

MOFFETT John Edward Address: 22 Adelaide Pk, Belfast. MB, BCh (QUB 1940). Flt Lt (M) RAFVR.

MOFFETT Joseph Herbert Address: 22 Adelaide Pk, Belfast. MB, BCh (QUB 1935), MD (QUB 1935), DPH (QUB 1936). Lt Col. RAMC. OBE. MID.

MOFFIT Hamilton Fleming L.LM (RCPI 1935), L.LM (RCSI 1935). Lt RAMC 1943.

MOGEY George Alexander Address: 36 Charlotte St, Ballymoney, Co. Antrim. MB, BCh (QUB 1940). Maj. RAMC.

MOLLAN Francis Robert Henry b. 20th Jun. 1893, Straffan, Co. Kildare. Educ. RCSI LRCPI (1915), LRCSI, LM. Lt RAMC SR 20th May 1914. Mobd 16th Jul. 1915. Capt. 16th Jan. 1915. PC Capt. 1st Apr. 1919. A/Maj. 20th Jul. 1918. Maj. 16th Jul. 1927. A/Lt Col. 1st Feb. 1940. T/Lt Col. 21st May 1940. Lt Col. 13th Oct. 1941. A/Col. 1st Jul. 1942. T/Col. 1st Jan. 1943. Col. 7th Apr. 1946. A/Brig. 20th Nov. 1944. T/Brig. 20th May 1945. Brig. 1st Nov. 1947. T/Maj. Gen. 11th Dec. 1948. Maj. Gen. 26th Jun. 1951. r.p. 20th Jun. 1953. Served France 2nd Oct. 1915–19. RMO 2nd Foresters 1916–18. India 1919–24. Shanghai Jan.–Sept. 1927. India ENT Spec. N. Comd 1929–34. OC 7th Indian Fd Amb. NWF Mohmand Jan.–Oct. 1933. R. Herbert Hosp. Woolwich 1934–37. Egypt MEF 1938–44: Citadel Mil. Hosp. Cairo 1939. OIC Surg. Div. 2/10 Gen. Hosp. 1940–41. CO 24 CCS Feb.–Jun. 1941. ADMS

HQ 84 L of C Sub area 1941–42. ADMS HQ 4th Indian Div. 1942–44. CO 109 Gen. Hosp. Apr.–May 1944. Australia 223 Mil. Mission May–Nov. 1944. Insp. of Army Med. Services 1944–46. BAOR 1946. ADMS HQ 51 (Highland Div.) Feb.–Mar., ADMS HQ 43 Div. Mar.–May. DDMS HQ 30th Corp Dist. Jun.–Sept. 1946. W. Africa Comd DDMS 1946–47. ADMS 1947–48. DMS HQ BAOR 1948–50. Comdr and Dean of Studies RAM Coll. 1950–53. KHS 21st Mar. 1950. QHS 1st Apr. 1952. Medals: CB (1st Jan. 1950), OBE (25th Nov. 1943). Colonel Mollan has been Assistant Director of Medical Services of the 4th Indian Division and was responsible for medical organisation in the battle of El Alamain, the Matmata Hills, Akarit of Garei and Medjez-el-Bav. In these operations each one quite different from the others, he was faced with the problem of organising at a few hours' notice, systems of medical treatment and evacuation in most difficult mountain country where, in many places, no track even existed. By brilliant improvisation and by most expert medical layout he succeeded in each case in solving his problem and in organising a system that worked without a flaw in spite of the heavy casualties with which the division organisation had to cope. By his energy, his wide military knowledge, his resolute decisions, and his resourceful talent for improvisation, he succeeded completely. Throughout, he inspired the medical personnel of the division with his own energy, devotion, cheerfulness and undaunted determination to conquer all difficulties, MC (3rd Jun. 1918), 1915 S., BWM, VM, GSM 1 cl. NWF, 1939–45 S., Africa S. with 8th Army cl. DM, WM. MID 29th May 1917, 24th Dec. 1917, 3rd Jul. 1934, 1st Apr. 1941, 5th Dec. 1942, 31st Jan. 1944.

MOLONEY Thomas Joseph MB, BCh, BAO (UCD 1931). Lt RAMC.

MOLONY John George MB, BCh, BAO (UCD 1925). Flt Offr RAF.

MONTGOMERY Alexander Rentoul MB, BCh (QUB 1927). Capt. RAMC.

MONTGOMERY Desmond Alan Dill Address: 22 Deramore Pk, Belfast. Campbell College. MB, BCh (QUB 1940). Maj. RAMC. MBE.

MONTGOMERY Douglas Wellington Address: Roebuck Castle, Roebuck Rd, Dundrum, Co. Dublin. b. 1913, Fort Wayne, Indiana. s. T.W. Montgomery, Roebuck, Dundrum. MB, BCh (TCD 1940). President RCSI 1968–70. Lt RAMC. D-Day Normandy landings. Specialist Surg.

MONTGOMERY Lancelot Craig Address: Ballycairn, Lisburn, Co. Antrim. MB, BCh (QUB 1933). Capt. RAMC. MID.

MONTGOMERY Susan (née Holland) Address: 6 Osborne Gdns, Belfast. MB, BCh (QUB 1940). Capt. IMS.

MONTGOMERY Thomas MB, BCh (QUB 1918). Group Capt. (M) RAF.

MONTGOMERY William Noel MB, BCh (QUB 1916). Wing Comdr (M) R. AUX. AF. Efficency Medal.

MOODY Thomas Edwin Address: Cashel, Coleraine, Co. Londonderry. MB, BCh (QUB 1939). Capt. RAMC.

MOONEY Robert St Clair Address: 26 Upr Fitzwilliam St, Dublin. MB, BCh (TCD 1940). Surg. Lt RNVR. POW Italy and Germany. Released 1945.

MOORE Brendan Address: Killough, Downpatrick, Co. Down. MB, BCh (NUI 1938). Lt RAMC 13th Apr. 1940.

MOORE Brian Ormond Address: 81 Marlborough Pk, Belfast. MB, BCh (QUB 1934), DPH (QUB 1937), MD (QUB 1938). Maj. RAMC.

*****MOORE** Charles Address: Ballinacarrick, Ballintra, Co. Donegal. s. William and Sarah Moore, Ballintra, Co. Donegal. MB, BCh (QUB 1942). Capt. 185th Fd Amb. RAMC. KIA 16th Nov. 1945 aged 26. Buried in Kilbarron C. of I. churchyard.

MOORE Edward Lewis b. 19th Sept. 1916, Ahoghill, Co. Antrim. MB, ChB (Liverpool, 1941), DOMS (England 1950). Lt 31st Jan. 1842. Capt. 31st Jan. 1943. A/Maj. 1st Aug. 1945. T/Maj. 1st Nov. 1945. Maj. 12th Mar. 1946. A/Lt Col. 12th Dec. 1945. T/Lt Col. 12th Mar. 1946. PC Capt. 31st Jan. 1947. Maj. 31st Jan. 1950. r.p. 2nd Feb. 1953. 4 Cdo 1942. 3 Cdo 1942–45. BANF/MEF 1943–44. NWE 1944 & 45. India/ALFSEA 1945–46. CO 15th Indian CCS 1945–46. Opthal. Spec. W. Comd Med. Pool Mil. Hosp. Chester 1950–51. BAOR 1951–53. BMH Hamburg 1951–52. BMH Hanover 1952–53. Medals: MC (21st Oct. 1943) & Bar (12th Jul. 1945), 1939–45 S., Africa S., Italy S., France and Germany S., WM.

MOORE George Leslie Address: Main St, Baltinglass, Co. Wicklow. L.LM (RCPI 1942), L.LM (RCSI 1942). Surg. Lt RNVR 1943.

MOORE James Herbert Campbell College. MB, BS (QUB 1903). Ship's Surg. MN. Deceased.

MOORE John Address: Grange Lower, Portadown, Co. Armagh. MB, BCh (TCD 1940). Maj. RAMC. Medals: MC.

MOORE John Charles MB (TCD 1938). Maj. RAMC 1940.

MOORE John Norman Parker Address: 4 Glena Tce, Wexford. MB, BCh (TCD 1935), MD (TCD 1937). Maj. RAMC.

MOORE Lillian Gertrude (née Bullick) Address: Monaville, Levaghoy, Portadown, Co. Armagh. MB, BCh (QUB 1941). Sq. Ldr (M) RAFVR. MID.

MOORE Reginald Thomas b. IFS. s. Thomas and Ellen Moore, husband of Mona Rosina Moore of Dun Laoghaire. MRCS (England 1939), LRCS (London 1939). Capt. RAMC. d. 8 Jun. 1946 aged 32. Buried in Yaba Cemetery Plot 4, Row M, Grave 4.

MOORE Richard Henry b. 9th Dec. 1897. Eldest s. Mr R.H. Moore, Dublin. Enlisted in the R. Irish Rifles during WWI at the age of 17. Transferred to the R. Flying Corps in 1917. MB, BCh (QUB 1925). Served in the RAF during WWII 1940–42 when ill health forced him to relinquish his commission. d. 10th Aug. 1960 at his home in New Southgate.

MOOREHEAD Robert Allison MB (QUB 1938). Sq. Ldr (M) RAFVR. OBE.

MORGAN William Malachy Address: 18–20 Iveagh St, Belfast. MB, BCh (QUB 1938). Flt Lt (M) RAFVR.

MORRIS Hugh McEvoy MB, BCh (QUB 1921), MD (QUB 1926). Maj. RAMC.

MORRIS John Vincent MB, BCh (TCD 1925). 1923. Capt. RAMC.

MORRIS Leslie Ephraim Address: Sitan, Knocksinna Rd, Blackrock, Dublin. MB, BCh (TCD 1939). Flt Lt RAF.

MORRISSEY John Declan Address: Green Ridge, Montenotte, Cork. MB, BCh, BAO (UCC 1943). Flt Offr RAF.

MORRISSEY Patrick Joseph Address: Loughatorick, Woodford, Co. Galway. MB, BCh, BAO (UCD 1940). Flt Offr RAF. 6th Mar. 1942.

MORRISON Daniel McVicker Address: Strand View Gdns, Ballycastle, Co. Antrim. MB, BCh (QUB 1930). Maj. RAMC. MBE.

MORRISON Eric Francis Saunderson MB, BCh (TCD 1929). Lt Col. RAMC. Wounded W. Desert. MC, MID (4).

MORRISON Ernest Address: Drumaduan, Coleraine, Co. Derry. MB, BCh (QUB 1942). Capt. RAMC.

*__MORROW__ Martin McAuley MB, BCh (QUB 1936). Lt Col. RAMC. KIA.

MORTON William Blair MB, BCh (QUB 1928). Capt. RAMC.

MORTON William Reynolds Macartney Address: 42 Rugby Rd, Belfast. MB, BCh (QUB 1930). Maj. RAMC.

MORWOOD James Bryan MB, BCh (QUB 1934), DPH (QUB 1939), FRCSI (1937). Maj. RAMC.

MORWOOD John Morrison Bell Address: 4 Malone Pk, Belfast. MB, BCh (QUB 1938). Flt Lt (M) RAFVR.

MOSHAL Bernard MB, BCh (TCD 1920), MD (TCD 1921). Maj. S. African Med. Corps.

MOSS Cecil Address: Glenmaroon, Wandsworth Rd, Knock, Belfast. MB, BCh, BCh, DPH (QUB 1936). Capt. RAMC.

MOSS John Edmund Address: 66 Wandsworth Rd, Belfast. MB, BCh (QUB 1939). Capt. RAMC.

MUCKLE Thomas Aubrey Address: Breeze Mount, Millisle Rd, Donaghadee, Co. Down. MB, BCh (QUB 1925). Lt Col. RAMC.

MULCAHY Edmond Francis Address: 3 Elderwood, College Rd, Cork. MB, BCh, BAO (UCC 1938). Flt Offr RAF.

MULDOON Patrick Bernard Llewellyn Address: Ardbear, Clifton, Co. Galway. MB, BCh, BAO (NUI 1940). Lt RAMC 8th Nov. 1941.

MULHOLLAND Henry Holmes b. 2nd Jun. 1887, Donaghadee, Co. Down. s. James Henry (house merchant and embroidery manu.) and Jeannie Mulholland, 19 Warren Rd, Donaghadee, Co. Down. Educ. Campbell College. RUI (QUB). MB (1912), BCh, BAO, DPH (Liverpool 1913). R. Presbyterian. Lt RAMC SR 29th May 1913. Mobd 15th Sept. 1914. Capt. 1st Apr. 1915. PC Lt (T/Capt.) 1st Jan. 1917. Capt. 15th Mar. 1918. T/Maj. 13th Feb. 1919. r.p. 2nd Jun. 1923. Rempld 3rd Sept. 1939. A/Lt Col. 1st Jan. 1942. T/Lt Col. 1st Apr. 1942. r.p. Hon Col. 24th Aug. 1945. Served in Gallipoli from 15th Jun. 1915. India 1916–21. Afghanistan 1919. Waziristan 1919–21. BEF France 1939–40. CO Mil. Hosp. Abergele 1942–44. Medals: 1915 S., BWM, VM, IGS Waz. (1919–21), Afghanistan NWF (1919), 1939–45 S., DM, WM. MID 10th Jun. 1921, 1st Jun. 1923.

MULLAN John Joseph Address: Dublin Rd, Maryboro, Co. Laois. (RCSI 1940) Lt RAMC Apr. 1943.

MULLEN Cecil Jameson Address: Killaloo, Co. Londonderry. MB, BCh (TCD 1932). RN.

MULLIGAN James Alexander Savage Address: The Manse, Jarrett's Pk, Newry, Co. Down. MB, BCh (QUB 1936). Capt. RAMC. MID. **MULLINS** Timothy Joseph MB, BCh, BAO (UCC 1935). Lt RAMC.

MUNN Norman Barry Campbell College. MB, BCh (QUB 1924). Lt RAMC. MC.

MURDOCK James Ronald Address: 31 Achill Rd, Whitehall, Dublin. MB, BCh (TCD 1938). RAMC.

MURPHY Daniel Francis Address: Lauriston House, Mardyke, Cork. MB, BCh, BAO (UCC 1937). Flt Offr RAF.

MURPHY Francis Dominick MB, BCh, BAO (NUI 1926), FRCS (England 1935). OBE.

MURPHY Frederick John Educ. TCD. MB (1916), BCh, DPH, RCPS (Eng. 1935). Lt RAMC 1916. Capt. 1917. Air Vice Marshal RAF. CBE, KHS.

MURPHY Jeremiah Joseph MB, BCh, BAO (UCC 1919). Lt RAMC 14th Nov. 1939.

MURPHY John MB, BCh, BAO (UCC 1928). Flt Offr RAF.

MURPHY John Address: Ballycotton, Co. Cork. MB, BCh, BAO (UCC 1928). Lt RAMC.

MURPHY John MB, BCh, BAO (UCC 1923). Flt Lt RAF.

MURPHY John MB, BCh, BAO (UCD 1922). Lt RAMC. First enlisted 17th Apr. 1942.

MURPHY John Francis Desmond b. 22nd May 1913, Kilrane, Co. Wexford. MB, BCh, BAO (NUI 1936), LM (1937). DPM (Bristol 1947), MD (NUI 1954). Lt 1st Feb. 1939. Capt. 1st Feb. 1940. PC Capt. 1st Feb. 1944. A/Maj. 31st Oct. 1940. T/Maj. 29th Apr. 1941. Maj. 1st Jul. 1946. T/Lt Col. 11th Feb. 1948. Lt Col. 31st Jul. 1953. r.p. 1st Apr. 1961. Rejoined 1st Sept. 1962. Lt Col. 4th Jul. 1962. Col. 4th Jul. 1962. A/Brig. 8th May 1967. BEF France 1939–40. NWE 1944–45. BAOR 1947–51: ADV in Psych. 1948–51. 94 (Hamburg) BMH 1947–49. Asst Prof. of Army Psych. RAM Coll. 1953–56. FARELF Adv in Psych. and BMH Singapore 1956–59. BAOR: Cons. Psych. and BMH Munster 1963–64. CO Royal Victoria Hosp. Netley 1964–67. DA Psych. and Cons. Psych. to the Army 1967. Medals: 1939–45 S., France and Germany S., DM, WM, GSM with cl. Malaya. MID 8th Nov. 1945.

MURPHY John Joseph Address: 4 Main St, Enniscorthy, Co. Wexford. MB, BCh (NUI 1938). T/Surg. RNVR 28th Feb. 1942.

MURPHY John Morgan Address: Lissodigue Spa, Tralee, Co. Kerry. MB, BCh, BAO (UCD 1935), DPH (NUI 1937). Lt RAMC.

MURPHY Leo b. 8th Oct. 1886, Midleton, Co. Cork. s. J. Murphy. Educ. Edinburgh Uni. LRCP (Edin. 1907), LRCS (Edin. 1907), LRFPS (Glasgow 1907), MSC (RUI). Married Millicent Fetherstonhaugh. Lt RAMC 4th Feb. 1908. Capt. 4th Aug. 1911. Maj. 4th Feb.1920. Lt Col. 19th Apr. 1933. Col. 5th Nov. 1936. r.p. 5th Nov. 1940. Rempld Lt Col. 13th Dec. 1940. A/Col. 19th Oct. 1942. Col. 19th Apr. 1943. r.p. 16th Sept. 1946. Served India 1910–15. Mesopotamia 27th Aug. 1915–18. POW 1916–18. BAOR 1922–23. India 1923–28. Palestine 1930–32. Egypt 1932–34. OIC Surg. Div. Cambridge Hosp. Aldershot 1934–46. India 1936–40. CO BMH Bangalore 1936–37. A/ADMS HQ Madras Dist. Apr.–Sept. 1937. ADMS HQ Waziristan Dist. 1937–40. ADMS HQ Lahore Dist. 1940. ADMS HQ Yorks Dist. HQ E. Riding Coastal Area. HQ Catterick Div. 1941–43. ADMS HQ 15th Scottish Div. 1943–44. ADMS HQ E & W. Riding Dist. 1946. Medals: DSO (19th Oct. 1916), 1915 S., BWM, VM. WM. MID 13th Jul. 1916, 23rd Oct. 1919, 30th Jan. 1920. d. 4th Dec. 1957, Weymouth, Dorset.

MURPHY Martin James MB, BCh, BAO (UCD 1933). Lt RAMC.

MURPHY Maurice Sylvester Address: Glash, Kiskean, Co. Cork. MB, BCh (NUI 1940). Lt RAMC 3rd Jun. 1944.

MURPHY Patrick Address: Broadview, Mallow, Co. Cork. MB, BCh, BAO (UCC 1928). Flt Offr RAF.

MURPHY Patrick Joseph Address: 8 Mount Prospect, Glasheen Rd, Cork. MB, BCh, BAO (UCC 1940). Lt RAMC.

MURPHY Patrick Joseph MB, BCh, BAO (UCD 1930). Lt RAMC.

MURPHY Patrick Noel Address: Asburn Villa, Waterfall, Cork. MB, BCh, BAO (UCC 1939). Flt Offr RAF.

MURPHY Philip Paine b. 23rd Aug. 1910, Co. Wexford. Address: Coolnagloose, Inch, Co. Wexford. MB, BCh (TCD 1932). Colonial Med. Service in British Somaliland Aden 1939. d. 7th Apr. 1960.

MURPHY Richard Esmonde b. 2nd Aug. 1896, Donnybrook, Dublin. MB, BCh, BAO (TCD 1920). T/Lt RAMC 14th Nov. 1920. T/Capt. 14th Nov. 1921. PC Lt 16th Mar. 1923. Capt. 14th May 1924. Maj. 14th Nov. 1932. A/Lt Col. 1st. Dec. 1940. T/Lt Col. 1st Mar. 1941. Lt Col. 18th Oct. 1944. A/Col. 7th Apr. 1942. T/Col. 14th Jan. 1943. Col. 11th Nov. 1948. T/Brig. 12th Mar. 1951. Brig. 28th Jul. 1952. T./Maj. Gen. 5th Feb. 1953. Maj. Gen. 5th Mar. 1953. r.p. 5th Aug. 1956. Served Iraq 1923–24. India 1924–48 and 1933–37. CO 1st Fd Amb. 1940–42. MEP: ADMS GHQ 1943–44. DDMS 1844–46. CO Connaught Hosp. 1946–48. Comdt Depot and Trg estab. RAMC 1948–51. DMS GHQ FARELF 1951. DDMS HQ Scottish Comd 1952–53 and HQ S. Comd 1953–56. Col. Comdt RAMC 1956. Medals: CB (10th Jun. 1954), CBE (8th Jun. 1950). IGSM (with cl. NWF 1936–37), 1939–45 S., Africa S. DM, WM, GSM and cl. Malaya, QEII Corn Medal 1953. OStJ (1955). MID 6th Apr. 1944.

MURPHY Thomas Kiely Address: The Pharmacy, Mitchelstown, Co. Cork. MB, BCh, BAO (UCC 1937). Lt RAMC.

MURPHY William MB, BCh, BAO (UCC 1923). Flt Lt RAF.

MURPHY William MB, BCh, BAO (UCC 1920). Lt RAMC.

MURRAY Charles Joseph L.LM (RCPI 1939), L.LM (RCSI 1939). Lt RAMC 1939.

MURRAY Cyril Victor Stanislaus Address: 13 Merlyn Pk, Ballsbridge, Dublin. MB, BCh, BAO (UCD 1942). Flt Offr RAF.

MURRAY Ernest Joseph Gerard MB, BCh, BAO (UCD 1935). Flt Offr RAF.

MURRAY Francis Joseph b. 4th Dec. 1912 in Belfast, above his father's shop on Oldpark Road. Educ. Interdenominational Jaffe School, Cliftonville Rd; St Patrick's CBS, Donegal St; St Mary's CBS Barrack St. MB, BCh (QUB 1937). Mater Hosp. Belfast, GP Birmingham. RAMC

1939, 29th Fd Amb. Indian Army. Captured by the Japanese at the fall of Singapore February 1942. POW at Changi Prison Singapore. Hokkaido Japan and Muroran 1944. OC and CMO. Married Eileen O'Kane, Feb. 1946 and had five children. GP Oldpark Road, Belfast until his surgery was burnt down in 1972. MBE 1946, 1939–45 S., Pacific S., Defence Medal and BWM. d. Sept. 1993.

MURRAY James Joseph Address: Co. Roscommon (RCSI 1941). RAMC Mar. 1941.

MURRAY John Malachy MB, BCh (QUB 1927). Maj. RAMC.

MURTAGH Gerald Paul Address: Altmore House, Clones, Co. Monaghan. MB, BCh (QUB 1942). Capt. RAMC.

MUSSEN Robert Walsh Address: 22 Windsor Pk, Belfast. MD (QUB 1922). Surg. Capt. RN.

N

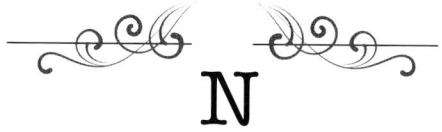

NAIRNSEY Colman (formerly Narunsky Soloman) MB, BCh (TCD 1923). Capt. RAMC. POW Malaya 1942. Released 1945.

*****NAPIER** William b. Belfast 1896. s. Alexander and Hester Napier. Husband of Katherine Margaret Napier. MB, BCh (QUB 1918), FRCSI (1921) and BAO. Maj. 100465 RAMC. KIA 3rd Jan. 1945, aged 49. Buried in Ballee C. of I. Cemetery Co. Down. MID.

NASH Edgar Llewellyn Foot b. 7th Jul. 1890, Dublin. s. William Henry (MD) and Louisa Nash, 8 Rathdown Tce, Nth Circular Rd, Dublin. Educ. St Andrews Coll. Dublin 23rd Mar. 1905–Sept. 1906. TCD (1913), MB (1914), BCh, BAO. R. C. of I. Lt RAMC SR 5th Aug. 1914. Mobd 1st Dec. 1914. Capt. 1st Jun. 1915. PC Capt. 1st Apr. 1919. Maj. 1st Dec. 1926. Lt Col. 2nd Sept. 1939. r.p. (disability) 25th Oct. 1945. Served in France 29th May 1915–19. POW Nov. 1917–Feb. 1918. India 1919–24 (NWF 1919–20) and 1927–32. Bermuda 1935–39. Physician and Surg. R. Hosp. Chelsea 1939–41. CO 7th CCS 1941–42. CO Mil. Hosp. Treverton 1942–43. CO Mil. Hosp. Glasgow 1943–45. Medals: MC (1st Dec. 1919), 1915 S., BWM, VM, IGS (cl. Afghan. 1919). d. 5th Jan. 1965 at Sandgate, Folkstone, Kent.

NASH John Address: Glynwood, Athlone, Co. Westmeath. MB, BCh (TCD 1940). Capt. RAMC. WA Forces.

NEELY Matthew Robert Address: Beneden, Derrykeeghan, Co. Fermanagh. MB, BCh (QUB 1942). Surg. Lt RNVR.

NEILL George Albert William Address: Slieve Moyne, Helen's Bay, Co. Down. MB, BCh, DPH (QUB 1936), MD (QUB 1937). Maj. RAMC.

NELSON Harry MB, BCh (TCD, 1925). Lt Col. S. African Med. Corps.

NELSON Ivan Douglas Magill Address: Drumcorran, Carnduff, Larne. MB, BCh, DPH (QUB 1941). Surg. Lt RNVR.

NELSON Maurice Gerald Address: 55 Richmond Pk, Stranmillis, Belfast. MB, BCh (QUB 1937), MC (QUB 1940). Sq. Ldr (M) RAFVR.

*****NESBITT** Robert Wallace s. Alexander and Elizabeth Nesbitt. Husband of Ethelreda Mary Nesbitt (née Coolican) of Chilslehurst, Kent. MB, BCh (TCD 1923), FRCPI. Surg. Comdr RN. KIA Sept. 1941, aged 47, on HM Hosp. Ship *Maine*. Buried in Alexandria (Hadra) War Memorial Cemetery, Plot 2.D.14.

NEVILL Gerald Edward Address: The Vicarage, Abbeyleix, Co. Laois. Campbell College. MB, BCh (TCD 1938). Captain East Africa. MC.

NEVIN Henry Millar MB, BCh (TCD 1926), DPH (1921 TCD). Pathologist. Medical Research FMS. POW.

NEVILLE Kathleen MB, BCh, BAO (UCC 1940). Lt RAMC.

NEWMAN Eldred Maurice MB, BCh, BAO (UCC 1935). Flt Offr RAF.

NEWMAN Noel Address: 3 Carriglea, Western Rd, Cork. MB, BCh, BAO (UCC 1938). Flt Offr RAF.

NEWMAN Sydney Lionel MB, BCh, BAO (UCC 1928). Lt RAMC.

NEYLON Joseph Anthony MB, BCh, BAO (UCD 1922). Lt RAMC. First enlisted 30th Sept. 1939.

NICHOLLS Cecil George Jasper MB, BCh, BAO (UCC 1924). Flt Lt RAF.

NICHOLSON John Campbell Address: 30 Hamilton Rd, Bangor, Co. Down. MB, BCh (QUB 1933). Surg. Lt Comdr RNVR.

NICHOLSON William Arthur MB, BCh (TCD 1908). Capt. RAMC.

NIGHTINGALE George McDowell Address: 15 Eastleigh Dr., Belfast. MB, BCh (QUB 1941). Flt Lt (M) RAFVR.

NIXON John Moylett Gerard MB (TCD 1937) Surg. Lt RNVR 1940.

*****NOLAN** Colm s. John James Nolan and Teresa Nolan, 14 Avoca Rd, Blackrock, Co. Dublin. Educ. Blackrock College and Belvedere College. LAH (Dublin 1943). Surg. Lt RN. HMS *Flamborough Head*. Killed in an aeroplane crash at Marcot Aerodrome Sydney, Australia aged 26, 19th Jul. 1945. Buried in Sydney War Cemetery, Plot 27 A 6.

NOLAN Joseph Gabriel Address: St Cecilias, St Anthony's Rd, Rialto, Dublin W.5. L.LM (RCPI 1940), L.LM (RCSI 1940). Flt Lt RAF 1941.

NYHAN Patrick John MB, BCh, BAO (UCC 1927). Flt Lt RAF.

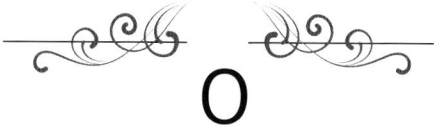

O

OAKES Robert Leslie MB, BCh (TCD 1936). Surg. Capt. RNVR.

O'BRIEN Horace Donough Address: 63 Fitzwilliam Sq., Dublin. MB, BCh (TCD 1934). Maj. RAMC. Served in N. Africa. MID.

O'BRIEN John Address: Drumaness, Belfast. L.LM (RCPI 1939), L.LM (RCSI 1939). Civil Surg. IMS 1941.

O'BRIEN Patrick MB, BCh (TCD 1934). Surg. Comdr RN 1938. MID.

O'CALLAGHAN Patrick Aloysius MB, BCh (TCD 1934). RAF.

O'CONNELL John Henry Address: Lisanore, Newcastle, Co. Down. MB, BCh (QUB 1938). Flt Offr RAF 6th Feb. 1940. Sq. Ldr (M) RAFVR.

O'CONNOR Anthony Address: 9 Rockboro Rd, Cork. MB, BCh (NUI 1939). Flt Lt RAF 2nd Apr. 1941.

O'CONNOR Charles Aloysius Conleth Address: Borton House, Straffan, Co. Kildare. MB, BCh (UCD 1935).

O'CONNOR Patrick Joseph Address: Borton House, Straffan, Co. Kildare. MB, BCh (NUI 1936). Flt Offr RAF 27th Aug. 1940.

ODBERT Arthur Noel Burchell b. 28th Dec. 1900, 8 Trafalgar Tce, Seapoint, Co. Dublin. LM LS (Dublin 1926). MB, BCh, BAO (TCD 1927). PC Lt 30th Jul. 1929. Capt. 30th Jan. 1933. Maj. 30th Jul. 1939. A/Lt Col. 26th Feb. 1941. T/Lt Col. 26th May 1941. Lt Col. 12th Aug. 1946. A/Col. 5th Jan. 1945. T/Col. 5th Jul. 1945. Col. 16th Oct. 1951. r.p. 28th Dec. 1957. Served India 1930–36. Palestine/MEF 1938–43. ADH W Force Greece 1941. ADH Alexandria 1941–42. ADH Palestine 1942. ADH HQ 8th Army 1943–44. Sicily 1943–44. NWE: ADH/DDH HQ 21st Army Group 1944–45. DDH HQ S. Comd 1945. ADH War Office (AMD 5) 1945–49. ADAH GHQ MELF 1950–52. CO Cambridge Hosp. Aldershot 1953–55. ADMS HQ Aldershot Dist. 1955–57. HQ London Dist. 1957. Medals: OBE (25th Nov. 1943). 'During the period February to May 1943. Lieutenant Colonel Odbert has been indefatigable in the performance of his duties, and it has been largely due to his efforts that the phenomenally low sick rate of the army has been attained. Over a vast area of difficult country he has supervised the hygiene arrangements with a complete disregard for anything else than the preservation of the health of the troops. He has personally investigated the important water supplies and arranged for their purification, while by prompt action and careful foresight he has prevented any outbreak of disease. Always one of the earliest on the spot in the many occupied towns and villages to anticipate and deal with hygiene problems, his preparation for the prevention of malaria was most comprehensive and machinery was immediately available should any epidemic have appeared likely. He is always cool and collected, ready with sound advice, while his devotion to duty has been an example and an inspiration to the whole hygiene tenor of the 8th Army and maintaining it fighting fit and at full strength.' GSM (with cl. Palestine 1936–39), 1939–45 S., Africa S (with cl. 8th Army), Italy S., France and Germany S., DM, WM, USA Legion of Merit 17th Oct. 1946. Anti-Gambia Memorial Medal, QEII Corn Medal 1953. MID 30th Dec. 1941, 24th Jun. 1943.

ODBERT Ernest Sydney Address: 8 Trafalgar Tce, Monkstown, Dublin. MB, BCh (TCD 1942). Flt Lt RAF.

O'DOHERTY Muriel Bridget Address: 37 Malone Rd, Belfast. MB, BCh (QUB 1934). Capt. RAMC.

O'DONNELL Godfrey Address: Cloonanure, Gurteen, Ballymote, Co. Sligo. MB, BCh (NUI 1938). Lt RAMC 20th Jan. 1940.

O'DONNELL Thomas Francis MB, BCh (TCD 1931). Maj. IMS 1932. Far East POW. MID.

O'DONNELL William Lyons Address: 8 Glentworth St, Limerick. L.LM (RCPI 1938), L.LM (RCSI 1938). Lt RAMC 1939.

O'DONOGHUE Desmond James Address: Goulnaspurragh, Idrone Tce, Blackrock, Co. Dublin. MB, BCh (NUI 1939). Surg. Lt RN 31st Mar. 1939.

O'DRISCOLL Daniel Edward L.LM (RCPI 1933), L.LM (RCSI 1933). Adm. RNVR. 1931. Order of the Bath 3rd class.

O'DRISCOLL Florence Joseph MB, BCh (NUI 1938). Maj. (Temp. Lt Col.) RAMC. b. Skerries, Co. Dublin. OBE Malaria Field Laboratory (advance party). 'Landed with corps troops and immediately set about surveying the country and procuring information regarding malaria from local sources. As the troops advanced, Lieutenant Colonel O'Driscoll and his men were never far behind and at great personal risk and under extraordinary difficult conditions brought back most valuable information showing details of malarial areas. Owing to the presence of numerous landmines, survey work along the banks of lakes, rivers and streams was extremely hazardous, and, in fact, two trucks were blown up and the occupants injured. In spite of this and due almost entirely to the leadership, drive and personal courage of Lieutenant Colonel O'Driscoll, the work went forward. It is necessary to stress the importance of this work from the army point of view, for it was on recommendations made by Lieutenant Colonel O'Driscoll that the whole fabric of anti-malaria work was built up. Had this information not been quickly obtained action would have been delayed and there is no question that malaria sick rates would have been much higher than they were.'

O'DRISCOLL Gerard Cornelius Vincent MB, BCh (TCD 1933). Maj. RAMC. Captured on fall of Singapore. POW for three-and-three-quarter years.

O'DRISCOLL Michael Pearse Address: 147 North Circular Rd, Dublin. MB, BCh (NUI 1939). Lt RAMC 3rd Apr. 1941.

O'DWYER John Joseph b. 10th Jun. 1902, Tipperary. MB, BCh, BAO (TCD 1927), DPH (England 1947). PC Lt RAMC 27th Jul. 1927. Capt. 30th Mar. 1931. Maj. 27th Jul. 1927. A/Lt Col. 25th Apr. 1941. T/Lt Col. 25th Jul. 1941. Lt Col. 29th Oct. 1945. A/Col. 20th Dec. 1944. T/Col. 20th Jun. 1945. r.p. Hon Col. 8th Mar. 1949. Served India 1928–33. Malaya /India SEAC 1939–45. ADH and P NW Army, HQ 14th Army 1943–44. ADH HQ 11th Army 1944. DDH Adv. HQ AALFSEA 1944–45 and 1945–46. Medals: CBE (6th Jun. 1946), 1939–45 S., Pacific S (with cl. Burma), DM, WM. MID 5th Apr. 1945.

O'FLANAGAN Harry Address: Castle Street, Roscrea, Co. Tipperary (RCSI 1939). RAF 1944.

O'FRIEL Arthur James Address: 54 Crumlin Rd, Belfast. MB, BCh (QUB 1938). Surg. Lt RNVR.

O'GRADY Emily Elizabeth Eleanor Ephanie (née Hill) Address: White Staunton, Portrush, Co. Antrim. MB, BCh (TCD 1938) RAF.

O'GRADY Patrick Joseph Standish b. 11th May 1887, Croom, Co. Limerick. Educ. NUI. MB, BCh (NUI 1913), BAO, LM. T/Lt RAMC 10th Dec. 1914. Capt. 10th Dec. 1915. Resigned 10th Dec. 1916. Rempld Capt. 19th Mar. 1917. PC Capt. 1st Jul. 1919. Maj. 19th Mar. 1927. A/Lt Col. 4th Jan.–15th Feb. 1940, T/Lt Col. 14th Nov. 1940. Retired, remained employed 1st Mar. 1941. r.p. Hon Lt Col. 14th Aug. 1947. Served France 1915–16 and 1917–19. India 1920–24 and 1928–33. Egypt 1935–39. Palestine Oct.–Nov. 1936. Sudan 1937–38. CO 126th Fd Amb. Jan–Feb. 1940. CO 23rd CCS 1940–41. Medals: 1915 S., BWM, VM, DM, WM. d. 9th Nov. 1960.

O'GRADY Richard Carew Address: Camzeen Hall, Tallow, Co. Waterford. MB, BCh (TCD 1935). Wing Comdr RAF.

O'GRADY Terence Patrick b. 1914 Dublin. Address: 131 Griffith Avenue, Drumcondra, Dublin. MB, BCh, BAO (NUI 1941). Flt Lt RAFVR 27th Jan. 1945. Served for three years. d. 31st Oct. 1960 at his home in Salford.

O'HARA Helena Address: Monument House, Mountmellick, Co. Laois. MB, BCh (NUI 1940). Lt RAMC 1st Nov. 1941.

O'HARE Hugh Ignatius Address: 20 Lindsay Rd, Dublin 9. L.LM (RCPI 1938), L.LM (RCSI 1938). T/Surg. RNVR 1939.

O'LEARY James Address: Ballymakeera, Macroom, Co. Cork. MB, BCh (NUI 1938). Flt Offr RAF 4th Jun. 1940.

OLIVERE Denis b. 20th Nov. 1918, Co. Cork. Address: 60 South Mall, Cork. MB, BCh, BAO (NUI 1943), DA RCS (England 1955). Lt RAMC 18th Nov. 1944. Capt. 18th Nov. 1945. Maj. 18th Nov. 1952. PC Lt 14th Oct. 1953. Capt. 14th Oct. 1953. Maj. 14th Oct. 1953. Lt Col. 10th Apr. 1960. India 1945–48: RMO 1st Gloucesters 1945–47. Mil. Hosp. Chester and Catterick. R. Herbert Hosp. Woolwich 1948–50. BAOR: BMH Berlin 1950–51. BMH Hanover 1951–54. Cambridge Hosp. Aldershot 1955–56. FARELF: BMH Singapore 1956–57. BMH Kinrara 1957–59. Mil. Hosp. Chester 1959–60. BAOR: MMH Rinteln 1960–65. Cyprus: BMH Dhekelia 1965. Medals: WM, GSM with cl. Malaya.

O'MAHONY John Brendan Address: Bay View House, Killorglin, Co. Kerry. L.LM (RCPI 1939), L.LM (RCSI 1939). Lt RAMC 1942.

O'MALLEY Alleyn Henry MB, BCh (TCD 1930). Lt Col. RAMC. IMF Colonial Medical Service Tanganyika.

O'MEARA Francis Joseph b. 4th Jul. 1900, Skibereen, Co. Cork. Educ. Clongowes Wood College. MB, BCh, BAO (TCD 1923), MA (1926), MD (RCPI 1926), MRCPI (1926), FRCPI (1926), DTM&H (Eng. 1932). British Army OTC 1918. PRAC. Lt RAMC 1st Aug. 1923, Capt. 1st Feb. 1927, Maj. 1st May 1934, Lt Col. 12th Nov. 1944, A/Col. 31st Mar. 1946, T/Col. 31st Sept. 1946, Col. 27th Nov. 1948, Lt/Brig. 21st Mar. 1946, T/Brig. 23rd Jun. 1952, Brig. 16th Feb. 1953, T/Maj. Gen. 11th Jul. 1954, Maj. Gen. 8th Jan. 1955. r.p. 8th Jan. 1959. Served in Egypt 1924–30 and India 1933–38. Casualty Clearing Station France 1939–40. Captured POW Germany 1940–44. Consultant Physician to the British Army of the Rhine (BAOR) 1945–50. Near and Far East Director of Middle East Land Forces 1954. DMS 1956–59 Western Comd. Retired to Hertfordshire. Medals: CB 2nd Jan. 1956, OStJ 1948, 1939–45 S., BWM, Gen. Service Malaya, UN SM with cl. Korea, QEII Corn Medal 1953. MID 21st Feb. 1946. d. 6th Oct. 1967.

O'NEILL Desmond Francis David Address: 99 Stockman's Lane, Belfast. MB, BCh (QUB 1939). Capt. RAMC. MC. MID.

O'NEILL John Lawrence b. 14th Nov. 1900, Athy, Co. Kildare. LRCP&SI and LM (1925). Lt IMS 3rd Feb. 1931. Capt. 3rd Feb. 1934. Maj. 3rd Aug. 1940. A/Lt Col. 29th Sept. 1941. T/Lt Col. 29th Nov. 1941. Lt Col. 14th May 1945. A/Col. 22nd Sept. 1942. T/Col. 14th May 1945. PC Maj. RAMC 8th Dec. 1947. T/Lt Col. 9th Dec. 1947. Lt Col. 28th Dec. 1947. r.p. disability 20th Jun. 1951. India/Burma/Singapore 1931–47. CO Trg. R/Amb. 1941. 23rd Fd Amb. 942. ADMS HQ 17th Div. 1942–43. CO 50th Fd Amb. 1943. ADMS HQ 202 L. of C. area 1944. CO 67th IGH (C) 1944–46. 93 IGH (C) 1946. CO 114th Mil. Con. Dep. Hereford 1947–49. CO Mil. Hosp. Waringfield 1949–50. FARELF 1950–51: CO BMH Kinrara 1950. Invalided. Medals: 1939–45 S. Burma S., WM, India Service M, GSM with cls SE Asia 1945–46 and Malaya.

O'NEILL Maurice Brendan MB (UCG 1940). Lt RAMC 17th May 1940.

O'NEILL Patrick Laurence MB, BCh (TCD 1930), L.LM (RCPI 1925), L.LM (RC SI 1925). Col. IMS. Burma 1941. O.C. 24th I.G.H. M.I.D.

O'NEILL Stephen Gerald L Med. LS (TCD 1933). Lt Col. IMS. POW at Tobruk.

O'NEILL-DONNELLION John Desmond TCD 1942. Surg. Lt RNVR.

O'REILLY Charles Joseph b. 9th Apr. 1891. s. Joseph O'Reilly (DL), Sans Souci, Booterstown, Co. Dublin. Address: Temora, Booterstown, Co. Dublin. Educ. TCD. MB (1913), BCh, BAO, LM (Rot. Hosp.). Occupation House Surg. St Patrick Dun's Hosp. T/Lt RAMC 16th Aug. 1914. Capt. 16th Aug. 1915. PC Lt (T/Capt) 1st Jan. 1917. Capt. 16th Feb. 1918. A/Maj. 4th Jan. 1918. Resigned 6th Jul. 1919. Rempld 2nd Sept. 1939. A/Maj. 20th Oct. 1939. T/Maj. 20th Jan. 1940. Maj. 7th Nov. 1941. A/Lt Col. 7th Aug. 1941. r.p. 16th Apr. 1943. Served with BEF France 1914–17. Italy 1917–19. CO 48th and 101st Mil. Con. Dep. 1941–43. Medals: DSO (3rd Jun. 1919), MC (2nd Nov. 1915), Bar (26th Nov. 1917), 1914 S., BWM, VM. MID 1st Jan. 1916, 5th Jun. 1919. d. 15th Jul. 1952.

O'REILLY Cyril Francis MB, BCh (QUB 1936). RAMC.

O'REILLY Michael Noel TCD 1939. Surg. Lt RNVR.

O'REILLY Patrick Joseph Address: 15 Vincent View, College Rd, Cork. MB, BCh (NUI 1939). Lt RAMC 5th Jun. 1941.

O'REILLY Patrick Vincent Address: Lisdonish House, Ballyjamesduff, Co. Cavan. L.LM (RCPI 1933), L.LM (RCSI 1933). Lt RAMC 1940.

O'RIORDAN John Patrick Address: 52 Kenilworth Pk, Rathgar, Dublin MB, BCh (NUI 1938). Lt IMS 1st Nov. 1938.

O'RIORDAN William Henry b. 8th Feb. 1885, Cork. L.LM (RCPI 1908), L.LM (RCSI 1908). Lt RAMC 30th Jan. 1909. Capt. 30th Jul. 1912. A/Maj. 28th Oct. 1917. Maj. 30th Jan. 1921. Bt. Lt Col. 20th Dec. 1932. Lt Col. 6th Dec. 1933. Col. 6th Jun. 1937. A/Brig. 22nd Jul. 1940. T/Brig. 22nd Jan. 1941. r.p. remained employed 6th Jun. 1941. r.p. Hon. Brig. 26th Nov. 1948. Served India 1912–14. France and Flanders 7th Nov. 1914–15. Mesopotamia 1915–19. India 1923–29 and 1931–36. CO Mil. Hosp. Catterick 1936–37. Comdt Depot and Trg. Estab. RAMC 1937–40. DDMS HQ 8th Corps. 1940–41. CO Cambridge Hosp. Aldershot 1941–45. MEF/NELF CO 12 Gen. Hosp. 1945–47. CO BAMH Bir Ya'acor 1947–48. Medals: MC (22nd Dec. 1916), 1914 S., BWM, VM, DM, WM. MID 1st Jan. 1916, 19th Oct. 1916, 21st Feb. 1919, 20th Dec. 1930. d. 7th Aug. 1963.

O'ROURKE Patrick Joseph Alfred (The O'Rourke), L.LM (RCPI 1922), L.LM (RCSI 1922). Flt Offr RN and RAF 1941.

ORR Charles James Kirkpatrick Address: Station View, Dunloy, Co. Antrim. MB, BCh (QUB 1939). Sq. Ldr (M) RAFVR.

ORR Charles Warden Address: Mondara, Kensington Rd, Knock, Belfast. LRCP (Edinburgh 1939), LRCS (Edinburgh 1939), LRFPS (Glasgow 1939). Captain RAMC.

ORR David Alexander Reginald Address: 15–19 Shankill Rd, Belfast. MB, BCh (QUB 1942). Capt. RAMC.

ORR James Wilson b. 12th Oct. 1909, Armagh. MB, BCh, BAO (QUB 1933). Lt RAMC 23rd Apr. 1936, Capt. 23rd Apr. 1937, PC Capt. 23rd Apr. 1941, Maj. 23rd Apr. 1945, A/Lt Col. 23rd Spt. 1939, T/Lt Col. 23rd Dec. 1939, Lt Col. 12th May 1949, A/Col. 24th Jul. 1945, T/Col. 24th Jan. 1946, Col. 4th Sept. 1958. Served India 1936–39, CO 3rd Armd Fd Amb. 1939–40, 1st Fd Amb. 1942–43. BNAF/CMF 1943–46, ADMS HQ N. Africa Dist. 1943–44, CO 2CCS 1944–45, ADMS HQ Sub. Areas 1945, CO 22nd Gen Hosp. 1945–56, ADMS HQ 56 (L Div) 1946, ADMS HQ Palestine 1948, ADMS HQ Malta Comd 1948, ADMS HQ Brit. Mil. Mission Greece 1950, ADMS GHQ MELF 1950–61, ADMS HQ W. Comd 1951–54, N. Africa 1954–56, CO BMH Tripoli 1954–55, ADMS HQ 25th Armd Brig. Dist/Tripolitania Dist. 1955–56, CO Mil. Hosp. Waringfield 1957, Mil. Hosp. Chester 1957–60, FARELF: ADMS HQ Singapore Base Dist. 1960–63, T/Duty SMO Brunei Dec. 1962, OIC Med. Servs. and WARC records 1963–68. Medals: MC 21st Sept.1937, IGSM with cl. NWF 1936–37, 1939–45 S., Africa S with cl. 1st Army, Italy S., DM, WM, GSM with cl. Palestine 1948 and Brunei 1962. MID 23rd Sept. 1943.

*ORR William Burnett Faris b. 24th May 1899, Templepatrick, Co. Antrim. s. James and Charlotte Orr. Husband of Maud Mary Orr of Morfa, Nevin, Caernarvonshire. MB, BCh (QUB 1921), DHP (QUB 1928). PC Lt 1st Aug. 1923 RAMC. Capt. 1st Feb. 1927. Maj. 26767 RAMC 1st May 1924. Served India 1924–30, Egypt 1933–38, Palestine 1936, BEF France 1939–40. d. 29th Jun. 1940 at Llandudno aged 41. Medals: 1939–45 S., WM. MID 29th Dec. 1940. Commemorated Liverpool (Anfield) Crematorium, Panel 2.

O'RYAN Innocent Address: 3 Clarinda Pk North, Dun Laoghaire, Dublin. L.LM (1937 RCPI), L.LM (1937 RCSI). Lt RAMC 16th May 1940.

OSBOURNE Thomas Stanislaus L.LM (RCPI 1926), L.LM (RCSI 1926) Flt Offr RN and RAF 1943.

O'SHEA Patrick b. 15th Jan. 1906, Killorglin, Co. Kerry. MB, BCh, BAO (TCD 1930). T/Lt 4th May 1933. PC Lt 1st Dec. 1933. Capt. 4th May 1934. A/Maj. 22nd Jan. 1940. T/Maj. 22nd Apr. 1940. Maj. 4th May 1943. A/Lt Col. 17th Apr. 1943. T/Lt Col. 17th Jul. 1943. Lt Col. 2nd May 1948. A/Col. 27th Feb. 1944. r.p. 30th Sept. 1954. Served India 1934–40. Sierra Leone 1942–44. India/Burma 1944–46. CO 1 (WA) Fd Amb. 1943–44 and 1945. ADMS HQ 82 (WA) Div. 1944–45. CO 10 IMFTU 1945. ADMS HQ N. Burma sub area 1945–46. MELF 1948–50. Comdt Base Depot RAMC 1948–49. CO BMH El Ballah 1949–50. E. Africa CO BMH Nairobi 1950–52. CO Mil. Hosp. Colchester 1953–54. Medals: IGSM (cl. NWF Mohmand 1935), 1939–45 S., Burma S., DM, WM, QEII Corn Medal 1953. d. 30th Aug. 1961.

O'SULLIVAN Bryan Michael MB, BCh (TCD 1935). Surg. Lt RNVR.

O'SULLIVAN Desmond Patrick Address: The Brea, Mount Charles, Co. Donegal. L.LM (RCPI 1937), L.LM (RCSI 1937). Flt Offr RAF 1941.

O'SULLIVAN Eoghan Thomas MB, BCh, BAO (UCC 1926). Flt Offr RAF.

O'SULLIVAN Francis Patrick Address: 27 Palmerston Pk, Dublin. MB, BCh (TCD 1939). RAF.

O'SULLIVAN John Vincent Address: The Laurels, Western Rd, Cork. MB, BCh (NUI 1940). Flt Offr RAFVR 1940.

O'SULLIVAN Timothy Alphonsus MB, BCh, BAO (UCC 1929). Lt RAMC.

O'TOOLE Cyril Paul L.LM (RCPI 1927), L.LM (RCSI 1927).

O'TOOLE Kevin L.Med. LCh (TCD 1934). Maj. RAMC.

O'TOOLE Michael Joseph MB, BCh (NUI 1926). Lt RAMC 17th Oct. 1942.

P

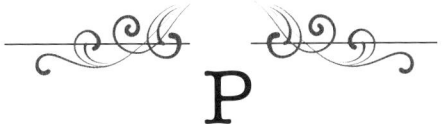

PAGE Ernest Victor TCD 1936. Lt RNVR. MBE.

PAGE John Allison Address: Melrose, Silchester Rd, Glenageary, Dublin. MB, BCh (TCD 1931). Surg. Comdr RN. POW Hong Kong 1941. Released 1946. MID.

PAGE Walter Ashley Address: 14 Railway St, Lisburn, Co. Antrim. MB, BCh (QUB 1932), MD (QUB 1936). Surg. Lt RNVR.

PAISLEY Dermod Patrick George Address: 23 University Ave., Belfast. MB, BCh (QUB 1936). Capt. RAMC. MID.

PALMER Philip Francis b. 8th Aug. 1903, Kroonstad, Orange Free State, South Africa. MB, BCh, BAO (TCD 1926), DPH and BHyg (Durham 1933). T/Lt 16th Jul. 1926. PC Lt 29th Jul. 1926. Capt. 29th Jan. 1930. Maj. 29th Jul. 1936. A/Lt Col. 15th Nov. 1940. T/Lt Col. 15th Feb. 1941. Lt Col. 5th Apr. 1945. A/Col. 7th Mar. 1943. T/Col. 7th Sept. 1943. Col. 1st Mar. 1949. T/Brig. 22nd Sept. 1954. Brig. 30th Aug. 1955. T/Maj. Gen. 22nd Feb. 1956. Maj. Gen. 6th Aug. 1956. r.p. 6th Aug. 1960. Served Shanghai 1927–28. India 1928–32 and 1937–40. CO 194th Fd Amb. 1940–41. CO 208th Fd Amb. 1941–42. BNAF/CMF/MEF 1942–46: CO 71st Gen. Hosp. 1943. ADMS HQ 4th Div. 1943–45 & 1945–46. BAOR 1946–69. ADMS HQ 5th Div. 1946–48. ADMS HQ Hanover Dist. 1948–49. ADMS HQ 7th Armoured Div. 1949. FARELF: ADMS HQ Malaya Dist. 1949–51. DDMS HQ BCFK 1954–55. DMS GHQ MELF 1955–57. DDMS HQ N. Comd 1957–60. Col. Comdt RAMC 1963. Medals: CB (13th Jun. 1957), OBE (19th Apr. 1945), IGSM (cl. NWF 1930–31), 1939–45 S., Africa S (cl. 1st Army), Italy S., DM, WM, GSM (cl. Malaya and Cyprus and Near East). MID 23rd Sept. 1943, 24th Oct. 1950. Greek Gold Cross of the Order of George I (10th Mar. 1950).

PANTRIDGE James Francis Address: Sion Hill, Hillsborough, Co. Down. MB, BCh (QUB 1939). Capt. RAMC. Served in Malaya MO attached to Gordon Highlanders. He was taken prisoner at the fall of Singapore in February 1942. For the next three-and-a-half years he endured dreadful hardships on the Thai/Burma railway. On returning to Belfast in October 1945, Pantridge resumed his medical career and began to specialise in diseases of the heart and was appointed consultant physician and cardiologist at the Royal Victoria Hosp. Belfast. He produced the world's first portable defibrillator in 1965, initially

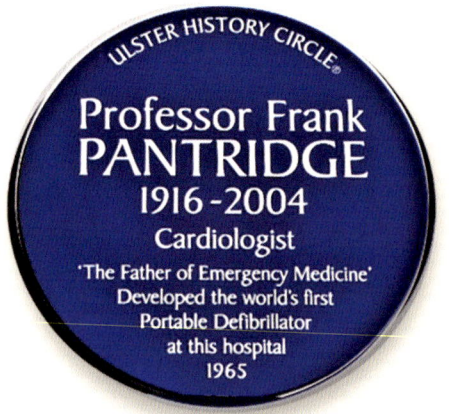

operating from a specially equipped ambulance, his prototype ran off car batteries and weighed in at around 70 kilos. His initial defibrillator gradually evolved into the small compact units so prevalent today, and subsequently into the mini-implantable devices placed into the chests of patients. American President Lyndon B. Johnston's life was saved by a Pantridge defibrillator in 1972 when he had a heart attack. Johnston said at the time: 'Almost certainly, only one cardiologist has conducted pioneering work that saved my life and those of thousands of others. This distinction goes to Dr James Francis 'Frank' Pantridge, a professor at Queen's University, Belfast, Northern Ireland. During a visit to Charlottesville, Virginia, I had a heart attack in 1972, which a mobile coronary care unit successfully treated with a Pantridge Portable Defibrillator. I owe my life to the invention of this former Japanese prisoner of war.' Medals: MC for remaining absolutely cool under the heaviest fire and completely regardless of his own personal safety at all times.

PARKE Frederick William Address: Cnoc Aluin, Coliemore Rd, Dalkey, Dublin. MB, BCh (TCD 1938). Flying Officer RAF. POW Java 1942.

PARKINSON George Singleton b. 1st Oct. 1880, Co. Dublin. Educ. MRCS (England 1906), LRCP (London 1906), DPH (London 1914), RCPS (England 1914). In the ranks 1900–01. Lt RAMC 1st Aug. 1908. Capt. 1st Feb. 1912. A/Maj. 25th Feb. 1918. T/Maj. 6th Nov. 1919. Maj. 1st Aug. 1920. A/Lt Col. 24th Jul. 1918. r.p. Lt Col. 1st Aug. 1928. Rempld 4th Sept. 1939. r.p. 30th Nov. 1940. Rempld A/Brig. 24th Aug. 1943. T/Brig. 24th Feb. 1944. r.p. Hon Brig. 23rd Oct. 1945. Served South Africa 1910–13. BEF France and Flanders from 15th Aug. 1914. ADMS HQ 1st Army 1918–19. Gibraltar DADH and MOH 1919–23. Asst Prof. of Hyg. RAN Coll. 1923–28 and Sept.–Nov. 1940. ADH HQ E. Comd 1939–40. Italy attd. Nat. HQ Armistice Control Comm. 1943–45. Medals: DSO (1st Jan. 1918), 1914 S., BWM, VM, 1939–45 S., Italy S., DM, WM, L de H War Cross (6th Nov. 1918), Mil. O. of Avis 5th Class (21st Aug. 1919), Silver M. de la Reconnaissance (2nd Mar. 1926), Typhus Comm. M (17th Oct. 1946). MID 1st Jan. 1916, 29th May 1917, 24th Dec. 1917. d. 17th Aug. 1953.

PARSONS Alfred Denis b. 1st Aug. 1914, Athlone, Co. Westmeath. s. George and Grace (née McClonaghan) Parsons. Address: Dromore, Greystones, Co. Wicklow. Educ. Aravon School, Bray, Co. Wicklow 1923 to 1928,

Portora Royal School, Enniskillen. TCD 1932. MB, BCh (TCD 1937). Capt. RAMC. Evacuation of Dunkirk 1st Jun. 1940. Egypt January 1941, 2nd Battle of Alexandria 1942. Thigh injury Battle of Alamein. Took part in the Anzio Landings. MC Nov. 1943. 'Captain A.D. Parsons is a medical officer attached to the Buffs. Throughout a period of almost continuous action from early August 1942 to March 1943 the personal bravery and determined initiative of this officer have been responsible for thesaving of a great many lives. On every occasion he was to be found at the spot where casualties were most likely to occur, and it is due to his complete disregard of danger, the calm skill and speed of his work, and his devotion to duty under fire that so many men owe their lives. The following are but a few examples of his consistent behaviour. On the morning of October 24th, 1943, he was with a company of Buffs behind the Miteiriya Ridge in a position which had just been captured by New Zealand battalions. A number of the New Zealanders had been lying for most of the night with severe wounds almost untreated. Under continuous shell and mortar fire, Captain Parsons collected about a dozen severely wounded men from an area exposed to direct small arms fire in the middle of a minefield. He would not have failed in his duty had he devoted himself to casualties nearer at hand and less exposed to fire. Throughout the twelve days of the Alamein battle he repeatedly recovered wounded men from forward slopes under fire, who must otherwise

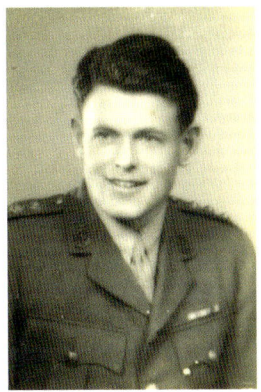

Alfred Denis Parsons

have lost their lives. On January 19th south of Tarhuna under heavy shellfire, a general was severely wounded. Captain Parsons at the time was characteristically returning in his jeep with a badly wounded man from the most shelled area, but on being informed he put the man in an ambulance and under continued fire went to the general, and there is little doubt that his calmed skill saved a valuable life. Again on the morning of January 22nd, in the Tarhuna pass at a time when four men had just been killed by close-range heavy mortar fire, after dressing several wounds Captain Parsons crawled out onto a forward slope under direct fire to rescue a man believed to be alive. West of Zavia on January 25th, 1943, his work under very heavy shelling while others were taking cover again saved several lives. It is in fact not possible to speak too highly of the sustained and unselfish courage of this officer in saving life throughout eight months of nearly continuous periods of action. After the war worked in Dublin and New Zealand. In

1955 he disappeared while on a medical mission with 24 others. The boat he had travelled in was found, but none of the passengers on board.'

PATON James Grogan Address: Imperial Hotel, Cobh, Co. Cork. MB, BCh, BAO (UCC 1938). Flt Offr RAF.

PATON John Walter Baxter Address: 94 Balmoral Ave., Belfast. MB, BCh (QUB 1937). Maj. RAMC.

PATRICK James Wilson Address: Dunaird, Broughshane, Ballymena, Co. Antrim. MB, BCh (QUB 1931), FPH (QUB 1934), Wing Comdr (M) RAF. MID.

PATRICK John Brian MB, BCh (TCD 1926), MD (TCD 1937). Surg. Comdr RN. MID.

PATTERSON Arthur Frederick Isbell b. 22nd Mar. 1891, Navan, Co. Meath. s. George Barnes and Mary Elizabeth Patterson, 7 Shipquay St, Londonderry. Educ. RCSI. LRCPI (1912), LRCSI (1912), LM (Rot. Hosp.). R. C. of I. Lt RAMC SR 23rd Sept. 1914. Mobd 6th Oct. 1914. Capt. 6th Apr. 1915. PC Lt (T/Capt) 1st Jan. 1917. Capt. 6th Apr. 1918. A/Maj. 1st Apr. 1920. Maj. 23rd Sept. 1926. r.p. 27th Mar. 1930. Rempld 2nd Sept. 1939. Served India 1915–16. Mesopotamia from 7th Apr. 1916–21. Malta 1924–26. r.p. ill health. Medals: DSO (17th Sept. 1917), BWM, VM, GSM (cl. Iraq), DM, WM. MID 15th Aug. 1917. d. 14th Feb. 1958.

PATTISON David Stanley Address: 30 Terenure Pk, Dublin. L.LM (RCPI 1938), L.LM (RCSI 1938). Flt Offr 1941.

PATTON George Address: 17 Queen's St, Ballymoney, Co. Antrim. MB, BCh (QUB 1937). Capt. RAMC. MC.

PATTON Kevin Francis b. Mullingar, Co. Westmeath. s. Henry and Annie Gertrude (Moore) Patton, Mullingar, Co. Westmeath. Address: Magloma, Mullingar, Co. Westmeath. As a medical student went to Spain with Eoin O'Duffy's group. MB, BCh, BAO (UCD 1938). Maj. 11780 RAMC. Posted to an artillery regiment. Served in Cairo 4th Field Regiment, capture of Amba Alagi in East Africa, with the Buffs at the Battle of Alam Hamza, overrun but escaped, taking 40 wounded with him. 1942 he was with the Cavalry Regiment living in the desert under severe conditions. Performed an operation with a blue Gillette razor blade. Tegna Gap under heavy gun fire. Suffered leg injuries and spent 15 months in hospital. Medals: MC. 'During the breakthrough of the enemy line towards El Hanna by an armoured division at first light on March 27th, 1943, the rear of the column was attacked by enemy tanks at close range. Despite experiencing a broken ankle as a result of a fall from a portee, Captain Patton tended to, and evacuated all wounded from the scene of action in face of very heavy and accurate shellfire and machine gun fire from the enemy tanks. During the approximate 30 minutes of the action, this officer not only showed complete disregard for his own personal safety, but also a very high standard of devotion to duty.' d. 29th Mar. 1947 aged 33. Buried in Termonfeckin C. of I. churchyard.

PAUL Robert Gordan Campbell College. LRCP (Edinburgh 1927), LRCS (Edinburgh 1927), LRFPS (Glasgow 1927). Captain RAMC.

PEACOCK Pryce Henry b. 14th Sept. 1907, Dublin. MB, BCh, BAO (TCD 1932). PC Lt RAMC 27th Jul. 1933. Capt. 1st Dec. 1934. Retired 12th Jun. 1939. Rejoined 2nd Sept. 1939. A/Maj. 25th Mar. 1940. T/Maj. 25th Jun. 1940. Served India 1934–38. Palestine 1938–39. BEF France 1939–40. E. Africa 1941–45, invalided. d. 9th Jul. 1950, France.

*****PEARSE** George Passmore s. Charles Perrin Pearse and Ellen Gertrude Pearse of Glenageary, Co. Dublin. MB, BS, BAO (NUI). Surg. Lt KIA 8th Jun. 1940, aged 31 on HMS *Glorious*. Commemorated on Plymouth Naval Memorial, Panel 36, Column 2.

PENNEFATHER Aubrey Lovelace b. 2nd Aug. 1908, Tipperary. Address: Marlow, Goold's Cross, Co. Tipperary. MB, BCh, BAO (TCD 1932). Lt RAMC 7th Jun. 1934. Capt. 7th Jun. 1935. PC Capt. 7th Jun. 1939. A/Maj. 20th Jun. 1940. T/Maj. 20th Sept. 1940. Maj. 7th Dec. 1943. A/Lt Col. 19th Aug. 1945. T/Lt Col. 19th Nov. 1945. Lt Col. 29th Nov. 1951. A/Col. 26th Jun. 1946. T/Col. 26th Jul. 1946. Col. 16th Sept. 1960. r.p. 31st Jul. 1965. Served Gibraltar 1934–48. Palestine 1938–39. India 1941–45: CO 5 and 24 Fd Amb. 1945. AFNEI: ADMS HQ 23 Indian Div. 1946. OC Mil Hosp. Bovington 1947–49. W. Africa: CO 68th (WA) Mil. Hosp. Lagos 1949–52. BAOR: CO 22nd Fd Amb. 1953–57. CO 5th Fd Amb. 1958 and Mil. Hosp. Shorncliffe 1958–59. FARELF 1959-62: CO 8th Brigade Gp Med. Coy. 1959–60 and BMH Singapore 1960–62. ADMS HQ NI Comd 1962–65. Medals: GSM (cl. Palestine 1936–39) cl. Malaya, 1939–45 S. and cl. SE Asia 1945–46. Burma S. DM, WM, QEII Corn Medal 1953, German O. Red Cross Cross of Merit 1937.

PERROT Henry Stanislaus Address: Millview, Malahide, Co. Dublin. MB, BCh (TCD 1923). RAMC.

PERRY Henry Marian Joseph b. 11th Mar. 1884, Cork. s. John Perry. L.LM (RCPI 1906), L.LM (RCSI 1906). Married Mary Eleanor dt. Edward Griffith, Cornwall. Lt RAMC 28th Jan. 1907. Capt. 28th Jul. 1910. T/Maj. 18th Sept. 1915. Maj. 28th Jan. 1919. Bt. Lt Col. 9th Feb. 1921. T/Lt Col. 6th Mar. 1931. Bt. Col. 26th Mar. 1933. Col. 28th Dec. 1934. Maj. Gen. 26th Sept. 1935. r.p. 25th Jun. 1941. Hon. Surg. to the King 1933–40. Hong Kong 1908–11. BEF France from 14th Aug. 1914 as Regt. MO. POW 1914–15. France and Belgium 1915–18. OC 65th Fd Amb 1915–16. RAM Coll. Asst Prof of Pathology 1919–21. Prof. of Pathology 1922. Seconded to the Foreign Office as Director of Egyptian

Public Health Lab. Services. Returned to the Army in 1930 Prof. At Millbank and Director of Pathology. Medals: CB (11th May 1937), OBE (3rd Jun. 1919), 1914 S., BWM, VM, KGV Silver Jub. Medal 1935. MID 1st Jan. 1916, 30th Dec. 1918, 10th Jul. 1919. d. 23rd Mar. 1955, Walton on Thames.

PERRY James Flack Address: Saintfield, Belfast. Campbell College. MB, BCh (QUB 1940). Capt. RAMC.

PERRY Samuel Address: Killans, Ahoghill, Co. Antrim. MB, BCh (QUB 1932). Sq. Ldr (M) RAFVR.

PETIT Gerard b. 18th May 1884, Sligo. Educ. RUI, RCSI. LRCPI (1906), LRCSI (1906), LM, Hon. MSc (RUI). Lt RAMC 29th Jul. 1907. Capt. 29th Jan. 1911. Maj. 29th Jul. 1919. r.p. 11th Aug. 1923. Rempld A/Col. 17th Dec. 1939. T/Lt Col. 17th Mar. 1940. A/Col. 1st Dec. 1941. T/Col. 1st Jun. 1942. r.p. 29th Sept. 1945. Served India 1910–14. France and Flanders from 9th Nov. 1914–16. India 27th Mar. 1916–17. Mesopotamia 1917–18. India 1918–20. BEF France 1939. PSMB Scottish Comd 1939–41 and 1944. ADMS HQ Central Mid. Area 1941–44. MEF: CO 27 Gen. Hosp. 1944–45. Medals: MC (14th Jan. 1916), 1914 S., BWM, VM, 1939–45 S., DM, WM. MID 1st Jan. 1916. d. 20th Aug. 1959, London.

PHELAN Theobald Denis MB, BCh, BAO (UCD 1933). Maj. (T/Lt Col.) RAMC. b. Clonmel, Co. Tipperary. OBE. 'During the period under review Lieutenant Colonel Phelan has commanded a field ambulance attached to an armoured brigade. He has consistently shown a very high degree of vision, foresight and initiative – the results of which have been manifest in the work of his unit. His field ambulance has won for itself a reputation second to none in the 8th Army and Lieutenant Colonel Phelan and the team of doctors working under him have inspired the confidence and affection of everyone in the brigade. The medical record of this brigade and of Lieutenant-Colonel Phelan's Field Ambulance is an impressive one, while the ratio of deaths to battle casualties dealt with by the main dressing station is most unusually low. The credit for the exceptionally fine work done by this unit must go to a large degree to its commanding officer.'

PHILLIPS Albert Edward MB, BCh (TCD 1922). Surg. Comdr RN.

PIKE William Archibald James Address: Clonoulty Rectory, Goolds Cross, Co. Tipperary. MB, BCh (TCD 1938). RAF.

PILKINGTON Arthur Chartres MB, BCh (TCD 1934). RNVR.

PINKERTON John Henry McKnight Address: 12 Hinton Pk, Londonderry. MB, BCh (QUB 1943). Surg. Lt RNVR.

PLEWS John Balfour b. 12th Jun. 1912, Blackrock, Co. Dublin. MB, BCh, BAO (TCD 1937). Lt RAMC 1st Feb. 1938. Capt. 1st Oct. 1939. PC Capt. 1st Feb. 1943. A/Maj. 13th May 1946. Maj. 1st Jul. 1946. Lt Col. 31st Jul. 1953. Col. 26th Apr. 1963. Served India 1939. MEF 1939–44. RMO 2nd Cameroon Highlanders 1939–40. NWE 1945–46. FARELF 1949–52. ENT Spec. Mil. Hosp. Catterick 1952–55. FARELF: BMH Singapore 1955–58. Cambridge Hosp. Aldershot 1958–61. BAOR: CO BMH Iserlohn 1963–66. ENT Spec. Mil. Hosp. Catterick 1966. Medals: 1939–45 S., Africa S., CM, WM, GSM (cl. Malaya).

PLUNKETT Harold Dudley L.LM (RCPI 1929), L.LM (RCSI 1929). OStJ 1937.

POLLOCK Robert Address: Knockaconny, Co. Monaghan. MB, BCh (TCD 1937). Capt. RAMC. POW France 1940. Released 1945.

POPHAM Cyril b. 13th Aug. 1890, Bantry, Co. Cork. s. Thomas (GP) and Kate French Popham, 1 Blackrock Tce, Bantry, Co. Cork. Educ. Edinburgh Uni. LRCP (Edinburgh 1914), LRFP (Glasgow), LRFS (Glasgow). R. C. of I. Lt RAMC SR 16th Sept. 1914. Mobd 30th Sept. 1914. Capt. 1st Apr. 1915. PC Capt. 1st Jun. 1918. A/Maj. 13th Sept. 1920. A/Lt Col. 1st May 1921. Lt Col. 1st Mar. 1938. A/Col. 1st Oct. 1940. T/Col. 1st Apr. 1941. Col. 11th Mar. 1944. r.p. 3rd Dec. 1947. Served with BEF France 22nd Oct. 1914–19. 11th Gen. Hosp. India 1919–22. Waziristan 1920–21. Malta 1926–31. India 1934–39. CO BMH Sialkot 1937–38 & BMH Ambala 1938–39. OIC Med. Div. Cambridge Hosp. Aldershot 1939. SMO R Mil. Coll. Sandhurst 1939–40. CO 14 CCS Jan.–Sept. 1940. Palestine Jun.–Nov. 1940. Egypt 1940–42. Palestine 1942–45. CO 26 Gen. Hosp. 1940–41. CO 32 Gen. Hosp. 1941–42. ADMS HQ 71 Sub Area 1942–43. DDMS HQ 21 area 1943–45. NWE 1945–46. CO 113 Gen. Hosp. Aug.–Sept. 1945 and 23 Scottish Gen. Hosp. 1945–46. CO Mil. Hosp. Chester 1946–47. Medals: OBE (30th Dec. 1941), 1914 S., BWM, VM, 1939–45 S., Africa S., DM, WM, MID 1st Jun. 1923, 30th Dec. 1941, 6th Apr. 1944. d. 9th Oct. 1958.

PORTER David Cuthbert MB, BCh (QUB 1933). Capt. RAMC.

PORTER Robert Alexander MB, BCh (QUB 1933). Surg. Lt RNVR.

POSNER Joseph (Joshua) L.LM (1919 RCPI), L.LM (1919 RCSI). RAF Jul. 1943.

POSTON Richard Irvine MB, BCh (QUB 1922), MD (QUB 1925). Capt. RAMC.

POWER Michael Patrick b. 15th Aug. 1889, Co. Cork. s. Bartholomew (farmer) and Frances Power, Castlemartyr, Co. Cork. Educ. Edinburgh Uni. LRCP (Edin. 1913), LRCS (Edin. 1913), LRFP (Glasgow 1913), LRFS (Glasgow 1913).

R. RC. T/Lt RAMC 4th Dec. 1914, Capt. 4th Dec. 1915. PC Capt. 1st May 1919. A/Maj. 14th Feb. 1920, Maj. 4th Dec. 1926. Bt. Lt Col. 17th Oct. 1939. A/Col. 27th Mar. 1941. T/Col. 27th Sept. 1941. r.p. Hon. Col. 15th Oct. 1948. Served in France 20th May 1916–17 and Apr.–May 1918. Italy 1917–18. India 1919–23 (Waziristan 1920–21), 1925–31 and 1934–39 (Mohmand Ops. 1935–36). BEF France 1939–40. CO 5 CCS Jan.–Oct. 1940. CO 10 Lt/Fd Amb. 1940–41. ADMS HQ 2 Div. 1941–42. India 1942–44. Insp. Hosps. GHQ (I) 1942–43, CO CIMH Quetta 1943–44, HQ C. Comd India Sept.–Dec. 1944. CMF 1945–46: CO 98 Gen. Hosp. Mar.–Apr. 1945. ADMS HQ 54 area 1945–46. MELF: EDMS HQ Canal S. Dist. 1945–47. CO 99 Nil. POW Hosp. Stafford 1947–48. Medals: OBE (3rd Apr. 1923), MC (3rd Jun. 1918), 1915 S., BWM, VM, IGS (cl. Waz. 1919–21), 1939–45 S., Italy S., WM. MID 1st Jun. 1923, 12th Jun. 1923, 8th May 1936, 17th Oct. 1939, 26th Jul. 1940. d. 27th Feb. 1952

POWER Richard Wood MB, BCh (1921), DPH (1923 TCD). Married Margary. Lt Col. RAMC.

PRATT Denis William Address: 102 Balmoral Ave., Belfast. MB, BCh (QUB 1934). Surg. Lt Comdr RN.

PRATT Robert Henry Address: Rossory Rectory, Enniskillen. MB, BCh (TCD 1935). Wing Comdr RAF. 1936.

PRENDERVILL James Thomas Address: 105 Grove Pk, Rathmines, Dublin. MB, BCh, BAO (NUI 1937). Lt IMS 6th Jun. 1939.

PRICE James Alan MB, BCh (QUB 1932), MC (QUB 1935), MRCP (London 1937). Lt Col. RAMC.

PRICE Sydney Henry Rhys Address: 4 Argyle Rd, Herbert Pk, Dublin. MB, BCh (TCD 1934). Surg. Comdr RN HMS *Lanba*.

PRINCE Gordon Stewart TCD 1940. Maj. RAMC. Served in India.

PRINGLE Alexander William Address: Aviemore, Monaghan. Campbell College. MB, BCh (TCD 1942). Captain RAMC.

PRINGLE George Morgan Address: Aughnacloy, Co. Tyrone. MB, BCh (QUB 1941). Flt Lt (M) RAFVR.

PRINGLE John Seton Michael Address: 33 Upper Fitzwilliam St, Dublin. MB, BCh (TCD 1933). Maj. RAMC.

PROCTOR Richard Louis Gibbon Address: 52 Wellington Rd, Dublin. MB, BCh (TCD 1924), MD (TCD 1936), DPH (TCD 1937), M (1931), F (RCPI 1936). Surg. Capt. RN.

PULVERTAFT Robert James Valentine MRCS (England 1923), LRCP (1923). b. Dublin. RAMC. OBE. 'Lieutenant-Colonel Pulvertaft arrived in the Middle East in September 1940, as pathologist on the staff of a 1,200-bed general hospital. In June 1942, he was appointed Officer-in-Charge Central Pathological Laboratory in Cairo, combining with this the duties of Deputy Assistant Director of Pathology, later upgraded to Assistant Director of Pathology in the Middle East. This officer is a distinguished pathologist in civil life on the staff of Westminster Hospital, London. He has brought to the army not only a rich store of experience but an original and inquiring mind. In addition to carrying out the routine work of his appointments he has interested himself in research work, especially in the treatment of infected wounds. His study of this treatment with chemotherapeutic substances has been accepted as of real value by the War Wounds Committee in the United Kingdom and especially his laboratory research into the substance now known as penicillin. By most industrious and painstaking investigations and experiments he has added considerable knowledge to the development of this substance. The introduction of penicillin into war surgery will undoubtedly revolutionise the treatment of septic wounds. In addition to his military duties, Lieutenant-Colonel Pulvertaft has rendered valuable aid to the British Council in Egypt under whose aegis he has given a series of lectures with highly commendable results.'

PURDON William Brooke b. 28th Nov. 1881, Donegal Pass, Belfast. s. Richard (physician) and Maud Mary Purdon, 8 Murrays Tce, Belfast, Co. Antrim. Educ. MB, BS (1906 RUI), BCh, BAO, DPH (QUB 1913). R. C. of I. Married Dorothy Myrtle dt. W. Coates. Lt RAMC 28th Jan. 1907. Capt. 28th Jul. 1910. T/Maj. 26th Apr. 1916. Maj. 28th Jan. 1919. A/Lt Col. 22nd Aug. 1916. T/Lt Col. 15th Jun. 1931. Lt Col. 30th Jun. 1931. Bt. Col. 1st Jul. 1934. Col. 1st Aug. 1935. Maj. Gen. 1st Mar. 1938. r.p. 28th Nov. 1941. Served in India 1908–13. BEF France and Belgium 1914–19. RMO 2nd Y and L 1914–15. CO 19th Fd Amb. 1916–17. Nos. 5, 6 and 16 Con. Dep. 1917–19. 1 Staty. Hosp. 1919. India 1923–27. ADH War Office 1930–34. ADH Egypt 1934–35. Prof. Hygiene RAM Coll. 1935–38. Comdt and Dean of Studies RAM Coll. 1938–40. KHS 15 Apr. 1938. BEF France: DMS HQ L of C area June 1940. DDMS HQ W.Comd 1940–41. r.p. 28th Nov. Med. Sup. Queen Mary's Hosp. Roehampton. Hon. Surg. to the King 1938–41. Gave up his medical career in 1946 to become the agent in London for the Northern Ireland government. A keen follower of rugby, he was in his younger days capped for Ireland. Medals: OBE (1st Jan. 1923), DSO (1st Jan. 1917), MC (18th Feb. 1915), 1914 S., BWM, VM, WM, KGV Silver Jub. Medal 1935, OStJ (22nd Jun. 1937). Medaille d'honneur du Service de Sainte Militaire-Chevalier de la Legion d'Honneur. MID 17th Feb. 1915, 4th Jun. 1916, 4th Jan. 1917. d. 1st Dec. 1950, London.

PYPER John Graham Address: 13 Windsor Ave., Bangor, Co. Down. MB, BCh (QUB 1935), MD (QUB 1938). Capt. RAMC. MID.

PYPER Robert Alexander Address: 13 Windsor Ave., Bangor, Co. Down. MB, BCh (QUB 1939). Maj. RAMC.

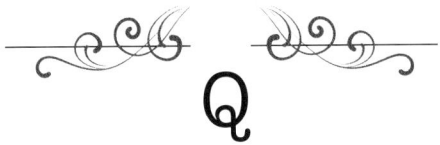

QUEALLY Francis James MB, BCh (TCD 1940). Capt. US Med. Corps.

QUIGLEY John b. 16th March 1898. Col. Indian Medical Service. MB, BCh (TCD 1926). Retired aged 50 years.

QUIGLEY Thomas Francis L.LM (RCPI 1931), L.LM (RCSI 1931). Lt RAMC 1940.

QUINLAN Gerald MB, BCh, BAO (UCD 1922). Lt RAMC.

QUINLAN Jerome Michael MB, BCh, BAO (UCC 1926). Lt RAMC.

QUINLAN Michael Finbarr Address: Loughrea, Co. Galway. MB, BCh, BAO (UCC 1928). Surg. RN.

QUINN Brian Stephen MB, BCh (NUI 1939). Lt RAMC.

QUINN John Vincent L.LM (RCPI 1931), L.LM (RCSI 1931). Flt Lt RAF 1941. Resigned Aug. 1943.

QUINN Patrick Joseph Gerard Address: Main Street, Drumquin, Co. Tyrone. L.LM (RCPI 1936), L.LM (RCSI 1936). Lt RAMC 1940.

QUINN Richard Butler MB (QUB 1922). Maj. RAMC.

R

RAINSFORD Seymour Grome MB, BCh (TCD 1922), MD (TCD 1932), DPH (TCD 1937). Surg. Capt. RN.

RAMSAY Robert Humphreys Address: Dunelm, Quay Rd, Ballycastle, Co. Antrim. MB, BCh (QUB 1942). Capt. RAMC with the 4th Army in Burma. Post-war GP Londonderry and served in the Territorials.

RAMSEY Andrew Shannon Address: 9 Glen Eden Villas, 15 Ballygomartin Rd, Belfast. MB, BCh (QUB 1939). Lt Col. RAMC. MBE. MID.

*****RANKEN** George Douglas MB, BCh (1924 TCD). b. Co. Donegal. Sudan Medical Service 1927. d. Cairo, 18th Oct. 1944.

RANKIN Matthew Neal Address: 11 Hopefield Ave., Belfast. MB, BCh (QUB 1941). Surg. Lt RNVR.

RAYMOND Michael Lt RAMC 4th Apr. 1942.

REA Eric Address: 130 Groomsport Rd, Bangor, Co. Down. MB, BCh (QUB 1941). Capt. RAMC. MID.

REA Martin Alexander MB (QUB 1926). Col. RAMC. OBE.

REA Samuel Brown MB, BCh (QUB 1926). Maj. RAMC.

READE Hilda Agnes Address: Excelsior, Portstewart, Co. Derry. MB, BCh (QUB 1943). Flt Offr RAFVR.

REDMOND Aidan MB, BCh, BAO (NUI 1925). Flt Offr RAF 28th Jan. 1941.

REES John Peter Raymond MB (TCD 1942) RAMC.

REEVES Anthony Joseph Address: Reevemount, Athy, Co. Kildare. MB, BCh (TCD 1937), DPH (U. Manchester 1942). Lt Col. RAMC. East Africa Comd.

REGAN Peter Leo MB, BCh, BAO (UCC 1920). Lt RAMC.

REGINALD Thomas Michael St John's, Malahide, Dublin. L.LM (RCPI 1938), L.LM (RCSI 1938). Lt RAMC 6th Apr. 1940.

*****REID** Adiel Elad Hazael Address: 24A Deramore Drive, Belfast. MB, BCh (QUB 1913). Capt. RAMC. Died on active service.

REID Robert Address: 79 Shankill Rd, Belfast. MB (QUB 1939). Maj. RAMC.

REID Robert Ian Gillespie Address: Little Castledillon, Armagh. MB, BCh (TCD 1928), DPH (TCD 1936). Maj. RAMC. Allied Land Forces s/e Asia 1942 to 1945.

REIDY Jeremiah MB, BCh, BAO (UCD 1933). Lt Col. IMS. Wife: Vera née Jones.

RENDLE-SHORT Angel Mary (née Jones) Address: Glenwilliam, Portrush, Co. Antrim. MB, BCh (QUB 1942). Lt RAMC.

RENTON Harold MB, BCh (TCD 1923). Lt Col. SAMC.

*****RETZ** Gilbert Charles b. 10th Sept. 1912. Address: Bannon Villa, Castlewood Pk Rathmines, Dublin. MB, BCh, BAO (TCD 1937). Entered the IMS Lt 1938. Capt. IMS. d. Malaya Mar. 1941.

REUBIN Isadore Address: 17 Strathmore Pk Sth, Belfast. MB, BCh (QUB 1937). Capt. RAMC.

REYNOLDS Kenneth Gordon Address: The Gables, St Lawrence Rd, Clontarf, Dublin. L.LM (RCPS 1934), L.LM (RCSI 1934). Flt Offr 1943. Resigned due to ill health.

RICE Henry James MB, BCh (1917), MD (1920 TCD). Lt RAMC Sept. 1917. Captain 1918. Served in France from 21st Jan. 1918. Col. IMS. Medals: MC (Jun. 1919), CIE, BWM, VM.

RICHARDSON Sir Albert Victor John b. 4th Sept. 1884, Monaghan. s. Mrs Richardson, 4 Victoria Villas, Morehampton Rd, Donnybrook, Dublin. Educ. St Andrews Coll. Dublin 7th Nov. 1901–30th Jun. 1902. Roebuck Masonic Sch. to 1901. MB, BCh (TCD 1908), DPH (TCD 1914). Director General Med. Services. R. C. of I. Surg. RN Nov. 1908. Surg. Lt Comdr Nov. 1914. Wing Comdr RAF. Maj. RAF Med. Sch. 1918. A/Lt Col. 1919. Air Marshal. Served in 1914–18 War RN and in 1935–45 War. Medals: KBE, CB, OBE.

RIGBY Claude Mallinson b. 29th Mar. 1882, Dublin. Married Mary Elaine Booth in 1920. Educ. Dulwich Coll. and The London Hosp. MRCS (England 1907), LRCP (London 1907), DMRE (Cambridge 1920). Lt RAMC 4th Feb. 1908. Capt. 4th Aug. 1911. A/Maj. 19th Mar. 1919. Maj. 4th Feb. 1920. r.p. 4th Feb. 1928. Rempld 27th May 1940. r.p. 24th Aug. 1945. From 1915–18 he was Surg. to the Governor of Bombay and from 1921–23 he was Surg. to Lord Rawlinson, the Comdr in Chief India. Served in India 1910–19 and 1921–23. Royal Cambridge Hosp. r.p. 1928. Recalled into the RAMC in 1940. Aldershot 1940–45. Specialist in radiology. Medals: BWM,VM. d. 29th Jan. 1960, Middleton on Sea.

RIORDAN Thomas Prior Address: Dunkerron, Model Farm Rd, Cork. MB, BCh, BAO (UCC 1936). Lt RAMC.

RITCHIE Desmond Thomas Crozier MB (QUB 1939). Surg. Lt Comdr RNVR.

RITCHIE Thomas Harold Wilson MB, BCh (QUB 1930), MD (QUB 1934). Surg. Lt Comdr RNVR.

ROANTREE William Bernard Address: Durham Lodge, Newbridge, Co. Kildare. MB, BCh (TCD 1925), FRCS (Edinburgh 1930). Lt Col. RAF 1942 Sq. Ldr.

ROBERTS Griffith Wyn MB, BCh (QUB 1941). Sq. Ldr (M) RAFVR.

ROBERTS (formally Rubinstein) Philip Harry Address: 24 Greenville Tce, South Circular Rd, Dublin. MB, BCh (TCD 1940). Capt. RAMC. NEF.

ROBERTSON William John b. 18th Feb. 1892, Curragh, Co. Kildare. Educ. Edinburgh Uni. MB (Edinburgh 1913), ChB, DOMS (England 1932). T/Lt RAMC 1st Jul. 1915. Capt 1st Jul. 1916. PC Lt (T/Capt) 1st Jun. 1918. Capt. 1st Jan. 1919. Maj. 1st Jul. 1927. A/Lt Col. 18th Feb. 1940. Lt Col. 30th Sept. 1940. T/Col. 25th Mar. 1942. Col. 15th Dec. 1945. r.p. 28th Apr. 1955. Served in France 21st Aug. 1915–18. India 1920–25 and 1929–35. Ophth. Spec. BMH Lahore and Kasauli 1929–32. BMH Rawalpindi 1932–35. Sierra Leone SMO Freetown 1938–39. CO 17 CCS Feb.–Jul. 1940. CO 7 Light Fd Amb. 1940–41. CO 47 Gen. Hosp. 1941–44. India 1942–46. CO 139 IBGH 1944–46. CO 232nd Mil. POW Hosp. 1946–47. ADMS HQ NI Dist. 1947–55. Medals: 1915 S., BWM, VM, 1939–45 S., Burma S., DM, WM, QEII Corn Medal 1953. d. 13th Oct. 1964, Musselburgh.

ROBINSON Alan Wellwood Wade LRCP (Edinburgh 1939), LRCS (Edinburgh 1939), LRFP (Glasgow 1939), MB, BCh (QUB 1939). Surg. Lt Comdr RN.

ROBINSON George MB, BCh (TCD 1924). Lt Col. RAMC. MC.

ROBINSON Harold Humphries TCD 1942. Lt RAMC.

ROBINSON Harold Hyman Address: 10 Fairfield Pk, Rathgar, Dublin. MB, BCh (TCD 1941). Lt RAMC.

ROBINSON Johnson Theodore b. 2nd Mar. 1908, Newry, Co. Down. MB, BCh, BAO (TCD 1930), MA, MD (TCD 1934), DTM&H (Eng. 1937), DPM (London 1949). PC Lt RAMC 29th Jul. 1930. Capt. 29th Jan. 1935. A/Maj. 1st Sept. 1939. T/Maj. 1st Dec. 1939. Maj. 29th Jul. 1940. A/Lt Col. 1st Jan. 1942. T/Lt Col. 1st Apr. 1942. Lt Col. 3rd Nov. 1946. A/Col. 20th Mar. 1944. T/Col. 20th Sept. 1944. Col. 13th May 1952. A/Brig. 18th Jun. 1945. T/Brig. 18th Dec. 1945. r.p. Hon. Brig. 1st Jun. 1956. Served Egypt 1932–45. SMO Trans Jordan Frontier Force 1935–39. ADGAMS War Office (AMD 1) 1942–43. CO 163 Fd Amb. 1943. CO 13th Light Fd Amb. 1943. BNAF/CLF 1944–45. ADMS (Ops) AF HQ 1944. ADMS HQ

1st Armoured Div. 1944. ADMS HQ LF Adriatic 1945 and Mil. Hosp Shaftesbury 1948–49. Adv Psych. HQ S. Comd 1949–50. OIC Psych. Wing R. Vic. Hosp. Netley 1950–51. Adv. Psych. HQ BAOR 1951–52. CO R. Vic. Hosp. Netley 1952–54. D Psych. Cons. Psych. to the Army 1955–56. QHP 1956. Medals: OBE (13th Dec. 1945), GSM (cl. Palestine), 1930–45 S., Italy S., DM, WM, QEII Corn Medal 1953, Order of El Nahda 3rd Class (Trans Jordan O. Merit 1939), OStJ. MID 19th Jul. 1945, 29th Nov. 1945.

ROBINSON Maurice MB, BCh (QUB 1921). Capt. RAMC.

ROBINSON Philip St George Address: Alma, Sandycove East, Dublin. MB, BCh (TCD 1935). Sq. Ldr RAF 1940.

ROBINSON William Arthur b. 2nd Mar. 1908, Newry, Co. Down. MB, BCh, BAO (TCD 1930), MD (TCD. 1934). PC Lt RAMC 11th Feb. 1931. Capt. 1st May 1934. A/Maj. 1st Sept. 1939. T/Maj. 1st Dec. 1929. Maj. 11th Feb. 1941. A/Lt Col. 21st Nov. 1941. T/Lt Col. 21st Feb. 1942. Lt Col. 3rd Mar. 1947. A/Col. 1st Nov. 1944. T/Col. 1st May 1945. Col. 5th Mar. 1953. Brig. 10th Apr. 1960. T/Maj. Gen. 13th Mar. 1960. Maj. Gen. 3rd May 1961. r.p. 20th Aug. 1965. Served Egypt 1932–37. MEF Italy 1941–44. NWE 1944–46: CO 200th Fd Amb. 1943–44. ADMS HQ 3rd Inf. Div. 1944–45. ADMS HQ 49th Div. 1945–46. ADGAMS War Office (AMD 1) 1946–49. E. Africa CO Mil. Hosp. MacKinnon Road 1950–51. MELF: ADMS HQ Cyrenaica Dist. 1951. ADMS HQ 1st Inf. Div. 1951–52. ADGAMS War Office (AMD 1) 1952–54. ADMS HQ Tps. Malta 1954–57. Comdt Depot and Trg. Establishment RAMC. 1958–60. DDGAMS War Office 1960–61. DDMS HQ S. Comd 1961–63. DMS HQ FARELF 1963–65. QHS 23rd Nov. 1960. Medals: CB (13th Jun. 1964), OBE (23rd Mar. 1944), 1939–45 S., Africa S. (cl. 8th Army), Italy S., France and Germany S., WM, QEII Corn Medal 1953. MID 4th Apr. 1946.

ROBINSON William Liddy Address: 25 Victoria Rd, Larne, Co. Antrim. MB, BCh (QUB 1941). Flt Lt (M) RAFVR.

ROCHE James MB, BCh, BAO (UCC 1926). Lt RAMC.

ROCHE James Joseph Dillon Knight b. 20th Jul. 1883, Donnybrook, Co. Dublin. s. Mary Knight Roche, Address: 29 Ailesbury Rd, Ballsbridge, Dublin. Educ. TCD. MB (1907), BCh, DPH (1913), BAO. Lt RAMC 30th Jan. 1909. Capt. 30th Jul. 1912. A/Maj. 13th Jun. 1916. Maj. 30th Jan. 1921. A/Lt Col. 28th Mar. 1918. Lt Col. 1st May 1934. Col. 13th Oct. 1937. r.p. 20th Jul. 1940. Rempld r.p. 4th Sept. 1946. Served Gibraltar 1911–15. Med EF Egypt 17th Mar. 1915–Aug. 1915, invalided. CO 50th Stat. Hosp. Mar–Jun 1918. N. Russia CO 86th Gen. Hosp. 1918–19. India 1922–27. Medals: 1915 S., BWM, VM, DM, WM. MID 5th Jun. 1919, 3rd Feb. 1920.

*RODDY Francis Augustus b. 21st Sept. 1891, Dublin. S. Michael and Ellen Roddy. Husband of Mary Roddy, Shankill, Co. Dublin. Educ. TCD. MB (1914), BCh, DPH (QUB 1925), BAO, LM (Rot. Hosp.). Lt RAMC SR 15th Oct. 1914. Capt. 18th Apr. 1915. PC Capt. 15th Apr. 1919. A/Lt Col. 30th Jun. 1917. r.p. Lt Col. 24th Dec. 1924. Rempld 2nd Sept. 1939 Lt Col. 27370 RAMC. Served France from 31st Jul. 1915–16, wounded. India 1917–21. Waziristan 1917. NWF 1919–20. Malta 1922–23. Constantinople May–Sept. 1923. BEF France 1939–40. SMO Hosp. Carrier *St Julien* 1939–44. Died on active service. Medals: OBE 1915 S., BWM, VM, IGS (Afghanistan and NWF 1919, Waz. 1919–20), 1939–45 S., Atlantic S., Italy S., WM. d. 15th Mar. 1944 at sea aged 52. Buried in Bari War Cemetery, Plot VI.C.4, Italy.

RODGERS John Stevenson Address: Maghereall Manse, Lisburn, Co. Antrim. MB, BCh (QUB 1941). Surg. Lt RNVR.

ROGAN Clara Mary Address: 65 Sandford Rd, Ranelagh, Dublin. L.LM (RCPI 1941), L.LM (RCSI 1941). Lt Indian Med. Service 3rd Mar. 1942.

ROGERS William Francis Address: 11 Grove Pk, Rathmines, Dublin. MB, BCh (TCD 1940), MD (TCD 1942). Surg. Comdr RNVR 1942.

RONALDSON John Gray b. 28th Jul. 1886, Holmpatrick, Co. Dublin. Educ. Oxmantown Sch. Lodge Dublin. TCD MB (1911), BCh, BAO, DPH (Cambridge 1924). R. C. of I. Lt RAMC SR 23rd Feb. 1914. Capt. 1st Apr. 1915. A/Maj. 4th Jan. 1918. PC Capt. 1st Apr. 1919. Maj. 10th Aug. 1926. Lt Col. 27th Jul. 1936. A/Col. 22nd Sept. 1940. r.p. Rempled 28th Jul. 1941. T/Col. 22nd Mar. 1941. r.p. 18th Jul. 1946. Served with BEF France 13th Sept. 1914–17 and 1918–19. RMO 11th Essex Regt. 1916–17. Italy 1917–18. India 1919–23. Waziristan 1920. China 1927–28. India 1928–32. DADH Deccan Dist. 1929–32. DADH NI Dist. 1932–35. Malaya 1935–39. DADH Malaya Comd 1936–39. ADH HQ Aldershot Comd 1939. CO 1st Armoured Div. Fd Amb. 1939–40. ADMS HQ 6th Armd Div. 1940–41. CO Mil. Hosp. Edinburgh 1941–42. CO 25th Gen. Hosp. 1942–44. CO Mil. Hosp. Morehampstad 1944–46. Medals: MC (18th Jan. 1918), Bar (1st Feb. 1919), 1914 S., BWM, VM, IGS (cl. Waz 1919–21 and Waz 1921–24) 1939–45 S., DM, WM. d. 7th Mar. 1966.

RONAYNE Maurice Francis Address: Ballyborishen House, Youghal, Cork. MB, BCh, BAO (UCC 1938). Lt RAMC.

ROONEY Daniel Address: 124 Antrim Rd, Belfast. MD (QUB 1939). Capt. RAMC.

*ROONEY John Joseph b. 27th Jan. 1890. s. James and Mary Rooney, Cork. MB, BCh, BAO (NUI 1920). Husband of Anne Rooney, East Hendred, Berkshire. Lt Lancashire Fusiliers 1915 to 1918. Commissioned IMS. Captain 1923. Major 1929, Lt Col. 1927. d. 5th Apr. 1941, Egypt, aged 51. Commemorated Alamein Memorial, Egypt, Column 237.

ROONEY Mervyn Stuart Carter Address: 107 Marlborough Rd, Donnybrook, Dublin. MB, BCh (TCD 1943). RAMC.

ROONEY Michael Robert Address: Howth Lodge, Howth, Co. Dublin. MB, BCh, BAO (UCD 1939). Lt RAMC.

ROSE Arnold Edwin MB, BCh (TCD 1930). Lt Col. RAMC 1939 with 8th Army in Egypt OC Surgical Division. MID.

ROSEFIELD Benjamin L.LM (RCPI 1933), L.LM (RCSI 1933). Lt RAMC 1942.

ROSEHILL Sydney Address: 9 Fernhurst Villas, College Rd, Cork. MB, BCh, BAO (UCC 1939). Flt Offr RAF.

ROSENFIELD Julius Louis Address: 53 Atlantic Ave., Belfast. MB, BCh (QUB 1934). Maj. RAMC.

ROSS Charles Duffin Address: 58 Sandymount St, Stranmillis Rd, Belfast. BCh, MD (QUB 1939). Sq. Ldr (M) RAFVR.

ROSS George Address: Breda Pk, Belfast. MB, BCh (QUB 1940). Capt. RAMC.

ROSS Thomas Lawrence Address: Fernville, Whiteabbey, Co. Antrim. MB, BCh (QUB 1937). Capt. RAMC.

ROSSITER Henry David Campbell College. MB, BCh, DPH (QUB 1941). Capt. RAMC. MID.

ROULSTON James Russell Address: 3 Moat St, Londonderry. MB, BCh (QUB 1938). Capt. RAMC.

ROUNTREE Joseph Germain Address: Thornford House, Castleblaney, Co. Monaghan. MB, BCh (QUB 1935). Sq. Ldr (M) RAF.

ROURKE Francis Louis Address: Kilcornan, Moate, Co. Westmeath. MB, BCh (NUI 1940). Lt RAMC 16th Sept. 1944.

ROWE John M. b. 10th Mar. 1888, Kingstown, Co. Dublin. s. Margaret Rowe, 1 Oval Rd, Rathmines, Dublin. Educ. Clongowes Wood Coll. MB, BCh, BAO, RUI (1912). R. RC. Lt RAMC 24th Jan. 1913. Capt. 30th Mar. 1915. A/Maj. 4th Jan. 1918. Maj. 24th Jan. 1925. Lt Col. 15th Jun. 1935. Col. 5th Nov. 1940. r.p. 24th Jul. 1947. Served with BEF France and Flanders 1914–19. CO 103rd Fd Amb. 1918–19. Mesopotamia 1920–22. Egypt 1922–25. Shanghai 1928, invalided. China 1930–33. India 1935–46. CO BMH Peshawar, Rawal Pindi and

Murree 1939–42. Medals: OBE (14th Jun. 1945), MC and Bar (3rd Jun. 1918), 1914 S., BWM, VM, DM, WM, Belgium War Cross (4th Sept. 1919). MID 15th Jan. 1916, 20th May 1917. d. 22nd Aug. 1959, Chester.

RUBIN Samuel MB, BCh (TCD 1937) USA MS.

RUDD Eric Thomas Sutherland MB, BCh (TCD 1925). Surg. Comdr RN. Served in Malta.

RUDDELL John Shegog b. 6th Jul. 1908, Lisnaskea, Ulster. MB, BCh, BAO (TCD 1933). Lt RAMC 7th Jun. 1934. Capt. 7th Jun. 1935. PC Capt. 7th Jun. 1939. Maj. 2nd Jul. 1943. A/Lt Col. 8th Apr. 1942. T/Lt Col. 8th Jul. 1942. Retired Hon. Lt Col. 13th Dec. 1946. Rejoined 27th Aug. 1956. Served India 1934–46. CO 44th Fd Amb. 1942–43. CO BMH Deolali 1945. ADMS GHQ (I) 1945–46. Medals: 1939–45 S., WM.

RUSSELL Alfred MacCarrison Address: Billis Rectory, Virginia, Co. Cavan. MB, BCh (TCD 1942). Flt Lt RAF.

RUSSELL John MB, BCh, BAO (UCC 1936). Lt RAMC.

RUSSELL John Gerald MB, BCh (TCD 1922). Group Capt. RAF.

RUSSELL John Noel Usher MB, BCh (TCD 1929). Lt Col. RAMC. BEF 1940, 8th Army 1943–45, Tripoli, Italy, Austria. MBE.

RUSSELL Mortimer McGee b. 16th Jun. 1893, London. s. Russell McGee Mortimer (bank clerk) and Myra McGee Russell, 49 Booterstown Ave., Blackrock, Co. Dublin. Educ. MB (TCD 1916), BCh, BAO, LM (Rot. Hosp.), MD (1920). R. C. of I. Lt Prob. RAMC SR 5th Aug. 1914. Mobd 9th Oct. 1916. Capt. 9th Apr. 1917. PC Lt (T/Capt.) 1st Apr. 1919. Capt. 9th Apr. 1920. r.p. 2nd Jun. 1923. Rempld 2nd Sept. 1939. A/Maj. 27th Apr. 1940. T/Maj. 27th Jul. 1940. Bt. Maj. 11th Jan. 1943. r.p. Hon. Maj. 12th Sept. 1945. Served in Mesopotamia 1916–19. NWF India 1919–20. Invalided. Hosp. Ship *Maid of Kent* 1930–40. BEF France May 1940. Medals: WM, VM, IGS (cl. Waz. 1919–21), 1939–45 S.

RUTHERFORD Ernest Davis Address: Woodlawn, Knock, Belfast. MB, BS (QUB 1900). Surg. Capt. RN.

RUTHERFORD Gordon Septimus L.LM (RCPI 1921), L.LM (RCSI 1921). RN.

RUTHERFORD Henry Ernest Address: Larne, Co. Antrim. MB, BCh (QUB 1938). Surg. Lt Comdr RNVR.

*****RYAN** Charles Youngest s. Dr J.F. Ryan, Mount Pleasant, Loughrea, Co. Galway. Educ. in Ireland. MB, BCh (QUB 1923), MD (QUB 1939). Married Susan Battock in 1939. Had one son. Short service commission in the RAMC. Served in Egypt, Palestine, Singapore and Shanghai. Returned to England at the beginning of 1940. KIA 13th Sept. 1943.

RYAN Francis Gerard L.LM (RCPI 1935), L.LM (RCSI 1935). Surg. Lt Comdr RNVR 1933.

RYAN Jeremiah Robert Address: Woodville, Blarney, Co. Cork. MB, BCh, BAO (UCC 1943). Flt Offr RAF.

RYAN John MB, BCh, BAO (UCC 1923). Lt RAMC.

RYAN John Address: High Park House, Cappawhite, Co. Tipperary. MB, BCh (NUI 1938). Lt RAMC 12th Sept. 1942.

RYAN Peter John b. 29th Jun. 1887, Rathmines, Dublin. Educ. NUI MB (1911), BCh, BAO, Hon. MSc (1919). Lt RAMC 31st Jul. 1914. Capt. 30th Mar. 1915. A/Maj. 4th Jan. 1918. Maj. 31st Jul. 1926. Lt Col. 11th Dec. 1935. A/Col. 16th Mar. 1940. T/Col. 16th Sept. 1940. r.p. Hon Col. 26th Jun. 1946. Served with BEF France 6th Nov. 1914–18. Egypt 1919–25. Mesopotamia 1921–22. India 1929–34 and 1936–38. CO BMH Delhi 1936–37. 16th Fd Amb. (Waziristan) 1937–38. BMH Jhansi 1938. OIC Surg. Div. R. Herbert Hosp. Woolwich 1939. BEF France CO 6th Fd Amb. 1939–40. ADMS HQ 12 Div. 1940. ADMS HQ 1st Div. 1940–41. CO Mil Hosp Shaftesbury May–Jul. 1941. ADMS HQ Cornwall Coast area 1942. ADMS HQ N. West Dist. 1942–46. Medals: MC (26th Jul. 1918), 1914 S., BWM, VM, DM, WM, Croix de Guerre 7th Jun. 1919, French Silver War Cross with swords 21st Aug. 1919, French War Cross 5th Nov. 1920. MID 24th Dec. 1917. d. 29th Jun. 1967, Rye, Sussex.

*****RYAN** William Astle Youngest s. William Astle Ryan, Cahore, Co. Wexford. MB, BCh, BAO (1932 TCD). Entered RN Surg. Lt soon after qualification. Surg. Lt Comdr RN 1938. Placed on retired list Jun. 1941. d. at Port of Spain, Trinidad 24th Aug. 1942.

RYLANCE Ralph Curzon MB, BCh (TCD 1942). Sq. Ldr RAF 1942.

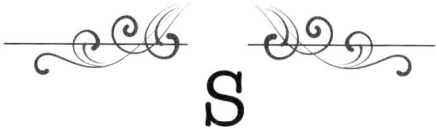

S

SACHS Albert b. 18th May 1904, Pretoria, South Africa. MB, BCh BAO (TCD 1926), MD (TCD 1931), MSc (Dublin 1935), MRCP (London 1953), FC Path. (TCD 1964). PC Lt RAMC 26th Jan. 1927. Capt. 26th Jul. 1930. Maj. 26th Jan. 1937. A/Lt Col. 8th Aug. 1942. T/Lt Col. 8th Aug. 1942. Lt Col. 2nd Dec. 1949. Col. 3rd Dec. 1949. T/Brig. 9th May 1949. Brig. 1st Jan. 1953. T/Maj. Gen. 1st Nov. 1953. Maj. Gen. 29th Nov. 1953. r.p. 10th Apr. 1956. Served India 1928–34 and 1935–41. MEF 1942–43. ADP HQ 10th Army 2nd Indian Div. ADP Scottish Comd 1944–45. ADP AFHQ Italy. CO 76 Gen. Hosp. 1945. MEF CO 1st Gen Hosp. 1945–46. India: ADP GHQ (I) 1946–47. ADP S. Comd 1948–49. D Path. and Cons. Path to the army 1949–53. KHP 1951/QHP 1st Apr. 1952. DDMS HQ E. Comd 1953–56. Col. Comdt RAMC 1964. Medals: CB (9th Jun. 1955), CBE (5th Jun. 1952), IGMS (cl. NWF Mohmand 1933), 1939–45 S. Africa S., Italy S., DM, WM, QEII Corn Medal 1953, OStJ (1956).

SACHS, Somah Boris MB, BCh (TCD 1935). Capt. RAMC 1939.

SALMOND James Readdie Campbell College. MB, BCh (QUB 1921). Maj. RAMC.

SALT Ida (née Campbell) Address: Lisnick, Dervick, Co. Antrim. MB, BCh (QUB 1940). Capt. RAMC.

SAMUELS Edward Soloman MB, BCh (TCD 1932). RAF.

SAMUELS Leslie Joseph L.LM (RCPI 1936), L.LM (RCSI 1936). Capt. RAMC from Dublin. MC. 'This officer has been employed as Regimental Medical Officer during several campaigns. His first consideration has always been the wounded and his succour has on many occasions been rendered with complete disregard to personal danger. During the attack across the river Trigno on October 27th, 1943, he tended the wounded under very heavy fire for five hours and there is no doubt he saved many lives. During this time he supervised evacuation across the river under continued enemy shellfire. His cheerfulness and courage under the worst conditions have been an inspiration and example to all.'

SANDERSON Noel Address: 5 The Glen, Limestone Rd, Belfast. MB, BCh (QUB 1943). Sq. Ldr (M) RAFVR.

SANDES John Drummond Educ. TCD (1904), MB (1906), BCh, MD (1924), FRCPI (1924). Lt IMS Feb. 1907. Capt. 1910. Maj. 1918. Col. SMO HMS *Harding* 1914. France 1915. Kitchener Hosp. Brighton 1915–16. India 1916.

SANDFORD William Address: Lyle, Portadown, Co. Armagh. MB, BCh (TCD 1939). RAMC.

SARSFIELD Thomas Herrick b. 14th Aug. 1891, Innishannon, Co. Cork. s. Dominick P. (land agent) and Phynia Sarsfield, Monkstown, Co. Cork. Educ. UCC. L.LM (RCPI 1915), L.LM (RCSI 1915). R. C. of I. T/Lt RAMC 9th Aug. 1915. Capt. 9th Aug. 1916. PC Lt 1st Jan. 1917. Capt. 9th Feb. 1919. A/Maj. 9th Dec. 1919. Maj. 9th Aug. 1927. A/Lt Col. 10th Nov. 1940. T/ Lt Col. 10th Feb. 1941. Lt Col. 15th Feb. 1942. A/Col. 7th Jul. 1941. T/Col. 3rd Jul. 1942. Col. 12th Aug. 1946. r.p. 12th Jan. 1947. Served in France 2nd Oct. 1915–16. India 1916–21. BAOR 1921–23. Egypt 1924–29. China 1932–36. India 1939–41.: CO Gen. Hosp. Nov.–Dec. 1940. CO CMH Poona 1940–41. Paiforce/MEF/N. Africa 1941–42. ADMS HQ Base sub area 1941–42. ADMS HQ 8 Indian Div. 1942–43. ADMS HQ 59 Area 1943–44. CO 8 Gen. Hosp. 1944–45: NWE/BAOR 1944–46: CO 105 Gen. Hosp. 1945–46. ADMS HQ Guards Div. Feb.–Oct. 1046. Medals: OBE 21st Jun. 1945, 1915 S., BWM, VM, IGS (2 cls Waz. 1919–21 and Mahsud 1919–20), 1939–45 S., Italy S., France and Germany S., DM, WM. MID 1st Jun. 1923, 20th Jun. 1941. d. 5th Aug. 1943.

SATCHWELL Ernest Edward Address: Fort Lodge, Enniskillen, Co. Fermanagh. MB, BCh (TCD 1926). Lt Col. RAMC. E. Africa Comd.

SAVAGE Stephen Julian MB, BCh, BAO (NUI 1928). Surg. Lt RN 19th Jun. 1928.

SAYERS Julius MB, BCh (TCD 1928). Capt. RAMC 1943.

SAYERS Louis Philip MB, BCh (TCD 1924). Surg. Comdr RNVR.

SCANLON Eileen Pearse Address: 53 Celtic Pk, Donnycarney, Dublin. MB, BCh (NUI 1940). Lt RAMC 17th Apr. 1943.

SCOTT Alexander Hill MB, BCh (QUB 1935). Address: Carncullagh, Dervock, Co. Antrim. Lt RAMC.

SCOTT George Albert Address: 34 Church St, Coleraine, Co. Derry. MB, BCh (QUB 1934). Surg. Comdr RNVR.

SCOTT James MB, BCh, BAO (UCC 1926). Lt RAMC.

SCOTT Kathleen Edith (née Smith) Address: Ye Nooke, Greystones, Co. Wicklow. MB, BCh (TCD 1938). Sq. Ldr RAF.

SCOTT Samuel Alan Address: Greenbank, Carr, Lisburn, Co. Antrim. MB, BCh (QUB 1942). Sq. Ldr (M) RAFVR.

SEAVER Charles Douglas Kingsley b. 30th Jul. 1887, Belfast. s. Rev. R.W. Seaver, The Rectory, Malone, Belfast. Educ. Campbell Coll. Belfast from Jan. 1900. QUB. RCSI LRCPI (1910), LRCSI, LM. R. Episcopalian. Lt RAMC 27th Jan. 1911. Capt. 29th Jul. 1914. A/Maj. 19th Aug. 1919. Maj. 22nd Jan. 1923. Lt Col. 1st May 1934. Col. 4th Jun. 1938. A/Brig. 27th Apr. 1941. T/Brig. 27th Oct. 1941. r.p. Hon. Brig. 26th Dec. 1946. Served India 1913–14. France and Belgium from 26th Sept. 1914, invalided, and 1915–16. Attd. 1st Manchester Regt. Egypt Mar.–Apr. 1916. India 1916–19, invalided, and 1922–27. Louise Margaret Hosp. Aldershot 1927–30. India 1930–35. BMH Rawalpindi and Murree 1933–35. CO Connaught Hosp. Aldershot 1936–37. India 1937–41. CO Connaught Mil. Hosp. Poona 1938–40. ADMS HQ Waziristan Dist. 1940. DDMS AHQ (I) 1940–41. DDMS HQ Malaya 1941–42. India ADMS HQ Rawalpindi Dist. 1942. Paiforce: DDMS HQ 10th Army 1942–43. BHS 1942. ADMS HQ Aldershot Dist. and Hants. Dist. 1943–46. Medals: 1914 S., BWM, VM, 1939–45 S., Pacific S., DM, WM. MID 5th Aug. 1943, 1st Aug. 1946.

SEAVERS James Albert MB, BCh, BAO (UCC 1939). Lt RAMC.

*SEAVERS Thomas Joseph b. IFS. MB, BCh, BAO (UCC 1936). Capt. RAMC. s. Thomas and Annie Seavers. Husband of Frances Seavers of St Luke's, Cork. Died Netherlands 22nd Oct. 1944 aged 33. Buried in Jonkerbos War Cemetery, Plot 9.D.4.

SEGERDAL John Adrian Wylie Campbell College. MB, BCh (QUB 1926). Lt Col. RAMC.

SELMAN David MB TCD (1938). Maj. US Army 1942.

SEVITT Simon Address: 115 Donore Tce, South Circular Rd, Dublin. MB, BCh (TCD 1939). Maj. RAMC 1943. UK., East Africa, Middle East.

SEYMOUR William Richard Dunham Address: 51 Clonmore Pk, Malone Rd, Belfast. MB, BCh (QUB 1939). Surg. Lt RNVR. MID.

SHAW George Frederick Address: 67 Terenure Rd East, Dublin. Campbell College. MB, BCh (TCD 1942). Capt. RAMC. Attached Paratroops.

SHAW James Brian Address: 13 Malone Rd, Belfast. MB, BCh, DPH (QUB 1936). Maj. RAMC. MID.

SHAW James Charlton Halliday MB TCD (1942). RNVR.

SHAW John Denis Reid Address: 39 Sans Souci Pk, Malone Rd, Belfast. MB, BCh (QUB 1940). Capt. RAMC.

SHAW Trevor Hamilton MB, BCh (QUB 1934). Maj. RAMC.

SHEE James Charles Address: Ardbrae, Ennis Rd, Limerick. MB, BCh (NUI 1935). Lt RAMC 2nd May 1940.

SHEEHAN Albert MB, BCh, BAO (UCC 1926). Flt Offr RAF.

SHEEHAN Daniel Address: Piltown, Co. Kilkenny. MB, BCh, BAO (UCD 1935). Flt Offr RAF.

***SHEEHAN** Jeremiah b. IFS. MB, BCh (NUI 1939). Lt 131327 RAMC 1st Apr. 1940. Capt. s. Edward and Catherine Sheehan. Husband of Julia Sheehan of Dundrum, Co. Dublin. d. 26th Jun. 1943, aged 27 in Libya. Buried in Tripoli War Cemetery, Plot 11. F.9.

SHEEHAN Michael Francis MB, BCh, BAO (UCD 1933). Surg. Lt RN.

SHEEHAN Michael Vincent Address: Curragh Camp, Co. Kildare. MB, BCh (NUI 1935). Lt RAMC.

***SHEILL** Gordon Spencer b. IFS. Address: Lismorna, Greenfield Pk, Donnybrook, Dublin. Only s. Dr and Mrs J. Spenser Shiell, Donnybrook, Dublin. Educ. Epsom College. MB, BCh (TCD 1939). The Black Watch 1939. After the evacuation of Le Havre, he was mentioned in dispatches for gallantry. He served in Gibraltar and the Mediterranean. Landed with the Paratroops in Normandy during the D Day Landing and was decorated with the MC by Montgomery. Engaged to Dr Mary Rennie of Dundee. Fd Amb. 6th Airborne Division. Capt. RAMC. KIA 24th Mar. 1945. MC. MID.

SHEIL Leonard James b. 26th Sept. 1887, Dublin. Educ. Clongowes Wood Coll. TCD. MB (1912), BCh, MD (1912). R. RC. Lt RAMC SR 4th Sept. 1914. Capt. 1st Apr. 1915. A/Maj. 27th Dec. 1918. PC Capt. 1st Apr. 1919. r.p. 30th Apr. 1924. Rejoined 1st Sept. 1939. Bt. Maj. 5th Jan. 1940. A/Maj. 23rd Apr. 1940. T/Maj. 23rd Jul. 1940. r.p. 26th Sept. 1942. Served with BEF France 12th Oct. 1914–15 No. 1 Gen. Hosp. later attd 8th DCLI. Served in Salonika 1915–19 and India 1919–22. Trooping Duties 1940–41. Ceased employment 26th Sept. 1942. Medals: MC (1st Jan. 1919), 1914 S., BWM, VM. MID 28th Nov. 1917. d. 25th Oct. 1962.

SHEPHERD Frederick Address: Lisnoble Manse, Raphoe, Co. Donegal. MB, BCh (QUB 1941). Surg. Lt RNVR.

SHEPHERD Irene (née Park) Address: Lislea, Belmont Pk, Londonderry. MB, BCh (QUB 1939). Flt Lt (M) RAFVR.

SHEPHERD William Henry Thompson Address: Lisnoble Manse, Raphoe, Co. Donegal. MB, BCh (QUB 1939). Sq. Ldr (M) RAFVR.

SHERIDAN Bertrand Cecil Owens b. 24th Dec. 1889, Dublin City. s. Francis Stephen (clerk Congested Dist. Board) and Marie Eliza Patricia Sheridan, 3 Belfast Tce, Nth Circular Rd, Glasnevin, Dublin. Educ. TCD. MB (1914), BCh, BAO, LM (Rot.). R. RC. Lt RAMC SR 6th Aug. 1914. Capt. 11th May 1915. PC Capt. 1st May 1919. A/Maj. 10th May

1921. Maj. 11th Nov. 1926. A/Lt Col. 30th Oct. 1919. Lt Col. 15th Jul. 1939. A/Col. 18th Mar. 1941. T/Col.18th Sept. 1941. r.p. 30th Aug. 1947. Served in BEF France from 15th Dec. 1914–19. India 1919–24. Waziristan 1920–23 and 1929–34. Mauritius SMO & CO Mil. Hosp. 1937–40. CO 6th Lt/Fd Amb. 1940–41. CO 5 Gen. Hosp. Mar.–Dec. 1941. ADMS HQ RM Div. Dec. 1941–Mar. 42. Madagascar ADMS HQ 121 Force Mar–Dec. 1942. ADMS HQ 48th Div. Jan.–Apr. 1943. MEF/Paiforce 1943–46. CO 43 Gen. Hosp. Jun–Nov. 1943. CO 3 and 30 Gen. Hosp. 1943. ADMS HQ S. Iraq area. CO Mil. Hosp. Nutsford, Cheshire Jul.–Nov. 1946. Medals: MC (26th May 1917), 1915 S., BWM, VM, IGS (cl. Waz. 1919–21, Waz 1921–24), WM. MID 4th Jan. 1917, 1st Jun. 1923, 12th Jun. 1923, 30th May 1924, 8th Jul. 1943. d. 22nd Oct. 1950.

SHERIDAN John Joseph MB, BCh, BAO (NUI 1930). Lt RAMC.

SHERIDAN (formerly Shreider), Matthew MB, BCh (TCD 1939). RAF.

SHERRARD Maurice MB, BCh (TCD 1927). Surg. Lt RNVR. MID.

SHIER Richard Ivers Address: Beagh, Maghera, Co. Derry. MB, BCh (TCD 1935). Sq. Ldr RAF.

SHIPSEY William Joseph MB, BCh, BAO (UCC 1925). Capt. IMS.

SHORT Cyril DeVere MD (TCD 1931). Lt Col. RAMC. MID.

SHORTALL Christopher Joseph Address: Laurel Lodge, Newry, Co. Down. MB, BCh, BAO (UCD), MD (1923), MCh (1932), FRCSI (1931). Flt Lt RAF 26th Jul. 1938.

SHORTEN Donal Address: Ard na Greine, St Francis's Ave., College Rd, Cork. MB, BCh, BAO (UCC 1943). Flt Offr RAF.

SHORTEN James Percy L.LM (RCPI 1910), L.LM (RCSI 1910). Sq. Ldr RN and RAF.

SHORTT Cecil de Lisle L.Med LS (1922), MB, BCh (1929), MD (TCD 1930). Maj. RAMC 1937.

SHORTT Francis Address: Dunsany, Co. Meath. MB, BCh, BSO (UCD 1937). Lt RAMC.

SHRIBMAN Irving Address: 2 Clifton Tce, Monkstown, Dublin. MB, BCh (TCD 1942). Capt. RAMC.

SIDEBOTTOM Desmond Holland Address: 15 Carlisle Tce, Londonderry. MB BCh (TCD 1943) Sq. Ldr RAF.

SIDES John Robert Address: Athelford, Ballycastle, Co. Antrim. MB, BCh (TCD 1936). Flt Lt RAF. Indian Comd.

SIEVERS Ivan Myer Address: 167 South Circular Rd, Dolphin's Barn, Dublin. L.LM (RCPI 1941), L.LM (RCSI 1941). Lt RAMC 1943.

SIMON Robert Henry Address: 55 Dufferin Avenue, Dublin. L Med Lch (TCD 1935). Lt Col. RAMC.

SIMPSON David Gordon Address: School Residence, Castlerea, Belfast. MB, BCh (QUB 1942). Sq. Ldr (M) RAFVR.

SIMPSON Elizabeth Davis Liken Address: Ardbana Crescent, Coleraine, Co. Derry MB, BCh (TCD 1941). Sq. Ldr RAF 1944.

SIMPSON Norman James Young Address: Union Pl., Dungannon, Co. Tyrone. MB, BCh (QUB 1935). Maj. RAMC. MID.

SINCLAIR Arthur Crawford MB, BCh (QUB 1921), MD (QUB 1924), DPH, RCPS (England 1930). Maj. RAMC.

SINCLAIR Samuel Ronald (QUB 1932). Lt RAMC Nov. 1939.

SINCLAIR William Address: Lr Main St, Bushmills, Co. Antrim. MB, BCh (QUB 1940). Flt Lt (M) RAFVR.

SINTON John Alexander s. Mrs Sinton. Address: Ulster Villas, Lisburn Rd, Belfast. MB, BCh, BAO (RUI 1908), MD, DSc (QUB 1908). IMS Lt 29th Jul. 1911. Capt. 29th Jul. 1914. Recalled as a reservist to the IMS in 1939 and was CO of a hospital in India. Brig. IMS and RAMC. VC (WWI), OBE, MID.

SLATTERY Mortimer Francis Xavier b. 4th Dec. 1913, Tralee, Co. Kerry. Address: 10 Elgin Rd, Ballsbridge, Dublin. MB, BCh, BAO (TCD 1938), MA, MD (Dublin 1940). Flt Lt RAF. 1st Nov. 1938, Capt. 5th Sept. 1940. A/Maj. 6th Nov. 1940. T/Maj. 16th Feb. 1941. PC Maj. 26th Nov. 1946. T/Lt Col. 12th Sept. 1949. r.p. 10th Nov. 1950. BAOR 1946–67. FARELF: CO BMH Hong Kong 1949, invalided. Medals: 1939–45 S., Atlantic S., WM.

SLOAN David Graham Address: 29 Mount Eden Pk, Belfast. MB, BCh (QUB 1942). Flt Lt RAFVR.

*****SLOAN** Harold Fitzgerald s. Harold Alexander Sloan & Mabel Fitzgerald Sloan, Bray, Co. Wicklow. BA, MB, BCh (TCD 1936). Surg. Lt RNVR 1940. HMS *Javelin*. KIA 29th Nov. 1940, aged 26. Commemorated Portsmouth Naval Memorial Panel 44, Column 2.

SLOAN Wolsey Cornwall MB, BCh (TCD 1926). Surg. Lt RNVR.

SLOANE James Morrow MB, BCh (QUB 1923), DPH (QUB 1935). Surg. Comdr RN.

SMALL William Alexander Werbiq MB, BCh (QUB 1942). Flt Lt (M) RAFVR.

SMART Robert Alexander Address: 249 Upr Newtownards Rd, Belfast. L.LM (RCPI 1939), L.LM (RCSI 1939). Surg. Lt RNVR 1939.

SMILEY Thomas Boyd Address: Castlewellan, Belfast. MB, BCh (QUB 1939). Capt. RAMC. Wounded during but survived the Alexandra Hospital, Singapore massacre, 14th–15th Feb. 1942 where the Japanese forces indiscriminately killed both medical staff and patients. Medal: MC. MID.

SMITH Edward Percival Allman MB, TCD (1909). Brig. RAMC. OBE, MC.

SMITH Frederick William Gordon MB, BCh (TCD 1923), MD (TCD 1924). Wing Comdr RAF.

SMITH Henry Ellis Address: Cheltenham Mount, Enniskillen. MB, BCh, DPH (QUB 1939). Lt Col. RAMC. MID.

SMITH Herbert John MB, BCh (TCD 1940). Capt. US Army Med. Corps.

SMITH Howard Alexander Address: 45 Malone Pk, Belfast. MB, BCh (QUB 1941). Surg. Lt RNVR.

SMITH John MB, BCh, BAO (UCC 1927). Lt RAMC.

SMITH Nevin Montgomery Address: Upton Pk, Templepatrick, Co. Antrim. MB, BCh (TCD 1940). Surg. Lt RNVR.

SMITH Noel Lewis Address: Upton Pk, Templepatrick, Co. Antrim. MB, BCh (TCD 1942). Capt. RAMC.

SMITH Roydon Turnbull MB, BCh (QUB 1938). Surg. Lt Comdr RN.

SMITH Sidney Graeme Address: 11 St Catherine's Ave., South Circular Rd, Dublin. L.LM (RCPI 1940), L.LM (RCSI 1940). Lt RAMC 1940.

SMITH Stanley Myer Address: 50 Landscape Tce, Belfast. MB, BCh (QUB 1942). Capt. RAMC.

SMITH William David Address: 7 Adelaide Pk, Belfast. MB (QUB 1940). Flt Lt (M) RAFVR.

SMITHWICK Harold Stanislaus MB, BCh (TCD 1928). Col. IMS. Lt Col. commanded 66th IGH (C) and subsequently 138 IBGH. OBE.

SMYTH Ernest Albert b. 30th Oct. 1938, Donaghmore, Laois. Address: Castletown, Donaghmore, Ballybrophy, Laois. MB, BCh, BAO (TCD 1933), FRCSI (1946), MCh Orth. (Liverpool 1948). Lt RAMC 23rd Oct. 1936. Capt. 23rd Oct. 1937. A/Maj. 3rd Sept. 1939. T/Maj. 3rd Dec. 1939. PC Capt. 23rd Oct. 1941. Maj. 23rd Oct. 1945. Lt Col. 27th Dec. 1949. r.p. 1st Dec. 1956. Served China 1937–40. Malaya 1940–42. POW Far East 1942–45. MELF 1949–51. BAOR 1953–56. Medals: OBE (31st May 1956), 1939–45 S., Pacific S., DM, WM.

SMYTH Gerald Spence MB, BCh (TCD 1927), MD (TCD 1932), M (1930), F (1931) RCPI. Lt Col. RAMC. Abyssinia 1940–41.

SMYTH James Coulter Address: 16 College Gdns, Belfast. L.LM (RCPI 1918), L.LM (RCSI 1918). Flt Offr RAF 1939.

SMYTH John Trevor b. 27th Jan. 1897, Holywood, Co. Down. MB, BCh, BAO (QUB 1924). Commissioned with INF 1916–18. PC Lt RAMC 29th Jan. 1925. Capt. 29th Jul. 1928, Maj. 29th Jan. 1935, A/Lt Col. 10th Mar. 1940, T/Lt Col. 8th Aug. 1940, Lt Col. 1st Mar. 1945, A/Col. 18th Nov. 1946, r.p. 27th Sept. 1952. Served India 1926–31, Gibraltar 1934–38, CO 184th Fd Amb. 1940–42, CO 4th CCS 1942–43, CMF 1943–45, OC TPS 1945–46, CO 231 Mil. PW Hosp. 1946–47, Burma/Malaya 1947–50, ADMS HQ Burma Comd 1947, ADMS HQ N. Malaya Sub. Dist. 1947–49, CO BMH Kluang 1949–50, BAOR BMH Wuppertal 1950–52. Medals: BWM, VM, 1939–45 S., Italy S., DM, WM, GSM with cl. Malaya, German O. Red Cross, Cross of Merit 1937.

SMYTH Joseph Francis Michael Address: The Chalet, Westminster Rd, Foxrock, Dublin. L.LM (RCPI 1940), L.LM (RCSI 1940). Flt Lt RAF 1941.

SMYTH Malachy Joseph Address: Fort Singleton House, Emyvale, Co. Monaghan. MB, BCh (UCD 1939). Married Ms Lucy O'Hara. Flt Offr RAF 4th Mar. 1943. Served North Africa, Middle East and Italy. Medical officer of POW camp in North Africa. Senior Fellow in orthopaedics at Univ. Hosp., Leeds and Royal Infirmary, Hull.

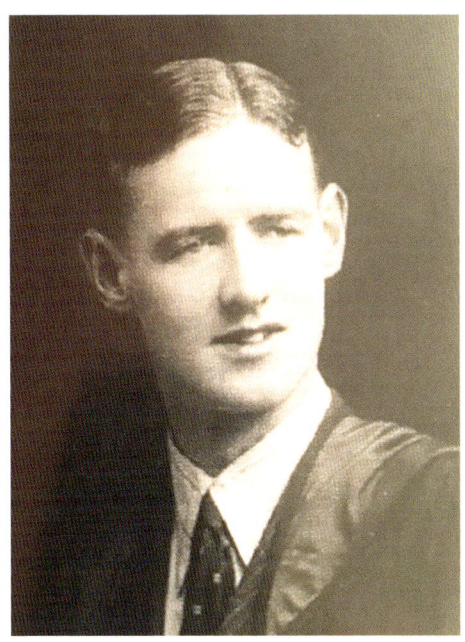

Malachy Joseph Smyth

In 1958, published with Vera Wright 'Sciatica and the Intervertebral Disk'. Research Fellow in Toronto, 1962 and later a private orthopaedic practice in New York State.

SMYTH Meredith George MB (TCD 1940). Maj. RAMC 1937. Served in India.

SMYTH Robert Patterson Address: 10 Cranbourne Pk, Belfast. MB, BCh (QUB 1930). Lt Col. RAMC. OBE. MID.

SMYTH William Francis Address: Ballydugan, Downpatrick, Co. Down. MB, BCh (QUB 1938). Maj. RAMC.

SMYTHE Robert Hastings Address: Bank of Ireland House, Athlone, Westmeath. L.LM (RCPI 1938), L.LM (RCSI 1938). Lt RAMC 1940.

SOLOMON Louis Address: 23 Lombard St West, South Circular Rd, Dublin. MB, BCh (TCD 1940). Capt. RAMC. Served North Africa, Italy and Greece.

SOLOMONS Bethel Eric Robert Address: 42 Fitzwilliam Sq., Dublin. MB, BCh (TCD 1940). Surg. Lt RNVR.

SOLOMONS Michael Joseph Maurice Address: 42 Fitzwilliam Sq., Dublin. MB, BCh (TCD 1941). Flt Offr RAF.

SOMERVILLE Walter Address: Laurleen, Clontarf Rd, Dublin. MB, BCh, BAO (UCD 1937), MC (UCD 1940), MRCP (London 1940). Lt RAMC.

SOMERVILLE-LARGE Lionel Becher Address: 7 Fitzwilliam Sq., Dublin. MB, BCh (TCD 1926). Col. RAMC.

SOMERVILLE-LARGE William Collis Address: Farmhill, Dundrum, Co. Dublin. MB, BCh (TCD 1925), FRCSI (1927). Lt Col. RAMC.

SPACEK Mortimer Rudolph William Address: Royal Marine Hotel, Kingstown, Co. Dublin. MB, BCh (TCD 1936). Maj. RAMC.

*****SPEEDY** William Dinwoodie b. Dublin 8th Jun. 1898. Eldest s. Thomas and Agnes (Patterson) Speedy. Address: 16 Clontarf Rd, Dublin. Husband of Doreen Constance Marguerite Speedy (née Archer) of Hurst Green, Surrey. R. Presbyterian. Educ. St Andrew's College, Dublin 1908 to 30th Jun. 1916. TCD 1916. MB (TCD 1922), BCh (TCD 1924), BAO, DPH (TCD 1931). Sgt Maj. St Andrew's OTC. TCD OTC. 2nd Lt 33rd Battery 6A Res. Bde. RFA 9th Apr. 1917. 2nd Lt RH & RFA 8th Mar. 1918. Lt RFA 'Special Reserve 8th Oct. 1918. Lt on Prob.' 29th Jan. 1925. Reg. Army Reserve of Officers RAMC. Lt 2nd Jul. 1930. Capt. Aux. Force Med. Corp 3rd Jun. 1932. Maj. 34073 RAMC. Occupation post-war, Gengal Magpur Railway, Calcutta. Medals: DM, WM. d. 7th May 1944, aged 45, India. Buried Kirkee War Cemetery India, Plot 3 E 6.

SPEEDY William James Yates Address: Dromore St, Rathfriland, Co. Down. LRCP (Edinburgh 1941), LRCS (Edinburgh 1941), LRFPS Glasgow (1941), MB, DPH (QUB 1946). Capt. RAMC.

SPEER James Address: Merrion, Newry Rd, Banbridge, Co. Down. (RCSI 1940). Lt RAMC Nov. 1940.

SPEIDEL Joseph Townley Address: 48 Merlyn Pk, Merrion Rd, Dublin. MB, BCh (TCD 1938). RAMC.

SPRONG William Arthur Temp. Lt Col. RAMC Oct. 1931.

SPROULE Alexander Bradley Address: Gilford, Co. Down. MB, BCh (QUB 1926). Sq. Ldr (M) RAFVR.

SPROULE James Chambers b. 28th Aug. 1887, Omagh, Co. Tyrone, 4th s. Alexander H.R. Sproule (JP), Fintona, Tyrone. Educ. R. Sch. Raphoe. L.LM (RCPI 1912), L.LM (RCSI 1912), DPH (QUB 1926), RCSI LRCPI&S LM (Rot.). R. Presbyterian. Married Clare Stewart dt. George F. Aldous FRCS (Edinburgh), Charlton House, Plymouth. Lt RAMC 26th Jul. 1912. Capt. 30th Mar. 1915. A/Maj. 21st Jul. 1919. Maj. 26th Jul. 1924. A/Lt Col. 3rd Mar. 1918. Lt Col. 6th Dec. 1934. A/Col. 18th Dec. 1934. Col. 15th Apr. 1940. A/Brig. 5th Mar. 1942. r.p. Hon. Brig. 10th Mar. 1947. War work France 9th Aug. 1914–Jan. 1920. 13th HAC. Invalided. India 1920–24. ADH Aldershot 1926–27. India 1927–33. Served through 1939–45 War. Egypt 1939–42. ADH HQ BF Egypt 1935–39. CO 2/10 Gen. Hosp. 1939–40. DDH GHQ MEF 1940–41. DDMS HQ 11 Corps. Dist. 1942–43. DDMS HQ 2 Corp 1943–44. DDH HQ Eastern Comd 1944–45 and 1946. DDH HQ Scottish Comd 1945–46. Spec. Hygiene 1926. Medals: CBE (30th Dec. 1941), OBE (12th Dec. 1919), 1914 S., BWM, VM, 1939–45 S., Africa S., DM, WM, Croix de Guerre France (16th Jan. 1920). MID 24th Dec. 1917, 10th Jul. 1919, 1st Apr. 1941. d. 15th May 1955, Somerton, Somerset.

STAFFORD John Ingham Address: 45 Terenure Rd East, Dublin. MB, BCh (TCD 1940). Flt Lt RAF.

STANLEY Herbert Vernon b. 3rd Jun. 1883, Donnybrook, Co. Dublin. Educ. TCD. MB (1908), BCh, BAO, LM (Rot Hosp.). Lt RAMC 31st Jul. 1909. Capt. 31st Jan. 1913. A/Maj. 17th Jan. 1919. Maj. 31st Jul. 1921. Lt Col. 1st May 1934. r.p. 31st Jul. 1935. Rempld Maj. 18th Apr. 1941. r.p. Lt Col. 30th Jun. 1948. Served Gibraltar 1912–15. MEF Gallipoli Apr. 1915–Oct. 1915. India 1916. Mesopotamia 1917, invalided. Gibraltar 1919–21. India 1923–26. Invalided and 1928. Medals: MBE, MC (24th Jan. 1917), 1915 S., BWM, VM, DM, WM. d. 29th Apr. 1960.

STANTON Thomas b. 20th Apr. 1892, Cork. s. John (solicitor) and Catherine Stanton, 47 South Mall, Cork. Educ. TCD. MB (1916), BCh, BAO, LM (Rot.). R. RC. Lt RAMC SR 1st Jan. 1917. Capt. 1st Jan. 1918. PC Lt (T/Capt.) 1st Jun. 1919. Capt. 1st Jul. 1920. Maj. 1st Jan. 1929. A/Lt Col. 4th Jan. 1940. T/Lt Col. 4th Apr. 1940. Lt Col. 13th Sept. 1943. A/Col. 1st Mar. 1943. T/Col. 1st Sept. 1943. r.p. Hon Col. 26th Jun. 1947. Served Malta 1917–18. Archangel Nov. 1918–Jan. 1919. N. Russia Aug.–Oct. 1919. Malta 1920–24. RMO 1st NF 1926–27. India 1928–33. Egypt 1935–39. Cyprus 1937–38. CO 2nd Fd Amb. 1940–42. W. Africa 1942–43. CO 2nd Fd Amb. 1942. W. Africa 1942–43. ADMS HQ 81 (WA) Div. 1943–44. India 1943–45. CO 31st Gen. Hosp. Jun.–Jul. 1945. CO CMH Quetta Jul.–Nov. 1945. CO 252 Mil. POW Hosp. 1946–47. Medals: BWM, VM, Burma S., WM and DM.

STAZ Leopold MB, BCh (TCD 1922). Maj. SAMC.

STEEDE Francis Desmond Fitzgerald b. 30th Oct. 1915, Dublin. TCD (1937). MB, BCh, BAO (Dublin 1938). Lt 1st May 1939. Capt. 1st May 1940. A/Maj. 29th Dec. 1941. T/Maj. 29th Mar. 1942. PC Capt. 1st May 1944. r.p. Hon Maj. 16th Feb. 1946. BEF France 1939–40. W. Africa 1943–44. India/Burma 1944–45. Medals: 1939–45 S. Burma S. DM. WM. MID 30th Dec. 1941.

STEEN James Ross MB, BCh (TCD 1937). Lt Col. RAMC 1939. MES, PAI Force, Burma. MID.

STEEN Philip Address: Inchna, Ballymoney, Co. Antrim. MB, BCh (QUB 1940). Flt Offr (M) RAFVR.

STEIN Maurice Address: 35 South Circular Rd, Portobello, Dublin. L.LM (RCPI 1939), L.LM (RCSI 1939). Flt Offr RAFVR 1939.

STEINBERG Myer Address: 59 Donore Ave., Dolphin's Barn, Dublin. MB, BCh (TCD 1941). Flt Lt RAF.

STEPHENSON George Vaughan MB, BCh (QUB 1924). Surg. Comdr RNVR.

*****STEVENSON** Alex King MB, BCh (QUB 1920). Surg. Comdr RN. d. Oct. 16th, 1947, Malta.

STEVENSON Alexander Leslie b. 27th Nov. 1883, Lisburn, Co. Antrim. s. Mary Stevenson, 19 Railway St, Lisburn, Co. Antrim. Educ. RUI MB (QUB 1907), BCh, BAO, BS. R. Methodist. Lt RAMC 4th Feb. 1908. Capt. 4th Aug. 1911. A/Maj. 22nd Oct. 1918. Maj. 4th Feb. 1920. Lt Col. 28th Oct. 1932. Col. 27th Jul. 1936. r.p. remained employed 27th Jul. 1940. r.p. 16th Jul. 1942. Rempld Maj. 17th Aug. 1942. r.p. Col. 15th Nov. 1944. Served India 1910–15. Mesopotamia 1st Sept. 1915–19, invalided. India 1923–28. Jamaica 1933–35. CO Mil. Hosp. Colchester. ADMS HQ E. Anglia area 1936–39. BEF France: ADMS HQ 4th Div. 1939–40. DDMS HQ 3rd Corps. Jan.–May 1940. ADMS HQ E. Anglia area. HQ Hertford area 1940. PSMB Scottish and Western Comd 1940–42. Medals: 1915 S., BWM, VM, 1939–45 S., DM, WM. d. 19th Apr. 1955.

STEVENSON Arthur Edwin Medlock Address: Daleholme, Ladysmile, Holywood, Co. Down. MB, BCh (QUB 1942). Flt Lt (M) RAFVR.

STEVENSON George Dougan Address: Grange Lodge, Dungannon, Co. Tyrone. MB, BCh (TCD 1938). Surg. Lt RNVR HMS *Anson*.

STEVENSON Howard Morris Address: 14 College Gdns, Belfast. MB, BCh (QUB 1943). Surg. Lt RNVR.

STEVENSON Walter Bernard b. 4th Jul. 1887, Londonderry. MB, BCh, BAO (QUB 1910), DPH, DTM. Lt 26th Jan. 1912. Capt. 30th Mar. 1915. T/Maj. 20th May 1918. Maj. 26th Jan. 1924. r.p. 26th Jan. 1932. Rejoined 1st Sept. 1939. A/Lt Col. 28th Mar. 1914. T/Lt Col. 28th Jun. 1940. A/Col. 23rd Oct. 1940. T/Col. 23rd Apr. 1941. Reverted to retired pay 12th Oct. 1945. Hon. Col. 21st Jun. 1949. Served India 1914–21. NWF Mar.–Apr. 1918. Hong Kong DADH and P. China Comd 1926–27. DADH 1927–28. DADH E. Anglia area 1929–31. BEF France DADH HQ 3 Corps. 1939–40. ADMS HQ 52 (Lowland Div.) 1940. ADMS HQ Orkney and Shetland Defences 1942. HQ South Wales Dist. 1942–43. CO 63 Gen. Hosp. 1943–45. Spec. Hygiene 1922. Medals: 1939–45 S., DM, WM.

STEWART Charles Douglas Address: Grange Rd, Ballymena, Co. Antrim. MB, BCh (QUB 1939). Capt. RAMC.

STEWART Donal Kenneth Address: 23 Ulverton Rd, Dalkey, Co. Dublin. MB, BCh (TCD 1938). Maj. RAMC. Served Sicily, Italy. MBE.

***STEWART** Henry Thorpe b. 1916. Belfast, Northern Ireland. s Rev David Stewart. Educ. Methodist College. MB (QUB 1939). Capt. RAMC. Invalided home Dec. 1940. d. 28th Mar. 1942, UK.

STEWART James Martin MB TCD (1942) Lt RAMC 1945.

STEWART Norman Hampton Address: 24 Newtownpark Ave., Blackrock, Co. Dublin. MB, BCh (TCD 1941). RAMC.

STEWART Robert William MB, BCh (QUB 1923). Sq. Ldr (M) RAFVR. MID.

STEWART William Muir b. 2nd Jun. 1913, Belfast. Address: 22 Ravenhill Pk, Belfast. MB, BCh (QUB 1935). Lt, RAMC 27th Oct. 1937, Capt. 27th Oct. 1938, A/Maj. 5th Nov. 1940, T/Maj. 5th Feb. 1941, PC Capt. 27th Oct. 1942, Maj. 1st Jul. 1946, T/Lt Col. 29th Nov. 1951, Lt Col. 5th Mar. 1953, T/Col. 23rd Jul. 1959, Col. 2nd Jun. 1961. Served India 1938–39, Malaya 1939–42, RMO 1st Gordons 1939–40, POW Far East 1942–45, Japan 1946, FARELF 1950–53: ADAH HQ Malaya Comd 1951–53, ADGAMS War Office 1953–57, W. Africa: CO Mil. Hosp. Accra 1957–59, DMS Ghana Army 1958–59, DDAH HQ W. Comd 1959–61, ADMS HQ 3rd Div. 1961–64, CMO HQ UNFICYP Feb.–May 1964, Norway: CMO (ADMS) HQ AFNE 1964–66, ADMS HQ S. Comd 1966. Snr Spec. In army health 1950. Medals: OBE 9th Jun. 1955, IGSM with cl. NWF 1937–39, 1939–45 S., Pacific S., DM, WM, GSM with cl. Malaya, UNSM with cl. Cyprus 1964. MID 17th Oct. 1939, 1st May 1953.

STOKES Harold William TCD 1899. Lt Col. RAMC. Home Guard.

STONE Louis (formerly STEIN Abraham) Address: 9 Patrick St, Dun Laoghaire, Co. Dublin. L.LM (RCPI 1930), L.LM (RCSI 1930). Surg. Lt RNVR 1939.

STRAHAN John Haslett MB, BCh (QUB 1924), DPH (QUB 1928). Lt Col. RAMC. MID.

STRAIN Robert William Magill Address: 9 University Sq., Belfast. MB, BCh (QUB 1930), MD (QUB 1933). Lt Col. RAMC.

STRINGER Charles Herbert b. 10th Apr. 1886, Armagh. Educ. RCSI L.LM (RCPI 1909), L.LM (RCSI 1919), DPH (RCPS England 1921). Lt RAMC 29th Jul. 1910. Capt. 29th Jan. 1914. A/Maj. 1st May 1919. T/Maj. 8th Aug. 1921. Maj. 29th Jul. 1922. A/Lt Col. 16th Dec. 1917. Bt. Lt Col. 1st Jul. 1933. Lt Col. 1st May 1934. Col. 1st May 1938. A/Brig. 26th Nov. 1940. T/Brig. 26th May 1941. r.p. Hon Brig. 23rd May 1947. Served Jamaica 1912–15. 1914–18 War France 4th Jun. 1916–19. CO 6th Cav. Fd Amb. 1917–19. BAOR 1921. India 1921–26. Waziristan 1922–24. ADH & P HQ E. Comd 1926. Egypt 1931–35. ADH HQ BTE 1930–31. ADH HQ S. Comd 1935–38. Malaya 1938–45. HQ Malaya Comd ADMS 1938–41. DDMS 1941. POW 1942–45. DDH HQ S. Comd 1945–46. Specialist in Hygiene 1921. Medals: DSO (26th Jul. 1918), CBE (1st Aug. 1946), OBE (13th Mar. 1925), BWM, VM, 1939–45 S., Pacific S., DM, WM, IGS (cl. Waz. 1921–24). MID 30th Dec. 1918, 30th May 1924, 13th Mar. 1925. d. 7th May 1961, Westminster, Middlesex.

STRONG John Anderson Address: Moate House, Kells, Co. Meath. MB, BCh (TCD 1937). Lt Col. RAMC. MBE.

STRONGE Robert Fawcett Address: 90 Cliftonville Rd, Belfast. MB, BCh (QUB 1934). Flt Lt (M) RAFVR.

STUART Charles Edward b. 21st Apr. 1910, Aughnacloy, Co. Tyrone. MB, BCh, BAO (QUB 1936), DTM&H (Eng. 1951). Lt R of O 31st May 1939. WS/Capt. 31st May 1940. A/Maj. 22nd Aug. 1941. T/Maj. 22nd Nov. 1941. WS/Maj. 28th Apr. 1943. A/Lt Col. 28th Jan. 1943. Capt. 10th Nov. 1944. PC Capt. 1st Sept. 1944. Maj. 1st Sept. 1947. Lt Col. 6th Aug. 1956. Col. 1st Sept. 1962. r.p. 1st Apr. 1965. BEF France 1939–40. India and Burma 1941–45. CO 72nd Indian Fd Amb. 1943. 67 Indian Fd Amb. 1943–45. 26th Indian CCS 1945. CO 178 Fd Amb. 1945. BTA 1951–53. OIC Comd Labs. 1956–60. BAOR ADP & OIC Central Path. Lab. 1960–62. RAM Coll. 1962–65. Sen. Spec. Pathology 1955. Medals: 1939–45 S., Burma S., DM, WM. MID.

STUBBS John William Cotter b. 30th May 1891, Dublin. s. William Cotter Stubbs (Irish Land Commission) and Mary dt. J.G. Gibbon (LLD). Educ. Portora and TCD MB (1913), BCh, BAO, LM (Rot. 1912). R. C. of I. Lt RAMC 30th Jan. 1914. Capt. 30th Mar. 1915. Maj. 30th Jan. 1926. A/Lt Col. 6th Jun. 1918. Lt Col. 26th Sept. 1935. Col. 1st Aug. 1941. A/Brig 24th Sept. 1943. r.p. 14th Mar. 1950. Served with BEF France 1914–17 and 1917–19. Seconded to Egyptian Army 1920–26. Iraq seconded under Colonial Office 1929–32. Kurdistan 1930–31. India 1935–42. CO BMH Kasauli 1936–41. 3 Gen. Hosp. Poona 1941–42. MEF/N. Africa 1942–44. DDMS HQ 3 Dist. 1943–44. CO 103 Gen Hosp. 1944–45. NWE 1944. CO 122 Mil. Com. Dep.

1945–46. ADMS HQ Mid-west Dist. 1946. PSBM 1946–50. Medals: DSO (3rd Jun. 1919), MC (23rd Jun. 1915), 1914 S., BWM, VM, GSM (cl. Iraq), 1939–45 S., France and Germany S., DM, WM. MID 22nd Jun. 1915, 10th Jul. 1919, 4th Apr. 1946.

STUTT John Charles Address: Epworth, Station Rd, Green Island, Co. Antrim. MB, BCh, DPH (QUB 1942). Capt. RAMC.

STYLES Sean Anthony MB, BCh, BAO (UCD 1943). Lt RAMC.

SUGARS John Colvan de Renzy Address: 15 Greenmount Rd, Terenure, Co. Dublin. MB, BCh (TCD 1938). RN.

SULLIVAN Robert Ievers b. 26th Jun. 1892, Co. Cork. s. Robert Ievers (Co. Insp. RIC) and Jane Dora Sullivan, 3, Finisklin Rd, Sligo. Educ. TCD (1913), MB (1914), BCh, MD (1916). R. C. of I. Lt RAMC SR 10th Nov. 1914. Capt. 11th May 1915. PC Lt RAMC (T/Capt.) 1st Jan. 1917. Capt. 11th May 1918. Maj. 10th Nov. 1926. r.p. 10th Nov. 1934. Rempld 1st Sept. 1939. Ceased R of O ill health 30th Dec. 1939. Served France from 15th Mar. 1915–18 21st Fd Amb. Wounded Apr. 1918. India 1919–23. Waziristan 1920–21. Iraq Levies 1925–30. Medals: MC (17th Dec. 1917), 1915 S., BWM, VM, GSM (cl. Iraq), IGS (cl. Waz and Mahsud). MID 24th Dec. 1917, 1st Jun. 1923. d. 22nd Jan. 1952.

SULLIVAN Thomas Address: 3 Dundela Gdns, Strandtown, Belfast. MB, BCh (QUB 1939). Lt Col. RAMC.

SUMM Julius Cecil b. Clones, Co. Monaghan 21st Nov. 1912. Address: 5 Eia St, Belfast. Educ. R. Belfast Academical Inst. and Queen's Uni. Belfast. MB, BCh (QUB 1936). Capt. (T/Maj.) RAMC. On mobilisation in 1939 he joined the 137th Fd Amb. and proceeded to France. Med. Campaign. 14th Lt Fd Amb. of the Armoured Div. (Desert Rats). Served through the invasion of Europe and the Low Countries. OBE. 'This officer has rendered invaluable services as my second-in-command throughout the whole period under review. The unit has on many occasions been "straffed" from the air and bombed. Major Summ has invariably been the first to go round the leaguer completely regardless of his own personal safety to see if the patients are safe and reassure them and to find and give medical treatment to the men of his own unit who have become casualties. Major Summ by his personal example and courage at all times has been an inspiration to the officers and men of this unit, serving with a forward brigade throughout the battle since Alamein. He has been directly responsible for maintaining the morale of the unit at a high level during many difficult times.' d. suddenly 21st Jul. 1951.

SUMMERS Henry Arthur Hamilton Address: 118 Somerton Rd, Belfast. MB, BCh, DPH (QUB 1942). Flt Lt (M) RAFVR.

SUPER Basil Address: 11 Eaton Rd, Terenure, Dublin. L.LM (RCPI 1942), L.LM (RCSI 1942). Lt RAMC 1944.

SUTCLIFFE John Forrest L.LM (RCPI 1934), L.LM (RCSI 1934). Lt RAMC 1942.

SUTTON Harold Brahan Address: Pinehurst, Blackrock, Co. Cork. MB, BCh (TCD 1935) MD (TCD 1939). RAF.

SWANN William George Address: 28 Beechwood Ave., Londonderry. MB, BCh (QUB 1934), DPH (QUB 1937). Maj. RAMC.

SWEENEY William Mason Address: 82 High St, Holywood, Co. Down. Campbell College. MB, BCh (QUB 1942). Capt. RAMC.

SWEETNAM Thomas William b. 25th Mar. 1893, Co. Londonderry. s. George (clerk in Holy Orders) and Sara Louisa Jane Sweetnam, Glebe, Tullykeeran, Londonderry. Educ. Campbell Coll. Belfast Sept. 1906–Jul. 1910. MB, BCh (TCD 1915). R. C. of I. Lt RAMC Oct. 1915. T/Capt. 18th Oct. 1916. Maj. Served France from 1st May 1916. Wounded France Sept. 1916. Served in 1939–45 War. Maj. RAMC. Medals: BWM, VM.

SWINSON Arthur Edward Percival Address: 5 Kilhorne Gdns, Knock, Belfast. MB, BCh (QUB 1942). Ship's Surg. RN.

SYMMERS William St Clair Address: 49 Wellington Pk, Belfast. BCh, MD (QUB 1939). Surg. Lt RNVR.

T

TABUTEAU Thomas Bousfield Herrick b. 14th Aug. 1894, Dunfanaghy, Co. Donegal. s. Mrs Tabuteau, Ormond, Chichester Pk, Belfast. Educ. Campbell Coll. Belfast Jan. 1906–Jul. 1911. MB, BCh (TCD 1917), BAO. Lt RAMC 1st Nov. 1917. Capt. 1st Nov. 1918. PC Lt (T/Capt.) 1st May 1919. Capt. 1st May 1921. Maj. 1st Nov. 1929. A/Lt Col. 15th Nov. 1940. T/Lt Col. 15th May 1940. Lt Col. 4th Feb. 1944. A/Col. 8th Sept. 1942. T/Col. 8th Mar. 1943. r.p. 15th May 1955. Served France 1917–19. China Jul.–Oct. 1919. India 1920–24 and 28–33. Malta 1935–40. CO 179 Fd Amb. 1940–41. CO 8 CCS May–Sept. 1942. BNAF/CMF 1942–46. CO 72 Gen. Hosp. 1942–44. CO 22 Gen. Hosp. 1942–45 and Apr.–Sept. 1946. ADMS HQ 52 area 1945–46. HQ Rome area Allied Comd Mar. 1946. HQ 86 area Sept.–Dec. 1946. CO Mil. Hosp. Lincoln 1947. ADMS HQ E. Anglia Dist. 1947–49. MELF 1949–50. ADMS HQ Canal N. Dist. Jul. 1949 and HQ 3rd Inf. Brig. Dist. 1949–50. DDMS HQ Malta Garrison 1950–53. CO David Bruce Mil. Hosp. Aug. 1951. PSMB W. Comd 1953–55. Medals: OBE (13th Dec. 1945), BWM, VM, IGSM (cl. Waz. 1919–21), 1939–45 S., Africa S (with 1st Army cl.), Italy S., DM, WM, QEII Corn Medal 1953. MID 23rd Sept. 1943.

TAGGART James McAllister Address: Capecastle, Ballyroth, Coleraine. MB, BCh, DPH (QUB 1939). Sq. Ldr (M) RAFVR.

TAIT Charles Edwin Address: 9 Seapark Rd, Mount Prospect, Clontarf, Dublin. L.LM (RCPI 1939), L.LM (RCSI 1939). Flt Lt RAF 1938.

TAPISSIER Maurice Edmund MB, BCh (TCD 1939). Maj. RAMC 1942.

TATE James MB, BCh (QUB 1914), DPH (QUB 1919), MRCP (London 1933). Wing Comdr (M) RAF.

TAYLOR Charles Morrison MB, BCh (TCD 1929). Maj. US Army Med. Corps.

TAYLOR Herbert Alexander Address: 128 Main St, Larne, Co. Antrim. MB, BCh (QUB 1931). Maj. RAMC.

TAYLOR James Address: 4 Victoria Rd, Bangor, Co. Down. MB, BCh (QUB 1938). Sq. Ldr (M) RAFVR. MID.

TAYLOR Robert George Address: Ballinacor House, Tinahely, Co. Wicklow, MB, BCh (TCD 1933), FRCS (England 1937). Maj. RAMC 1939. UK, Normandy, Belgium, Norway, Germany.

TAYLOR Roland Edward Address: Tinahely, Co. Wicklow. MB, BCh (TCD 1937). RAMC.

TAYLOR Susan Doris Dickson MB (QUB 1941). Maj. RAMC.

TAYLOR Victor Norman Address: 128 Main St, Larne, Co. Antrim. MB, BCh (QUB 1941). Capt. RAMC. MID.

TEASEY William Bennett Address: Hadeley, Avenue Rd, Lurgan, Co. Armagh. MB, BCh (QUB 1936). Surg. Lt RNVR.

TEEVAN Kevin b. IFS. Address: 82 St Mobhi Rd, Glasnevin, Dublin. MB, BCh, BAO (NUI 1939). Lt RAMC 11th Aug. 1941. Capt. D. 29th Nov. 1942, West Africa.

TEMPLE Robert Wilbur Address: Magherabeg House, Donegal. MB, BCh (TCD 1938). Capt. RAMC. MID.

THOMAS Garry Uttley Address: 437 Cregagh Rd, Belfast. MB, BCh (QUB 1942). Surg. Lt RNVR.

THOMPSON Adeline Howie MB, BCh (QUB 1943). Capt. RAMC.

THOMPSON Arthur Geoffrey Address: 36 Lower Baggot Street, Dublin. MB, BCh (TCD 1928), MD (TCD 1932), MRCPI (1931). Maj. RAMC 1940.

THOMPSON Eric Wilfred Lowther Address: The Rectory, Ballivor, Co. Meath. MB, BCh (TCD 1936). Maj. RAMC.

THOMPSON Noel James William Address: 52 Cabin Hill Gdns, Knock, Belfast. MB, BCh (QUB 1935), DPH, RCPS (England 1940). Flt Lt (M) RAFVR.

THOMPSON Thomas James Logan b. 17th Aug. 1889, Cork. s. Mrs Thompson, Mountain View, Rostrevor, Co. Down. Educ. St Andrews Coll. Dublin 1st Sept. 1902–Oct. 1907. TCD (1914), MB (1914), BCh, BAO. R. Presbyterian. Lt RAMC 20th Dec. 1914. T/Capt. 20th Dec. 1915. PC Lt (T/Capt.) 1st Jun. 1918. A/Maj. 8th Jan. 1918. Lt Col. 29th Mar. 1940. A/Col.30th Dec. 1941. T/Col. 30th Jun. 1941. r.p. Hon Col. 29th May 1958. Served in 1914–18 War Dardanelles and Gallipoli Jul–Oct. 1915. Egypt Dec. 1915–Jan. 1916. France 1916–19. Oct. 1915 Salonika. N. Russia May–Oct. 1919. Somaliland Dec. 1919–Aug. 1920. India 1920–23. Shanghai 1927–29. India 1931–37. ADMS Liverpool Sept.–Dec. 1940. ADMS Transport, NW Ports 1940–42. ADGMS War Office 1942–43. ADMS Medical Embka. HQ 1945–48. Medals: OBE (1st Jan. 1945), MC (26th Sept. 1917), Afr. GSM (cl. Somaliland 1920), 1915 S., BWM, VM, DM, WM, L. of Merit USA 14th Nov. 1947, OStJ 8th Jul. 1947.

THOMPSON Thomas Rolland Stewart MB, BCh (QUB 1916). Sq. Ldr (M) RAF.

THOMPSON Walter John Address: 12 James Street, Cookstown, Co. Tyrone. MB, BCh (TCD 1941). Surg. Lt RNVR.

THOMPSON William David Address: 1 Manor St, Belfast. MB, BCh (QUB 1936). Surg. Lt Comdr RNVR.

THOMSON Charles Samson Address: 50 Malone Pk, Belfast. MB, BCh (QUB 1936), DPH (London 1939). Lt Col. RAMC.

*THOMSON Humphrey Barron b. Belfast. Only s. Sir William Thomson, MD FRCP, JP and of Lady Thomson née Baron of Hillsborough, Co. Down. Educ. Elm Park and Campbell College. MB (QUB 1939). Married Miss Mary Glendinning of Island Reagh, Comber, Co. Down. Capt. 128238 RAMC (East Surrey Regiment). KIA Singapore, 14th Dec. 1941, aged 25. Commemorated on Singapore Memorial Column 103.

THORNBERRY Cyril Joseph Address: Mullaglass, Newry, Co. Down. L.LM (RCPI 1941), L.LM (RCSI 1941). Surg. Lt RNVR 1942.

THRIFT Geoffrey Berry MB, BCh (TCD 1929). Lt Col. RAMC. India Comd.

THRONE Basil McCrea Address: Matheragh, Ballymagorry, Strabane, Co. Tyrone. MB, BCh (QUB 1941). Flt Lt (M) RAFVR.

TIERNEY William Fitzgerald Address: L'Abri, Model Farm Rd, Cork. MB, BCh, BAO (UCC 1938). Flt Offr RAF.

TIMONEY Joseph Address: 19 Lea Rd, Sandymount, Dublin. MB, BCh, BAO (UCD 1937). Lt RAMC.

TINKLER Alfred Ernest Address: 4 Dolphin Ave., Dublin MB, BCh (TCD 1940), DPH RCPS (England 1943). RAF.

*TODD Andrew William Palethorpe b. Jul. 1892, Dublin. s. Judge Andrew Todd (KC) and Ellen Todd, 21 Hatch St, Dublin. Educ. St Andrews Coll. Dublin Sept. 1898–31st Dec. 1900 and Oct. 1901–Jun. 1908 and 11th Jan. 1910–30th Jun. 1910. MB (TCD 1915) , BCh, BAO. R. Presbyterian. T/Lt 25th Aug. 1915. T/Capt. 25th Aug. 1916. PC Lt (A/Maj.) 1918. PC Capt. 1st May 1919. A/Maj. 10th Nov. 1918. r.p. 9th Dec. 1939. T/Maj 11th Mar. 1940. Served 1914–18 War MEF from Oct. 1915. Gallipoli 25th Sept.–3rd Dec. 1915. Invalided. F and F 20th Sept. 1916–29th Nov. 1917 and 3rd Apr. 1918–11th Nov. 1918. Italy 29th Nov. 1917–3rd Apr. 1918. India 1919–21. BEF France 1939–40. Medals: MC (15th Oct. 1918), 1915 S., BWM, VM, 1939–45 S., WM. d. 15th Mar. 1942, aged 49. Buried in Brookwood Military Cemetery, Plot 5.J.6.

TODD Charles Patrick MB (QUB 1944). Lt RAMC.

TOMLINSON Sterling MB, BCh (TCD 1937). Colonial Med. Service. POW Hong Kong 1942. Released 1945.

TOOHEY Monty b. 13th Dec. 1914, Limerick. Address: 31 Westfield Rd, Harold's Cross, Dublin. Educ. Wesley Coll. MB, BCh (TCD 1936). Norman Conolly Medal, DPH (1938), MRCP (London 1939), MD (1941). Maj. RAMC. 88th Gen. Hosp. Served with the RAMC in India, France and the Far East. Lt Col. in charge of Medical Div. Post war consultant Physician to New End Hospital. Author of many medical articles and the standard work *Medicine for Nurses*. d. 21st Mar. 1960, survived by his widow and two daughters.

TOOLE Dermot Stephen Address: Park House, Killiney, Co. Dublin. MB, BCh (TCD 1937). Maj. RAMC. 8th Army.

TORRIE Edwin Cecil Address: 20 Enmore, Coleraine, Co. Derry. MB, BCh (QUB 1940). Surg. Lt RNVR.

TOWNLEY John Benedict Address: Crosshill, Crumlin, Belfast. L.LM (RCPI 1937), L.LM (RCSI 1937). Lt RAMC 1940.

TOWNSEND Attwell Allen MB, BCh, BAO (UCC 1924). Flt Offr RAF.

TOWNSLEY Norman Joyce MB, BCh (QUB 1930), FRCS (Edinburgh 1937). Lt Col. RAMC.

TRANT Hope MB, BCh (TCD 1925), MD (TCD 1933). Capt. E. Africa Med. Corps.

TRACY John Bernard Address: 2 Clonskeagh Tce, Clonskeagh, Dublin. L.LM (RCPI 1937), L.LM (RCSI 1937). Lt RAMC 1940.

TRIMBLE Arthur Philip b. 21st Aug. 1909, Holywood, Co. Down. MB, BCh (QUB 1931), MD (QUB 1951), MRCP (Edinburgh 1957), FRCP (Edinburgh 1961). PC Lt RAMC 1st Oct. 1931, Capt. 1st May 1934, A/Maj. 9th Sept. 1939, T/Maj. 9th Dec. 1939, Maj. 1st Oct. 1941, A/Lt Col. 23rd Apr. 1942, T/Lt Col. 23rd Jul. 1942, Lt Col. 8th Jul. 1947, T/Col. 19th Feb. 1953, Col. 6th Mar. 1956, T/Brig. 1st Jan. 1958, Brig. 21st Nov. 1960, r.p. disability 24th Jan. 1964. Served China 1933–36, MEF/N. Africa/CMF 1941–45: CO 12th Lt Fd Amb. 1942–43, CO 1st Lt Fd Amb. 1943–45, SMO Sandhurst 1947–48, MELF: OIC Med. Div. BMH Fayid 1948–51, OIC Med. Div. Cambridge Hosp. Aldershot 1951–53, GHQ FARELF 1953–56, OIC Med. Div. Mil. Hosp. Catterick 1957, ADMS HQ Northumbrian Dist. 1957, HQ BAOR 1957–62, HQ NEARELF 1962–63. Medals: CBE 1st Jan. 1961, 1939–45 S., Africa S. with cl. 8th Army, Italy S., DM, WM, GSM with cl. Malaya MID 6th Apr. 1944, 29th Nov. 1945

TROTTER Enid Beatrice (née Roulston) Address: 46 Edecumbe Gdns, Holywood Rd, Belfast. MB, BCh (QUB 1936). Maj. RAMC.

TROY Elizabeth Mary Address: 44 Dartmouth St, Dublin. MB, BCh, BAO (UCD 1940). Flt Offr RAF.

TULLY Brian Patrick Address: 21 High St, Enniskillen. MB, BCh, BAO (UCD 1939). Lt RAMC. Medals: MC.

TULLY Denis Redmond Address: St Anthony's, Carrigaline, Co. Cork. MB, BCh, BAO (UCC 1939). Lt RAMC.

TURNER Alfred Clough MB, BCh (QUB 1923), FRCS (Edinburgh 1923). Col. RAMC. OBE.

TURNER Arthur Francis Address: Oakley, Broughshane Rd, Co. Antrim. MB, BCh (QUB 1934), DPH (London 1937). Lt Col. RAMC.

TWEEDY Ernest Stewart b. 14th Nov. 1905, Dublin. MB, BCh, BAO (TCD 1930). PC Lt RAMC 15th Apr. 1932, Capt. 1st May 1934, A/Maj. 12th Jan. 1940, T/Maj. 12th Apr. 1940, Maj. 15th Apr. 1041, A/Lt Col. 23rd Jun. 1941, T/Lt Col. 23rd Sept. 1941, r.p. disability Hon. Lt Col. 22nd Sept. 1945. Served India 1933–39, BEF France 1939–40. Medals: 1939–45 S., WM.

TWEEDY Henry Richard Francis, s. of Richard Thomas and Henrietta Tweedy, Skerries, Co. Dublin. MB, BCh (TCD 1928). Maj. E. Africa Med. Corps.

TWEEDY Richard Thomas Pilkington, s. Richard Thomas and Henrietta Tweedy, Skerries, Co. Dublin. MB, BCh (TCD 1930). Capt. 1930 RAMC, Maj. 1937 RAMC.

TWIGG Thomas Hill b. 11th Nov. 1893, Limerick. s. William Robert (Bank of Ireland agent) and Anna M. Twigg, 95 George's St, Limerick. Educ. NUI (UCC). MB (1915), BCh, BAO. R. C. of I. T/Lr. RAMC 13th Dec. 1915. Capt. 13th Dec. 1916. Resigned 13th Dec. 1917. Rejoined Capt. 1st Jun. 1918. PC Lt (T/Capt.) 1st Jun. 1919. Capt. 1st Dec. 1919. Maj. 1st Jun. 1928. A/Lt Col. 3rd Apr. 1942. T/Lt Col. 3rd Jul. 1942. Lt Col. 29th Oct. 1942. A/Col. 27th Oct. 1945. Col. 3rd Mar. 1947. A/Brig. 2nd Sept. 1948. r.p. 20th Oct. 1951. Served France Feb.–May 1916 and Jun–Nov. 1918. Salonika 1917. Egypt 1919–24. Sec. Under Colonial Office Lagos and Nigeria 1926–28. Somaliland 1929–30 and 1931–33. Invalided. India 1938–45. DADP Madras Dist. 1938–42. GHQ (1) 1943–45. SMO HQ 157 Inf. Brig. Apr.–Oct. 1945. W. Africa ADMS HQ Gold Coast 1945–46. BAOR 1946–47. ADMS HQ 49 Div. Jun.–Oct. 1946. HQ 7th Armd Div. 1946–47. CO 29th (Hanover) BMH 1947. Palestine/Malta 1948–49. ADMS HQ 1st Div. 1948. DDMS HQ Malta 1948–49. ADMS HQ Aldershot Dist. 1949–51. Spec. in Pathology.

TWOHIG Jeremiah Nicholas Address: Reendesert, Bantry, Co. Cork. MB, BCh, BAO (UCC 1937). Lt RAMC.

TWOHIG William Joseph Address: Reendesert, Bantry, Co. Cork. MB, BCh, BAO (UCG 1938). Lt RAMC.

TWOHILL Jeremiah Patrick Address: Knock, Ennis, Co. Clare. MB, BCh, BAO (NUI 1925). Flt Offr RAF 13th Jul. 1926.

TYNDALL William Ernest b. 27th May 1891, Dublin. Educ. TCD (1913). MB (1914), BCh, BAO, LM (Rot. 1914), RCPS (England 1931), DPH (England 1931). Lt RAMC SR 31st Aug. 1914. Capt. 1st Apr. 1915. PC Capt. 1st Dec. 1918. A/Maj. 4th Sept. 1918. T/Maj. 22nd Sept. 1924. Maj. 26th Aug. 1926. Lt Col. 29th May 1937. A/Col. 29th Feb. 1940. T/Col. 21st Jun. 1941. Col. 14th Jun. 1943. A/Brig. 13th Mar. 1942. T/Brig. 13th Sept. 1942. A/ Maj. Gen. 7th Apr. 1945. T/Maj. Gen. 7th Apr. 1946. Maj. Gen. 1st Jun. 1947. r.p. 28th Jan. 1951. Rempld 5th Nov. 1956. r.p. Maj. Gen. 19th Feb. 1957. Served BEF France from 4th Oct. 1914–16 and 1917–19. Attd 11th Hampshire Regt. India 1919–23. BAOR: DADP 1924–25. W. Africa 1925–26 and 1927–28: DADP and H Sierra Leone 1925–26. China DADP China Comd 1932–35. CO Mil. Hosp. Shanghai 1937–38. TRG Officer (Anti-Gas) RAMC 1938–40. Norway ADMS HQ 6 Base sub-area Apr.–Jun. 1940. ADMS HQ E. Comd 1940–41. ADMS HQ 11th Armoured Div. Mar.–Jul. 1941. GHQ Home Forces: Med Adv 1941–42, DDMS 1942–43. DGAMS (Ops) War Office 1943–45. DMS GHQ ALFSEA/FARELF 1945–48. DDMS HQ S. Comd 1948–50. KHS 1st Mar. 1948. Spec. Duty as public health adv. CA HQ 2 Corps. 1956–57. Medals: MC (16th Sept. 1918), CB (6th Jun. 1946), CBE (2nd Jul. 1943), 1915 S., BWM, VM, 1939–45 S., Burma S., DM, WM, GSM (cl. S.E. Asia 1945–46), OStJ. MID 20th Dec. 1940.

TYNER Richard Colles MB, BCh (TCD 1934). Surg. Lt RNVR. HMS *Eagle* (Sunk Med. 1942). HMS *Londonderry* (torpedoed 1943).

TYRRELL Sir William b. 20th Nov. 1885, Belfast. s. John (army contractor) and Jeannie Tyrrell, 3 Antrim Rd, Clifton, Antrim. Educ. R. Belfast Acad. Inst. and QUB. MB, BCh, BAO (Belfast 1913), DPH (QUB 1922). Married 1929 Barbara Coleclough. Note: International rugby player for Ireland. Lt RAMC SR 18th Oct. 1912. Mobd 6th Aug. 1914. Capt. 1st Apr. 1915. A/Lt Col. 19th Mar. 1917. Capt. 1st Dec. 1918. Resigned on appointment to RAF MS 1st Oct. 1920. Wing Comdr RAF MS Nov. 1928. Air Com. 1935. T/Air Vice Marshal RAF MS 1939–44, r.p. Air Vice Marshal 1944. Served 1914–18 War attd 2nd Lancs. Fus. From 1st Oct. 1914 OC 76th Fd Amb. Served with RAF 1920–44, BEF France 1914–19, Somaliland 1919–20, seconded to RAF 1919. Medals: CBE, KBE, DSO (1st Jan. 1918), Bar (26th Jul. 1918), MC (18th Feb. 1915), 1914 S., BWM, VM, Belgium War Cross. MID 16th Jan. 1915, 1st Jan. 1916, 24th Dec. 1917, 30th Dec. 1918.

U

UPRICHARD William Leonard Address: 125 Marlborough Pk Sth, Belfast. MB, BCh (QUB 1939). Sq. Ldr (M) RAFVR.

UPTON James Barnes Address: Fairways, Magheraleave Rd, Lisburn, Co. Antrim. MB, BCh (QUB 1937), DPH (QUB 1939). Capt. RAMC.

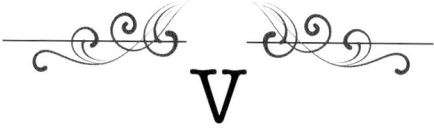

V

VAN MIERT Pieter James Address: 10 Beechwood Rd, Ranelagh, Dublin. MB, BCh (NUI 1943). Lt RAMC 2nd Nov. 1939.

VANCE Ernest Sydney George Killen Address: 52 Crumlin Rd, Belfast. MB, BCh (QUB 1918). Capt. RAMC.

VANCE Robert Lancelot MB, BCh (TCD 1915). Col. RAMC.

VARIAN Stephen Noel Address: 5 Richmond Hill, Monkstown, Co. Dublin. MB, BCh (TCD 1932). Maj. RAMC. MBE.

VAUGHAN Cyril Joseph Address: St Valerie, Bray, Co. Wicklow. MB, BCh (TCD 1934). Lt RNVR. DSC.

VAUGHAN Victor St George MB, BCh (TCD 1926), MD (TCD 1933). RAMC India Comd.

VICKERY George Edward Gordon b. 21st Feb. 1885. s. George Vickery (MD), Green Hill, Kinsale, Co. Cork and Ellen Frances Vickery. Educ. St Andrew's Coll. Dublin 1st Sept. 1898–31st Oct. 1901. TCD (1907), MB (1907), BCh, MA. Staff Surg. RN May 1915. Surg. Lt Comdr 14th May 1917. Surg. Comdr 30th Jun. 1933. Surg. Capt. Served in 1914–18 War, HMS *Ambrose*, and in 1939–45 War. Medals: OBE (1919). MID 1917.

VINCENT Samuel Anderson Address: 37 Malone Rd, Belfast. MB, BCh (QUB 1933). Capt. RAMC.

VINE Richard George Address: 337 Ravenhill Rd, Belfast. MB, BCh (QUB 1941). Flt Lt (M) RAFVR.

VINT Robert Washington b. 4th Jul. 1887 at Carrickfergus, Co. Antrim. MB, BCh, BAO (QUB 1910). Lt 26th Jan. 1912. Capt. 30th Mar. 1915. A/Maj. 4th Feb. 1918. Maj. 26th Jan. 1924. Lt Col. 4th Jun. 1934. Col. 15th Jul. 1939. r.p. 24th Apr. 1947. Serviced India 1914–16, Mesopotamia 1916–19. Persia 1919–20. Mil. Hosp. Catterick 1929–31. Malta Mil. Hosp. Imtarfa 1931–35 (CO from 1934). Mil. Hosp. Edinburgh 1935–38. India 1938–43. CO BMH Bombay 1938–39. CO BMH Meerut 1939–40. ADMS HQ Waziristan Dist. 1940–42. ADMS HQ 106 L. of C. area 1942–43. CO CIMH Palampur 1943. BHS 1942. ADMS HQ S. Midland Dist. 1944–45. PSMB Catterick 1945–47. Spec. in Surgery 1922. Medals: 1939–45 S., DM, WM. d. 2nd Mar. 1953.

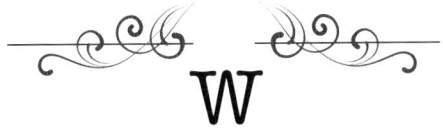

W

WALBY Alfred Leonard Address: 56 Dublin Rd, Belfast. MB, BCh, DPH (QUB 1940). Sq. Ldr (M) RAFVR.

WALDRON Daniel Hyacinth MB, BCh (NUI 1925). MD (NUI 1938), DPH, RCPS (England 1939). Lt IMS 29th Jul. 1929.

WALDRON Edward Augustine Address: 8 Mellifont Ave., Dun Laoghaire, Dublin. L.LM (RCPI 1941), L.LM (RCSI 1941). Flt Lt RAFVR 1945.

WALDRON Francis Raymond MB, BCh (UCG 1926), DPH (1929), MD (1935 NUI). T/Major 257963 RAMC. Belsen concentration camp.

WALKER Frederick George Connor Address: 6 Cherryvalley Pk, Belfast. Campbell College. MB, BCh (QUB 1938). Surg. Lt RNVR.

WALKER Joseph Henry Cranston b. 20th Jul. 1893, Dublin. Educ. TCD. MB (1915), BCh, BAO, DPH (Belfast 1930). Lt RAMC SR 21st Feb. 1914. Capt. 1st Apr. 1916. PC Lt RAMC 1st Jun. 1918. Capt. 1st Apr. 1919. T/Maj. 11th Feb. 1924. Maj. 1st Oct. 1927. A/Lt Col. 21st Mar. 1940. T/Lt Col. 21st Jun. 1940. Lt Col. 13th Apr. 1942. A/Col. 5th Nov. 1942. T/Col. 5th May 1943. Col. 9th Sept. 1946. r.p. 19th Sept. 1948. Served Egypt 31st Dec. 1915–16. France 1916–17. 94th Fd Amb. India 1917–18. E. Persia 1918–21. BAOR 1922–24. Egypt 1924–25. Malaya 1925–29. DADP 1925–26. Hong Kong Jan.–Nov. 1927. DADH and P Malta 1931–36. Physiologist Defence Experimental Station Porton 1936–40. Chief Inst. Chemical Warfare Sch. RAMC 1940–42. CO 102 Gen. Hosp. 1942–43. ADMS HQ 49 Div. 1943–44. NWE 1944–45. India 1945–46: CO 104 IGH (C) 1945, ADMS HQ 303 Bengal and Assam area 1945–46. ADMS HQ Singapore dist. 1946–47. ADMS HQ S. Western Dist. 1947–48. Specialist in pathology 1924. Medals: MC (1st Jan. 1918), BWM, VM, 1939–45 S., France and Germany S., DM, WM, IGS(Afghan NWF 1919), O. of Leopold, Croix de Guerre (Belgium). d. 30th Jan. 1964, Cambridge.

WALKER Lawrence MB, BCh (QUB 1923). Capt. RAMC.

WALKER Robert Fowler b. 21 Nov. 1890 at Galway. MB, BCh, BAO (QUB 1915), DPH (QUB 1928). 2nd Lt R.I. Fus. 15 Aug 1914. Lt 3 Jul. 1915. Trans. Lt RAMC SR 1 Sept. 1915. Capt. 1 Mar. 1916. PC Capt. 1 Apr. 1919. Maj. 1 Sept. 1927. Lt Col. 11 May 1940. A/Col. 21 Dec. 1940. Col. 1 Aug. 1945. A/Brig. 12 Feb. 1942. T/Brig. 12 Jul. 1942. r.p. Hon. Brig. 26 Dec. 1947. BEF France 1914–15, invalided. 1915–17 wounded and invalided. RMO to IG and 2nd Coldstream Gds 1916–17 and 1918–19. Hong Kong 1923–26. India 1929–34. Egypt 1938–44. CO 9 Gen. Hosp. 1940–41. Seconded to Egypt govt. 1939–40. DDMS GHQ MEF Apr.–May 1941. DDMS HQ Alexandria Area 1941–44. DDMS HQ 21 Army Group Mar.–Oct. 1944. NWE Jul.–Dec. 1944: DDMS HQ 30th Corps. Nov.–Dec. 1944. CO QA Mil. Hosp. Shenley 1945–46. ALFSEA: DDMS HQ Burma Comd 1946–47. Spec. in Hyg. 1928. OBE (9 Sept. 1942). CBE (6 Jan. 1944). MC (Nov. 1917). OStJ (1936), 1915 S., BWM, VM, 1939–45 S., France and Germany S., KGVI Corn Medal 1937. 'This officer, who is a Deputy Director of Medical Supplies in the Middle East, is mainly responsible to the Director of Medical Supplies for the many and difficult medical plannings to suit the 1,001 projects planned in the Middle East. Each plan necessitates the medical planning for the provision of the many large and small medical units required for the countries and climates through which the forces involved may pass. It also necessitates the planning of the type and quantity of medical stores required, special drugs, chemicals, clothing, medical and advance equipment, the provision and supply, and medical advice. It also necessitates the planning of the type of medical transport required in the different types of countries. Up to date, this officer's foresight, judgement and careful calculations based on his specialised knowledge have covered medical results in evacuation and nursing of casualties, which have brought nothing but praise from the highest authorities. His keenness, loyalty, devotion to duty and entire application to these many difficult problems have been an example to all.'

WALKER William Alexander Address: 2 De Molyen Pk, Londonderry. MB, BCh (QUB 1940). Surg. Lt RNVR.

WALLACE Caleb Paul Address: Rathmore, Palmerston Rd, Dublin. MB, BCh (TCD 1927). Capt. RAMC.

WALLACE David Wilson Address: Greenmount, Carnmoney, Co. Antrim. MB, BCh (QUB 1933), DPH (QUB 1937). Surg. Comdr RNVR. MID.

WALLACE Hugh Bryson Calwell MB, BCh (QUB 1929), MC (QUB 1935). Malayan Med. Service, POW.

WALLACE Quentin Vaughan Brooke b. 6th Jan. 1891, Dublin. s. Sir Arthur Wallace (CB DL Chief Sec. Office Dublin Castle), Ardnamona, Lough Eske, Co. Donegal. Educ. Shrewsbury Sch and TCD. MB (1914), BCh, BAO. Lt RAMC SR 19th Oct. 1914 mobilised 24th Oct. 1914. Capt. 19th Apr. 1915. PC Capt. 1st Jun. 1918. Maj. 19th Oct. 1926. Lt Col. 8th Mar. 1939. A/Col. 16th Mar. 1940. T/Col. 16th Sept. 1940. Col. 27th Nov. 1944. A/Brig. 3rd Jul. 1942. T/Brig. 3rd Jan. 1943. r.p. Hon. Brig. 8th Aug. 1948. Served France from 14th Jul. 1915–17, invalided, and 1917–18, wounded and invalided. RMO 7th Border Regt. 1915–16. Wounded Aug. 1918. 10th Bn.

Tank Corps. 1917–18. India 1919–21. Gibraltar 1927–32. Egypt 1936. Obst. Spec. Aldershot 1937–38. Egypt/MEF 1938–43. CO BMH Khartoum 1939–40. ADMS HQ 7th Armoured Div. 1940–41. ADMS HQ Suez sub area Aug.–Sept. 1941. CO 9 Gen. Hosp. 1941–42. ADMS 1942 43. DDMS HQ 1st Corps. 1943–45. NWE 1944–45. DDMS HQ London Dist. 1945–48. Medals: CBE (1st Feb. 1945), OBE (1st Apr. 1941), MC (14th Jan. 1916), 1915 S., BWM, VM, 1939–45 S., Africa S. with 8th Army cl., France and Germany S., WM. MID 1st Jan. 1916, 8th Nov. 1945.

WALLEN Otto Lancelot James MB, BCh (NUI 1938). Lt RAMC 22nd Jan. 1940.

WALMSLEY George Alexander b. 20th Sept. 1903, Dublin. MB, BCh, BAO (TCD 1926). T/Lt RAMC 16th Jul. 1926, PC Lt 26th Jan. 1927, Capt. 26th Jul. 1930, Maj. 10th Dec. 1943, Lt Col. 11th Jun. 1945, A/Col. 10th Jun. 1943, T/Col. 10th Dec. 1943, Col. 28th Nov. 1949, r.p. 20th Sept. 1960. Served India 1927–33, Egypt 1935–36, India 1937–39, Norway 1940, CO 3rd Fd Amb. 1940–42, 10th Fd Amb. 1942–43, BNAF/CMF 1943–45: ADMS HQ 59 area 1943, ADMS HQ 8th Inf. Div. 1943–45, India 1945–47: CO BMH Poona 1946–47, ADMS HQ LF Hong Kong 1948, ADMS HQ N. Midland Dist. 1949–50, BAOR: ADMS HQ 2nd Inf. Div. 1950–52, Gibraltar ADMS and CO Mil. Hosp. 1953–56, ADMS HQ Lowland Dist. 1956–58, ADMS HQ Mid W. Dist. 1958–60. Medals: OBE 29th Apr. 1945, 1939–45 S., Africa S. with cl. 1st Army, Italy S., DM, WM, QEII Corn Medal 1953. MID 27th Jan. 1944.

WALSH Dermot Francis TCD 1927. MB, BCh (1928), FRCS Edin. (1943). Surg. Lt Comdr 18th Jan. 1935, Surg. Rear Adm. Resided at Latona, Torquay Rd, Foxrock, Co. Dublin. Medals: OBE (Military) 5th Jun. 1952, CB 11th Jun. 1960, 1939–45 S., Atlantic S., Africa S., Burma S., Pacific S., Italy S., DM, BWM, QEII Corn Medal 1953. MID 11th Jun. 1946.

WALSH Harold Victor S. Campbell College. MB, BCh (QUB 1913). Lt Col. RAMC. MID.

WALSH Ian Alistair b. 28th Jul. 1911, Co. Tipperary. Address: Ard na Glaise, Stillorgan Pk, Stillorgan, Co. Dublin. MB, BCh, BAO (TCD 1934). Lt RAMC 31st Jan. 1940. Capt. 31st Jan. 1941. PC Capt. 31st Jan. 1945. A/Maj. 25th Apr. 1945. T/Maj. 25th Jul. 1945. Maj. 31st Jan. 1948. T/Lt Col. 9th Feb. 1954. Lt Col. 27th Jan. 1959. Col. 31st Jan. 1963. MEF 1941–45. MELF 1948–50 & 1954–55. CO 5th Fd Amb. 1954–57. Chief Inst. Trg. Wing Depot and Trg Est. RAMC 1957–60. Caribbean area ADMS and CO Mil. Hosp. 1960–62. CO 15th Fd Amb. 1962–63. ADMS HQ S. Comd 1963–66. FARELF: ADMS HQ S. Comd 1963–66. FARELF: ADMS HQ LF Hong Kong 1966. Medals: 1939–45 S., Africa S., DM, WM, OStJ 1957.

WALSH James MB, BCh, BAO (NUI 1925). Lt RAMC 24th Apr. 1940.

WALSH John b. 17th Feb. 1906, Cork. MB, BCh, BAO (UCC 1933). PC Lt 14th Jan. 1933, Capt. 14th Nov. 1934, A/Maj. 11th Mar. 1940, T/Maj. 11th Jun. 1940, Maj. 24th Jan. 1943, A/Lt Col. 27th Jul. 1946, T/Lt Col. 27th Oct. 1946, r.p. disability 13th Jun. 1949. Served India 1935–40, Trooping duties 1945–46, NELF: CO 78 Gen. Hosp. 1946, invalided. d. 24th Feb. 1952. Medals: DM, WM.

WALSH John James Address: Cael, Meadoan, Bishopstown, Co. Cork. MB, BCh (NUI 1940). Flt Lt RAF 5th Mar. 1940.

WALSH Nannie Christina Address: Templeorum, Piltown, Co. Kilkenny. MB, BCh (NUI 1942). Flt Offr RAF 1941.

WALSH Neil Forbes Address: Ard Na Glaise, Stillorgan Pk, Stillorgan, Co. Dublin. MB, BCh, BAO (UCD 1943). Lt RAMC.

WALSH Stanley Denmede Address: Limerick. MB (TCD 1942). Youngest s. Wm. and Mrs W.H. Walsh, Berwyn, O'Connell Avenue, Limerick. Married Margaret, younger dt. Mr L.W. Stiven, Mountown Pk, Dun Laoghaire, Co. Dublin. Surg. Lt RN. He dived from the deck of his ship the Destroyer *Constance* to rescue a naval airman, Ernest Leonard Lindsay, of Newcastle-on-Tyne who fell overboard from the light Fleet Carrier *Theseus* during operations off Korea. The Admiralty stated that during an attack a Sea Fury aircraft unshipped a rocket when landing on the *Theseus* and the 80lb missile hurdled along the deck at 60 miles an hour. Lindsay jumped to avoid it and fell 40 feet into the Yellow Sea. A lifebuoy was thrown to him but he was carried past it. Surg. Lt Walsh saw the rating was in difficulties and he dived in and supported him for several minutes until the destroyer's boat arrived.

WALSH Stephen Joseph Address: Tren Lewis House, Kilmallock, Co. Limerick. MB, BCh (NUI 1938). Flt Offr RAF 9th Apr. 1940.

WALSH William Maurice MB, BCh (NUI 1939). Lt RAMC 22nd Apr. 1940.

WALSHE Patrick Joseph Address: Kilkee, Co. Clare. MB, BCh, BAO (UCD 1922). Lt IMS.

WALSHE Sarsfield James Ambrose Hall b. 12th Jun. 1881, Ballyclough, Co. Cork. Educ. Edinburgh Uni. MB (1912), ChB. Married. Lt RAMC SR 4th Aug. 1910. Capt. 15th Feb. 1914. Mobd 8th Aug. 1914. PC Capt. 1st May 1919. A/Maj. 29th May 1918. Maj. 8th Aug. 1926. Lt Col. 4th Jun. 1936. r.p. 12th Jun. 1936. Rempld Maj. 29th Jun. 1940. r.p. Lt Col. 7th Sept. 1941. Served 1914–18 War with BEF France 18th Aug. 1914–17 and Mar.–Sept. 1919. Italy 1917–19. India 1921–26. Egypt 1926–31 and 1933–36. Medals: DSO (18th Feb. 1915), 1914 S., BWM, VM.

MID 17th Feb. 1915, 1st Jan. 1916, 6th Jan. 1919. d. 11th Jul. 1959, Sheppey.

WARD David Address: Dromtrasna, Abbeyfeale, Co. Limerick. MB, BCh, BAO (UCD 1936). Lt RAMC.

WARREN Henry Robert L.LM (RCPI 1937), L.LM (RCSI 1937). Flt Offr RAF 1937.

WARRINGTON William Oswald MB, BCh (TCD 1925) RAMC.

WARICK Wilfred James Greer Address: 3 Cowper Rd, Rathmines, Dublin. MB, BCh (TCD 1937). RAMC.

WARRINER Thomas Joseph Clarke Address: 34 Terenure Rd, East, Rathgar, Dublin. MB, BCh (TCD 1943). Lt RAMC. Served in Burma.

WASS Norman Harwin MB, BCh (QUB 1939). Capt. RAMC.

WATERS Gerard Joseph MB, BCh, BAO (UCD 1926). Flt Offr RAF 27th Feb. 1940. 18th Mar. 1941 relinquished commission due to ill health.

WATERS Maurice Hubert MB, BCh (TCD 1939). Capt. RAMC. Served in North Africa.

WATSON Albert Address: 63 Avenue Rd, Lurgan, Co. Armagh. MB, BCh (QUB 1937). Capt. RAMC.

WATSON Anna Address: The Hamlet, Earlwood Rd, Belfast. MB, BCh, DPH (QUB 1924). Maj. RAMC.

WATSON Harry Christian MB, BS (QUB 1905). Capt. SAMC.

WATSON James Derek Address: Kenmuir, Castlerock, Co. Derry. MB, BCh (QUB 1942). Surg. Lt RNVR.

WATSON John Address: The Asylum House, Londonderry. MB, BCh (QUB 1941). Capt. RAMC.

WATSON John Charles Address: Dervaghroy, Beragh, Co. Tyrone. MB, BCh (TCD 1941). Capt. RAMC. Served in Sierra Leone.

WATT Thoms McGowan Address: 11 Grasmare Gdns, Belfast. MB, BCh (QUB 1940). Surg. Lt Comdr RNVR.

WAUCHOB David William Address: Laraghs, Newtownstewart, Co. Tyrone. MB, BCh, DPH (QUB 1941). Flt Lt (M) RAFVR.

WEBSTER Edwin William Address: 60 Serpentine Ave., Ballsbridge, Dublin. L.LM (RCPI 1940), L.LM (RCSI 1940). Lt RAMC 1942.

WEINSTEIN Nathan MB, BCh (TCD 1934). US Army Med. Corps. Served North Africa.

WEIR Desmond Alexander Address: Streid Mills, Gracehill, Ballymena, Co. Antrim. MB, BCh, DPH (QUB 1942). Surg. Lt RNVR.

WEIR Matthew McCauley Address: 44 Clonlee Dr., Belfast. MB, BCh (QUB 1939). Surg. Lt RNVR.

WELDON Samuel Gerald MB, BCh (TCD 1922), DPH (TCD 1923). Surg. Comdr RN. HMS *Medway* 1939–42.

*****WELLS** Hayter Arnett b. IFS. Address: St Mary's, Templeogue Rd, Terenure, Dublin. MB, BCh, BAO (TCD 1934). s. Hardy Heyter William and Mary Norman Wells, of Terenure, Dublin and husband of Delia Wells. Capt. 111839 RAMC. KIA Normandy 19th Jul. 1944, aged 33. Buried Ranville War Cemetery Calvados, France, Plot IVA.M.3. MID.

WELLWOOD John Thomas Address: 7 Fitzwilliam Sq., Dublin. MB, BCh (TCD 1935). Surg. Comdr RN.

WELPLY William Brian Address: Shippool, Innishannon, Co. Cork. MD, BCh (TCD 1939). Lt RAMC. 115th Gen. Hosp.

WEST Edward William MB, BCh (TCD 1931). Capt. RAMC. 105th Gen. Hosp.

WEST George Francis MB, BCh (TCD 1930). Lt Col. Malay States Volunteer Force. POW Sumatra 1942–45. OBE.

WEST John Weir b. 27th Aug. 1875, Antrim. MB (QUB 1899), BS (RUI 1899), BCh, BAO, DPH (1910), RCPSI (1910), FRInstPH, MCh (QUB 1917). Lt RAMC 29th Nov. 1900. Capt. 29th Nov. 1903. Maj. 29th Nov. 1911. A/Lt Col. 3rd Feb. 1917. Lt Col. 26th Dec. 1917. Bt. Col. 15th Apr. 1922. T/Col. 1st May 1924. Col. 26th Dec. 1927. h.p. 26th Dec. 1931. f.p. 1st Mar. 1932. Maj. Gen. 15th Jun. 1932. r.p. 27th Aug. 1935. Served South Africa 1901–06. India 1910–14. BEF France 17th Aug. 1914–17. CO 3rd Cav. Fd Amb. 1914–16. OIC Surg. Div. 13th Gen. Hosp. 1918–19. Surg. Spec. QA Mil. Hosp. Millbank. Asst Mil. Surg. RAM Coll. 1919. Prof. Mil Surg. 1920–27. Burma ADMS HQ. Burma Dist. 1927–31. Prof. Mil. Surg. and Consultant Surg to Army 1932–35. Medals: CBE (20th Dec. 1932), CB (3rd Jun. 1935), CMG (1st Jan. 1919), QSA (4 cls), 1914 S., BWM, VM, IGSM (cl. Burma 1930–32), L de H, Croix de Chev. (24th Feb. 1916), Italian Silver M. De la Salute Publica (29th Oct. 1920). MID 22nd Jun. 1915, 1st Jan. 1916, 24th Dec. 1917, 30th May 1918, 30th Dec. 1918. d. 6th Mar. 1949.

WHEELER Donald Reid MB, BCh (QUB 1918), FRCSI (1922), FRCS (England 1923). Maj. RAMC.

*****WHEELER** William Ireland DeCourcy b. 8th May 1879, Dublin. s. William Ireland DeCourcy Wheeler (Past Pres. RCSI 1883) and Frances Victoria Wheeler (née Shaw). Educ. Strangeways School, Dublin, High Sch. Dublin. TCD

(1899). MB (1912), BCh, MCh (Hon.), MD (1902), FRCSI (1905), FACS Hon. Married 1909 Elsie eldest dt. 1st Baron Craigmyle. Hon. Maj. RAMC Mar. 1916. T/Hon. Lt Col. May 1917. Surg. R Adm and Consultant Surg. to Admiralty 1939–43. War work Surg. to Hosp. for Officers, Dublin. Hon. Surg. to Forces in Ireland. Medals: MID Jan. 1917, Sept. 1917. d. 11th Sept. 1943, suddenly in Aberdeen aged 64. Cremated and interred in Deansgrange Cemetery Blackrock, Co. Dublin, Plot No. 34C, St Nessans. Commemorated on Roll of Honour RCSI. Note: President RCSI 1922–24, MID for distinguished service during the 1916 Easter Rebellion in Dublin.

WHELTON Michael James b. 17th Jun. 1892, Macroom, Co. Cork. MB, BCh, MD (1926), DPH, RCPS (England 1926). Lt RAF Med. Branch 15th Jul. 1918. Capt. 15th Jul. 1919. Demobbed 5th Nov. 1919. PC RAMC Capt. 6th Mar. 1920. Lt RAMC 1st Jun. 1920. Capt. 13th May 1922. Maj. 13th Nov. 1930. A/Lt Col. 4th Oct. 1940. T/Lt Col. 4th Jan. 1941. Lt Col. 12th Nov. 1941. A/Col. 12th May 1942. T/Col. 12th Nov. 1942. Served France 1919. Egypt 1920. India 1920–25. Shanghai 1927–28. BAOR 1928. India 1929–34, Egypt 1935–36, Palestine 1936–37, BEF France 1939–40, MEF/CMF: CO 70th Gen Hosp. 1942–45. Medals: IGS (cl. Waz. 1921–24), 1939–45 S., Africa S. (8th Army cl.), Italy S., DM, WM. MID 1943. d. 17th Jan. 1946, UK. Remembered St Finbarr's Cemetery, Cork, Grave 10/19.

WHITE Harry Ernest Bantry MD. TCD (1935). Military Registrar Bangor North Wales 1940. Maj. SMO HM. Troop Ships 1941. MO RA. (A.A.) 1943, SMO HM Troop Ships 1945, MC.

WHITE Micheal b. 2nd Feb. 1882, Macroom, Co. Cork. Educ. RUI. MB (1908), BCh, BAO. Lt RAMC 30th Jan. 1909. Capt. 30th Jul. 1912. A/Maj. 28th May 1918. Maj. 30th Jan. 1921. A/Lt Col. 20th Nov. 1918. Lt Col. 1st May 1934. r.p. 2nd Feb. 1937. Rempld Maj. 3rd Apr. 1940. r.p. disability Lt Col. 9th Apr. 1948. Served India 1911–17. Mesopotamia May 1916–17. Invalided. France 1918–20. CO 61st Fd Amb. 1918–19. India 1924–29. Egypt 1933–35. India 1935–37. Medals: MC (8th Mar. 1919), BWM, VM, DM, WM. d. 26th Sept. 1956.

WHITE Patrick James Address: Carndonagh, Co. Donegal. MB, BCh (NUI 1938). Lt RAMC 12th Jun. 1941.

WHITE Thomas Kyran MB, BCh, BAO (UCC 1928). Lt IMS.

WHITESIDE John Donald Address: Thwaite, Castle Pk, Rathfarnham, Dublin. MB, BCh (TCD 1938), MD (TCD 1941) MRCPI (1941). Sq. Ldr RAF.

WHITESIDE William Noel Address: Montana, Whitechurch Rd, Rathfarnham, Dublin. MB, BCh (TCD 1934). Sq. Ldr RAF. MID.

WHITFIELD Charles Alexander b. 29th Mar. 1891, Lambeg, Co. Antrim. Address: Hillbrook, Dunmurray, Co. Antrim. s. Henry Stewart (head bleacher) and Mary Jane Whitfield, Lambeg Town, Co. Antrim. Educ. MB, BCh (QUB 1918), BAO, MRCOG (1934). R. Presbyterian. T/Lt ASC SR 14th Aug. 1914. T/Capt. 1st Sept. 1915. Resigned Hon. Capt. 21st Aug. 1917. T/Lt RAMC 5th Sept. 1918. PC Lt 1st May 1919. T/Capt. 5th Sept. 1919. Capt. 5th Mar. 1922. Maj. 5th Sept. 1930. A/Lt Col. 11th Feb. 1940. T/Lt Col. 11th May 1940. Lt Col. 1st Jun. 1944. A/Col. 30th May 1945. T/Col. 30th Nov. 1945. r.p. Hon. Col. 17th Dec. 1946. Served France 1st Oct. 1915–17 and 1918–19. Germany 1919. Mesopotamia 1920–21. India 1921–23 invalided and 1924–30. OC and Spec. Obst. MFH Shorncliffe 1931–33. Louise Margaret Hosp. Aldershot 1933–34. MFH Tidworth 1934–36. MFH Gibraltar 1936–40. CO 195th Fd Amb. 1940–41. ADGMS War Office (AMD 2) 1941–45. India 1945–46: CO 33 Gen Hosp. May–Dec. 1945. 70 IGH (C) 1945–46. 81 IGH (C) Apr.–Aug. 1946. Medals: 1915 S., BWM, VM, DM, WM, KGV Silver Jub. Medal 1935, GSM (cl. NW Persia). MID 29th May 1917. d. 29th Jun. 1962, Chatham.

WHITSITT Thomas Hoskins Address: Sterling Lodge, Clones, Co. Monaghan. L.LM (RCPI 1940), L.LM (RCSI 1940). Flt Offr RAF 1941.

WHYTE Augustine Patrick MB, BCh (TCD 1943). RAMC.

WHYTE Desmond Gilbert Cromie b. 20th Sept. 1913, Belfast, Co. Antrim. Address: Laurels, Helen's Bay, Co. Down. MB, BCh, BAO (Belfast 1937), MD (Belfast 1951), DMRD (England 1951), MRCP (London 1952), MRCP (Edinburgh 1952), FRFPS (Glasgow 1952), FRCP (Edinburgh 1958), FFR (1958), FFR RCSI (1962). Lt 14th Oct. 1939. Capt. 14th Oct. 1940. A/Maj. 14th Jul. 1943. T/Maj. 14th Oct. 1943. PC Capt. 14th Oct. 1944. Maj. 22nd Mar. 1945. WS Maj. 22nd Mar. 1945. Maj. 14th Oct. 1947. A/Lt Col. 22nd Dec. 1944. T/Lt Col. 22nd Mar. 1945. R. 13th Jun. 1954. Recalled 12th Aug. 1956. Served RMO 9th Worc. Regt 1939–40. 24th LAA Regt RA 1941–43. Paiforce 1941–42. India 1942–47: CO 11th Indian R/Amt. 1944–45. 17th Indian Para Fd Amb. 1945–47. CO 23 Para Fd Amb. 1947–48. BAOR 1948. MELF: BMH Fayid 1953–54. MELF Cyprus 5th Gen. Hosp. 1956. Recommended for a VC while serving with the Chindits, Burma, but received a DSO instead. Medals: DSO 5th Oct. 1944, 1939–45 S., Burma S. DM, WM, GSM with cl. Cyprus. MID 16th Dec. 1943.

WHYTE Frank De Burgh Address: The Cottage, Greystones, Co. Wicklow. MB, BCh (TCD 1939). Maj. RAMC. Served in Western Desert, Iraq, Italy. MID.

WICHT Johan Fredrik TCD 1918. Surg. Comdr S. African Navy Reserve.

WIER Henry Wood Campbell College. MB, ChB (1914 Uni. Edinburgh). Captain SAMC.

WIGODER Robert Godfrey Bradlaw Address: 4 Harrington St, Dublin. L.LM (RCPI 1935), L.LM (RCSI 1935). T/Surg. Lt RNVR 1941.

WILDE John Frederick MB, BCh (TCD 1925), MD (1941). Col. RAMC. 32nd British Gen. Hosp.

WILEY Ian Trevor Fitzmaurice Address: Shantonagh Lodge, Castleblayney, Co. Monaghan. MB, BCh (TCD 1933). Lt RAMC. Discharged ill health.

WILKIN William Mitchel MB (QUB 1944). RNVR.

WILLIAMS Cecil Edward Address: Grove House, Malahide, Co. Dublin. MB, BCh (TCD 1941). RAF.

WILLIAMS John Joseph Address: Beechmount, Toomarane, Nenagh, Co. Tipperary. L.LM (RCPI 1937), L.LM (RCSI 1937).

WILLIAMS Norman Ernest Hamilton Powell Address: Sandys Pl., Downshire Rd, Newry, Co. Down. MB, BCh (TCD 1923). Capt. RAMC.

WILLIAMSON Norman Alexander Address: The Fort, Ballooley, Katesbridge, Co. Down. MB, BCh (QUB 1938). Capt. RAMC.

WILLINGTON Frederick Lane MB, BCh (TCD 1939). Maj. RAMC. MEF.

*****WILSON** A.V. S.M. Pilot Officer RAFVR. KIA.

WILSON Charles Brian Address: Carnbeg, The Spa, Ballynahinch, Co. Down. MB, BCh (TCD 1943). Surg. Lt RN 1943.

WILSON Dennis Aird Orr b. 1st Oct. 1905, Pembroke, England. MB, BCh, BAO (QUB 1929), MA (Cambridge 1933), DPH (Wales 1937). PC Lt 30th Jul. 1929 RAMC, Capt. 30th Jan. 1933, Maj. 30th Jul. 1939, A/Lt Col. 21st Mar. 1941, T/Lt Col. 21st Jun. 1941, Lt Col. 1st Aug. 1946, A/Col. 13th Dec. 1943, T/Col. 1st Jul. 1944, Col. 22nd Aug. 1951. Served India 1930–36, BEF France 1939–40, CO 10th Light Fd Amb. 1941–42, ADMS HQ 1st Corps. 1942–43, BNAF/CMF 1943–44, ADMS HQ Force 141/15 Army Group 1943, US Army British Increment 1943, AF HQ 1943–44, ADGAMS War Office 1944–45, SEAC 1945–47, ADMS HQ 1st Area/S. Burma area 1945–46, ADH HQ E. Africa Comd 1947, DDH HQ S. Comd 1949, BAOR 1949–51, CO BMH Hanover 1949–51, CO 28th Fd Amb. 1950–51. Medals: 1939–45 S., Africa S., Italy S., DM, WM, USA Legion of Merit. MID 20th Dec. 1940. d. 28th Nov. 1951 at Hanover W. Germany.

WILSON Edward Lewis MB, BCh (QUB 1937). Lt Col. IMF.

WILSON Gordon Neill Address: 43 Wellington Pk, Belfast. MB, BCh, DPH (QUB 1937). Maj. RAMC.

WILSON Hilary (née Crymble) Address: 7 College Gdns, Belfast. MB, BCh (QUB 1940). Capt. RAMC.

WILSON James Jordan Stewart Address: 2 Harbeton Ave., Belfast. MB, BCh (QUB 1940). Flt Lt (M) RAFVR.

WILSON James Victor Address: Ballygowan, Belfast. MB, BCh (QUB 1933), MD (QUB 1937). Maj. RAMC.

WILSON John Dundee Address: 10 Malone Rd, Belfast. MB, BCh (QUB 1940). Capt. RAMC.

WILSON Joseph Andrew Lawther b. 16th Dec. 1885. Educ. MB (QUB 1912), BCh, BAO (QUB 1912), LM (Tot. Hosp.). Lt RAMC SR 4th Sept. 1914. Mobd 30th Sept. 1914. T/Capt. 1st Apr. 1915. PC Capt. 1st May 1919. Maj. 4th Sept. 1926. Lt Col. 13th Sept. 1937. A/Col. 19th Mar. 1940. r.p. remained empld. 16th Dec. 1940. r.p. Hon Col. 26th Sept. 1945. Served BEF France from 5th Nov. 1914. India 1915–16. Egypt 1919–24. India 1931–35. Palestine: CO Mil. Hosp. Haifa 1938–39. OIC Surg. Div. Royal Victoria Hosp. Netley 1939. BEF France 1939–40. CO 6 Gen. Hosp. 1940. ADMS HQ 42nd Div. 1940. ADMS HQ E. Central Area. Medals: 1914 S., BWM, VM, 1939–45 S., DM, WM. d. 21st Aug. 1966 at Tunbridge Wells, Kent.

WILSON Kenneth Smith Address: Nottinghill, White Abbey, Co. Antrim. MB, BCh (QUB 1937), DPH (QUB 1939). Maj. RAMC.

WILSON Malcolm Orr b. 27th Oct. 1879, Cushendall, Co. Antrim. s. John (bank manager) and Margaret Malcolm R. Wilson, 6 George St, Ballymena, Co. Antrim. Educ. QUB. MB (1904), BCh, BAO. R. Presbyterian. Lt RAMC 28th Jan. 1907. Capt. 28th Jul. 1910. A/Maj. 20th Apr. 1918. Maj. 28th Jan. 1919. A/Lt Col. 24th Jan. 1918. T/Lt Col. 15th Apr. 1931. Lt Col. 15th May 1931. r.p. 15th Aug. 1934. Served India 1909–14. France and Belgium 15th Aug. 1914–15 invalided attd. RFA. Gallipoli 1915–16. Egypt EEF 1916–19. Egypt 1919–20. BAOR 1922–23. Egypt Nov.–Dec. 1924. Gibraltar 1924–28. India 1931–34: CO BMH Agra and Jubbalpore. Specialist in Dermatology and VD. Medals: 1914 S., BEM, VM. MID 25th Sept. 1916. d. 19th Jan. 1963, Plymouth, Devon.

WILSON Martha Neill Algie Address: Straid, Ballyclare, Co. Antrim. MB, BCh (QUB 1942). Capt. RAMC.

*****WILSON** Norman b. Antrim, Northern Ireland. Capt. RAMC. d. 21 Oct. 1943, North Africa.

WILSON Robert Irvine Address: 36 Ardenlee Ave., Belfast. MB, BCh (QUB 1938). Lt Col. RAMC. MBE.

WILSON Robert John Spence Address: 262 York St, Belfast. MB, BCh (TCD 1940). Flt Lt RAF. Malaya, Java, Singapore. POW Java 1942.

WILSON Terence Reginald MB, BCh (Uni. Leeds 1938). RAMC. Capt. (T/Maj.). b. Dublin M.C. 'This officer established an advanced dressing station in a gully on February 27th, 1942. This station is still in position. He was responsible for evacuation of casualties from the area around St De Ksar Mezouar, and the high ground north and north-west of it. During this time he has handled his company with consummate skill, maintaining a close liaison with regimental aid posts and taking over responsibility from the regimental aid posts when they, of necessity, had ceased to function. He has inspired his men with zeal and devotion which has taken them beyond their normal role and pushed them forward to the limit of endurance with one intention, to get the wounded off the ground at all costs, and back quickly to skilled surgical hands. On the night of March 4th–5th, 1943, he organised three of his stretcher squads to go forward to positions still held by a few platoons. These squads took up rations with them on open stretchers for the infantry and brought back casualties on the return journey. He has perfected his system of evacuation so well from that ground and has disposed his squads so well tactically, including a continuous staffing of the tunnel at St Ksar Mezouar, that all casualties recoverable from our lines on that sector have been back at Beja on the operating table in three to four hours, a factor which has undoubtedly saved the lives and limbs of many badly wounded men and which has only been achieved by constant and tireless devotion to duty, carried out at times in face of heavy mortar and shellfire.'

WILSON Thomas MB, DPH (QUB 1927). Capt. RAMC.

WILSON Thomas Scott Address: 17 Arvliston Dr., Belfast. MB, BCh (QUB 1940). Sq. Ldr (M) RAFVR.

WILSON Thomas William L.LM (RCPI 1924), L.LM (RCSI 1924). RAF Medical Services.

WILSON William MB, DPH (QUB 1939). Capt. RAMC.

WILSON William McConaghy MB, TCD (1948). US Army.

WILSON William Thomas Cregeen MB TCD (1942). RAMC.

WINDER Alexander Stuart Monck b. 3rd Oct. 1883, Kingstown, Co. Dublin. s. Henry Monck (civil servant) and Emily Frances Winder, 28 Upr Leeson St, Dublin. Educ. TCD MB (1908), BCh, BAO, LM (Rot.). R. C. of I. Lt RAMC 30th Jan. 1909. Capt. 30th Jul. 1912. Maj. 30th Jan. 1921. Lt Col. 1st May 1934. r.p. 3rd Oct. 1938. Rempld 2nd Sept. 1939. r.p.

4th Apr. 1944. Served India 1911–18. Mesopotamia 1915–17. India 1922–28. Amara, Persian Gulf OC Central Dermatological Lab. Poona. DADP Home Counties Area E. 1928–31. DADH and P Malaya 1931–35. ADP E. Comd 1935–38 and 1939–44. Specialist in Pathology 1921. Medals: 1915 S., BWM, VM, DM, WM. Comm. on Roll of Hon. St Patrick Dun's Hosp.

WINTERS Maurice Ernest (formerly Weiner) MB BCh (TCD 1940). Surg. Lt RAMC 1942. West African Frontier Force 1942. Royal Indian Naval Volunteer Reserve 1945. Capt. Surg. Lt.

WOLFE Frances Mary Christine Address: Ilen House, Skibbereen, Co. Cork. MB, BCh (TCD 1939). RAMC.

WOLPE Irving Theodore MB TCD (1939). Capt. SAMC 1942.

WOOD George (Charles) Harold b. 6th Sept. 1901, Ballina, Co. Mayo. MB, BCh, BAO (TCD 1914). Lt RAMC 13th Apr. 1915. Capt. 13th Apr. 1916. PC Capt. 1st Oct. 1919. Retired 10th Oct. 1923. Rejoined 1st Sept. 1939. A/Maj. 17th Aug. 1942. Reverted to R of O. Hon. Maj. 31st Aug. 1945. Served BEF France. Served Gallipoli 1915. Invalided. Mesopotamia 1918–19. India 1919–21. BAOR 1922. BEF France 1939–40.

WOOD John Stuart Address: North Street, Skibbereen, Co. Cork. MB, BCh (TCD 1932). Surg. Lt Comdr RN 1943.

WOOD Michael Charles Address: Cullinagh, Newcastle West, Co. Limerick. MB, BCh (TCD 1937), MD (TCD 1941). Surg. Lt RNVR.

WOODS Frederick Brian Baird MB, BCh (TCD 1943). RN.

WOODS Thomas Frederick Mackie b. 14th Jul. 1904, Pekan, Pahang, Malaya. MB, BCh, BAO (TCD 1926), MC (TCD 1932). MRCPI (TCD 1934). PC Lt 17th Oct. 1927. Capt. 28th Jun. 1930. Maj. 28th Dec. 1936. A/Lt Col. 8th Jun. 1940. T/Lt Col. 8th Feb. 1941. Lt Col. 20th Jun. 1945. A/Col. 29th Nov. 1942. T/Col. 29th May 1941. Col. 6th Jun. 1949. Brig. 10th Apr. 1956. T/Maj. Gen. 9th Jul. 1956. Maj. Gen. 25th Jul. 1957. r.p. 17th Oct. 1961. Served India 1929–32 and 1933–34. Malta 1935–40. CO 164th Fd Amb. 1940–42 India/Paiforce/MEF/India/SEAC 1942–45. ADMS HQ 31st Indian Div. 1942–44. ADMS HQ 10th Armoured Div. 1944. ADMS HQ 5th Indian Div. 1944–45. ADGAMS War Office (AMI) 1946. E. Africa BAOR: ADMS HQ 2nd Inf. Div. 1949–50. Comdt Depot and Training Estab. RAMC 1951–54. ADMS HQ London Dist. 1954–56. BAOR: DDMS HQ 1st Br. Corps 1956. DDMS HQ S. Comd 1956–61. QHP 6th Jan. 1959. Medals: CB (1st Jan. 1960), OBE (19th Sept. 1945), 1939–45 S., Burma S., DM, WM, QEII Corn Medal 1953.

WRAY George Arthur Address: 85 Magdalen St, Kilkenny. MB, BCh (TCD 1931). RAMC.

WRIGHT Alan Glynn b. 1894, Dublin. s. Albert M. Wright (mem. Dublin Stock Exchange) and Arabella Lane Wright, 3 Clyde Rd, Ballsbridge, Dublin. Educ. Portora Sch. Enniskillen. TCD. BA (1915), BCh, MB (1917), DPH (1921). R. C. of I. 2nd Lt ASC Feb. 1915. Lt RAMC 1st Nov. 1917. Capt. 1918. Served 1914–18 War attd. 127th Beluch Inf. Mesopotamia from 3rd Dec. 1917. 2nd WW Lt Col. Served Greece, Crete Cairo and Tripolitania. Medals: BWM, VM. Commemorated on Roll of Hon Sir Patrick Dun's Hosp.

WRIGHT Henry Bunting Address: 8 St James's Tce, Clonskeagh, Dublin. MB, BCh (TCD 1932). Maj. IMS Indian Comd. MC.

WRIGHT Henry John Address: 2 York Rd, Rathgar, Dublin. MB, BCh (NUI 1939). Lt RAMC 1st May 1941.

WRIGHT Richard James MD (QUB 1938). Capt. RAMC.

WRIGHT Trevor MC (QUB 1940). Capt. RAMC. MID (2).

WULFSOHN Max MB, BCh (TCD 1923). Capt. SAMC.

Y

YOUNG Augustus Henry Owen b. 18th Jan. 1874, Portarlington. Educ. RCSI. L.LM (1896) RCPI, L.LM (1896) RCSI. Lt RAMC 28th Jan. 1898. Capt. 28th Jan. 1901. Maj. 28th Oct. 1909. Lt Col. 1st Mar. 1915. Served South African War 1902. Served in 1914–18 War from 12th Aug. 1914. Served WWII. Lt Col. 1943. Medals: 1914 S., BWM, VM, SWB, OStJ.

YOUNG Oliver Gordon Campbell College. MB, BCh (QUB 1939). Address: 86 Maryville Pk, Malone Rd, Belfast. Maj. RAMC.

YOUNG Robert James MB (QUB 1942). Flt Lt (M) RAFVR

Acknowledgements

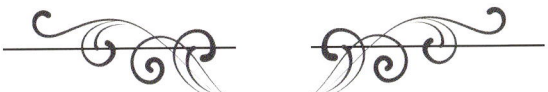

The research that informed this directory of *Irish Doctors in the Second World War* has been made possible by the assistance and guidance of a number of people. In particular we would like to thank Emer Purcell of the National University of Ireland for assistance in accessing the annual college calendars. Thanks also to Joy Guthrie of the Queen's University Services Club and the archivists at both the Queen's University and the Trinity College libraries for arranging access to the colleges' Rolls of Honour for the Second World War. Special thanks are due to Harriet Wheelock of the Royal College of Physicians in Ireland for arranging access to the college's archives and its Kirkpatrick Files.

Sincere thanks are owed to all the relatives of those Irish doctors who took part in the Second World War and who contacted us offering to share their family histories. Wewould especially like to thank Carl Murray and Adrienne MacCarthy for sharing information and images relating to their fathers' experiences as Japanese prisoners of war.

We owe a special thanks to Cathal Kelly, CEO, and the Council of the Royal College of Surgeons in Ireland for their sponsorship of this publication. Thanks also to Kevin Myers for writing the foreword to our book.

We are indebted to Merrion Press for the design of our publication, to Kevin O'Sullivan for the maps and to Wendy Logue for ensuring that the detail of the publication is a fitting record of the Irish doctors who served in the Second World War, especially of those who suffered such deprivations as Japanese prisoners of war.

We extend our thanks to Eileen, Ann and Eilis for their support throughout the past five years. In particular, we would especially like to thank Eileen for her remarkable patience and resilience in the production and editing of the directory.

INDEX

Note: Military ranks of doctors refer to the rank they held at that time discussed in the text. Page locators in bold refer to photographs and maps.

Advanced Dressing Station, **74**
affidavits by medical POWs, 84–7
aircraft, 8, 11, 88; PBY Catalina (US), 51, 52
Alardyce, Capt. Ransome McNamara, 65
Alexandra Military Hospital, Singapore, 65
Allied strategy, 18, 27–8, 42, 57; invasion of Italy, 49–50; landings in Northwest Africa, 48; in North Africa, 44–6; in the Pacific, 66–7 (*see also* British strategy and actions)
American Red Cross, the, 76 (*see also* International Red Cross, the)
Anderson, T/Lt Col. William, 57
annexation of Sudetenland, the, 13
Anschluss, the, 13
antibiotics, 9
antimicrobials, 10
Anzio landings, the, 47, 49
Araki, Sgt Maj. Kuniichi, 84, 87
Armistice (November 1918), the, 32
Asari, Q.M. Sgt Eiji, 86, 87
  atomic bomb drops, the, 67, **85**; on Nagasaki, 89–90

Barber, Maj. John Morgan, 43
Bataan Death March, the, 66
Battle of Britain, the, 16, 39, 40
Battle of France, the, 34–8, **35**
Battle of Kursk, the, 56
Battle of Normandy, the, 57
Battle of Singapore, the, 65
Battle of Stalingrad, the, 56
Battle of the Atlantic, the, 9, 27, 50–4
Belfast bombing raids (1941), the, 5
Belsen concentration camp, 57–8, 59
Beveridge, Lt Col. Arthur Joseph, 34
blitzkrieg warfare, 8, 34
blood and plasma transfusions, vii, 9, 10, **11**, 67, 74

Bluett, Col. Douglas, 44
British Army, the, 4; 8th Army, 44, 46, 47; Devonshire Rgt, **30**; Royal East Kent Rgt (Buffs), 47, 48; Royal Norfolk Rgt, 80 (*see also* British Expeditionary Force (BEF), the)
British Expeditionary Force (BEF), the, 13, 16, 31, 34, 35, 36, 38, 47, 75, 80, 87 (*see also* British Army, the)
British Medical Association, the, 6
British Red Cross Society, the, 75
British strategy and actions, 44, 51, 62–3, 66, 88
burn wounds, 9
Byrne, Capt. Aiden, 94

Camps Stalag Luft system, the, 38, 43, 78 (*see also* POW camps)
Caraher, Capt. Edward Francis More, 46–7
casualties, **3**, **12**, **33**, **46**, **47**, 48, **49**, **53**, 73, **74**, **76**, 110–11
Casualty Clearing Stations (CCS), 10, 36
Cavanagh, Surg. Lt William Anthony, 62
citations for bravery and decorations, 46–8, 93–8
Clancy, Flt Lt Martin, 59
Collis, Dr Robert, 59
Concannon, T/Maj. John Noel, 36
concentration camps, the, 57–9, 73
conscription, 3
Conway, Capt. Stephen, 96
Corry, Capt. Samuel, 26
Curran, Brig. Edward Joseph, 64

D-day landings, the, **56**
D'Arcy McCrea, Dr Edward, 39
Davis Cup, the, 40
De Panne Communal Cemetery, Belgium, 36
de Valera, Éamon (Jr), 78

INDEX

Deane, Dr Hastings Fitzmaurice, 43
deaths, 5, 7, 18, 32, 36, 37, 38, 39, 40, 48, 51, 52, 54, 56, 57, 58, 68, 74, 84
Derry as safe harbour for the Allied fleet, 5, 52
Dieppe raid, the, 26
diplomacy between the Vichy government and Britain, 51
'Draffin Bipod', the, 80
Draffin, Capt. Alexander, 80–1
Draffin (née Lyle), Margaret R., 80
Dublin bombing raids (1941), 5
Duggan, Surg. Lt Dermot Harry Tuthill, 52
Dunkirk evacuation, the, 23, 26, 36–7, 47, 72, 87
Dutch East Indies, the, 61, 64

Eastern Front, the, 54–6, **55**
Eaves, Lt Col. Thomas Preston, 54
emigration, 2, 4
employment for doctors after demobilisation, 1–2
employment opportunities in the British Army, 4
endotracheal intubation, 9
evacuation procedures, 10–11

Ferguson, Dr Ion, 43, 74, 77–9; *Doctor at War* (memoir), 77
Field Dressing Station, Western Desert, **19**
Field Surgical Unit, Italy, **viii**, **20**, **73**
first aid post, Calcutta, **70**
First Battle of El Alamein, the, 45
First World War, the, 6, 32, 38
food rations, 57, 86, 87
French Army, the, 13, 31, 34
French Navy, the, 51

Geneva Convention, the: Article 10 and the inspection of POW camps, 72; Article 12 and medical personnel, 71–2; and conditions of labour, 72; and the treatment of POWs, 71
George IV, King, 88
German Army, the, 33, 37, 39, 43, 56, 57, 87; Afrika Korps, **44**, **47**

German Navy, the, 50; ships: Admiral *Graf Spee* (battle cruiser), 51; *Bismarck* (battleship), 9, 51, 54; *Prinz Eugen* (battleship), 54; *Scharnhorst* (battle cruiser), 52; U-boats, 9, 37, 50, 51, 52
German strategy and actions, 13, 16, 33, 34–6, 40, 42; invasion of Greece, 41, 42–3, 77; and the invasion of Russia, 54–6; invasion of Yugoslavia and Greece, **41**; in North Africa, **44**, 44–6, 47; at sea, 50–1, 52–4
German treatment of POWs, 75–9
Glover, Sapper, 84
graduate records of military enlistments in the First World War, 6
Gray, Capt. John Astley, 88
Greek Army, the, 40, 42
Greek evacuation, the, 43
Greene, Col. Charles Westland, 43
Griffin, Sq. Ldr William Patrick, 43
Guadalcanal campaign, the, 66

Hackett, Dr Edward William, 64
Haft Neurosis (detention neurosis), 79
Harland & Wolff, Belfast, 5
Hearn, Capt. James, 57
Hirate, Kaichi, 87
Hirohito, Emperor, 61, 67
Hitler, Adolf, 13, 33, 34, 40, 42
hospital ships, 54
Hughes, Capt. Greg Doyly, 52
Hughes, Dr William, 59
Hunt, Surg. Rear Adm. Frederick George, 68
Hurst, Cdr Surg. Henry, 27, 54

Indian Medical Service (IMS), the, 1, 6, 7, 38
intramedullary nailing, 10
intravenous fluids, 9
Irish doctors and medical students in the Allied forces, 3–5, 6, 7, 18, 39–40, 68; with the BEF, 32; in the Far East, 65, 65, 66; in the Greece campaign, 43; in North Africa, 44, 46–8; in the Norway Campaign, 34; as POWs, 63, 64, 65, 66, 68, 74–90
Irish Free State Medical Union, the, 6

307

Irish National Army Medical Corps (NAMC), the, 2
Irish neutrality, 5
Italian actions, 16, 49; invasion of Egypt, 43–4; invasion of Greece, 40–2; in North Africa, 46
Italian Army, the, 40; 10th Army, 43–4
Italian Campaign, the, 28

Japanese Air Force, the, 62
Japanese strategy and actions, 16, 62, 64, 65–6; attack on Hong Kong, 62, 64; and the invasion of China, 61; and Java, 66, 88; and occupation of the Malaysian Peninsula, 64, 65, 81; and Singapore, 65, 72; and treatment of POWs, 66, 71, 72, 73, 81, 84–7, 88–9
Jordan, Surg. Lt John, 23

Kelly, Dr Thomas Bernard, 38
Kerr, Capt. Ralph, 54
Kinnear, Dr Nigel, 59
Kranji War Cemetery, Singapore, 65

lightweight sub-machine gun, the, 9
Lindsay, Ernest Leonard, 98
Luftwaffe, the, 5, 8, 33, 34, 40
lunacy certification and repatriation, 79

MacArthur, Gen Douglas, 89
MacCarthy, Flt Lt Joseph Aidan, 25, 33, 36, 66, 68, 87–90, **88, 91**; *Doctor's War, A* (memoir), 33, 89–90
MacCarthy (née Wall), Kathleen, 90
Maginot Line, the, 13, 16, 34
Malayan Medical Service (MMS), the, 1, 6, 63
maps of Main Theatres of War: Europe (1939–45), **14–15**; Pacific and South-east Asia (1939–45), **17**
Marks, Surg. Lt Hugh, 54
Martin, Capt. John, 95
Martin, T/Surg. Lt Miles, 26
matériel losses, 37, 50, 51, 52, 54, 62, 63
May, Maj. Peter, 96
McMahon, Dr John Ernest, 63

medals and awards for gallantry, 21–9, 22, 23, 24, 25, 27, 28, 29, 31, 34, 46–8; 8th Army Bar, 27; 1939–1945 Star, 25, 26; Africa Star, 25, 27; Atlantic Star, 25, 27, 29; Bar, 21, 23, 24, 27, 29, 54; Burma Bar (Clasp), 29; Burma Star, 25, 29; Commander of the Most Excellent Order of the British Empire (CBE), 24; Distinguished Service Order (DSO), the, 23, 23, 26, 31, 38, 54; France and Germany Star, 25, 29; George Medal (GM), 25, 87–8; Italy Star, 25, 28, 28; Member of the Most Excellent Order of the British Empire (MBE), 24, 83; Military Cross (MC), 24, 24, 31, 46–7; Médaille d'honneur du Service de Sainte Militaire-Chevalier de la Legion d'Honneur, 31; Mentioned in Dispatches (MID), 25; Norwegian Military Cross, 34; Officer of the British Empire (OBE), 24, 31, 90; Pacific Star, 25, 29; Victoria Cross (VC), 23; War Medal (WM), 25, 26
medical advances and care of casualties, 9–11
Medical Directory, the, 2
Merchant Navy (MN), the, 6, 27, 38, 47; SS *Madura*, 38
Mers-el-Kebir and Royal Navy attack on the French fleet, 51
metal plates and heal fractures, 10
Metaxas, Gen. Ioannis, 40
military strengths, 31
military training for medical undergraduates, 4, 47
mobile neurosurgical care, 10
Montgomery, Field Marshal Bernard, 27, 45–6
Moore, Maj. Edward Lewis, 24
Munich Conference, the, 13
Murray, Maj. Frank, 81, 81–7, 82, 85, 86
Murray (née O'Kane), Eileen, 83
Mussolini, Benito, 16, 40, 49

Nairnsey, Capt. Colman, 63
North African Campaign, the, 43–7, 44–5, 48
Norway Campaign, the, 34

Oberkommando der Wehrmacht (OKW), the, 78
O'Connor, Flt Lt Anthony, 33
Odbert, Lt Col. Arthur Noel, 43, 96–7
O'Driscoll, Lt Col. Florence Joseph, 97
O'Dwyer, T/Col. John Joseph, 29
Officer Training Corps, the, 4
O'Meara, Maj. Francis, 74, 75–6
O'Neill, Lt Col. Stephen Gerald, 44
Operation Barbarossa, 54–6
Operation Torch, 48
orthopaedics, 10, **92**
Officers' Training Corps (OTC), the, 75

Pacific Steam Navigation Company, the, 38
Pacific theatre, the, 66–7
Page, Surg. Cdr John Allison, 64
Parke, Flt Offr Frederick William, 66
Parsons, Capt. Alfred Denis (Andy), 46, 47–8
Patton, Maj. Kevin, **26**, 94
peacetime reduction in the armed forces, 1
Pearl Harbour attacks, the, 16, 62
Pearse, Surg. Lt George Passmore, 52
penicillin, 10
Phelan, Lt Col. Theobald, 97
Phoney War, the, 13–16, 33
POW camps, **81**, 86; Bad Sulza, Germany, 75; Camp Fukuoka 14B, Nagasaki, Japan, 89; Changi POW camp, Singapore, 81; Colditz Castle, Germany, 77–8, 80; Corinth, 77; Muroran, Hokkaido, Japan, 81, 83; Spangenberg, Germany, 75; Stadtroda, Germany, 75–6; Stalag 18A, Wolfsberg, Austria, 77; Stalag IVd, Torau, Germany, 79 (*see also* Camps Stalag Luft system, the)
POWs (Prisoners of War), **26**, **37**, 38, **39**, 43, 44, 46, 48, **53**, 64, 65, 66, 67–8, 71–2; affidavits by, 84–7; and escape attempts, 80; and Japanese treatment of, 66, 71, 72, 73, 74, 81, 84–7, 88–9; and members of the medical services, 71–3, 75–90
Protectorate of Bohemia and Moravia, the, 13
Purdon, Maj. Gen. William Brooke, 31

Queen's University Belfast (QUB), 4, 5, 6, 7, 21, 34, 43, 65, 68, 80, 81

records of Second World War medical graduates, 6
Red Cross, the, **53**, 59, **59**, 72, 83, 87
registered doctors in Ireland, 2
Ringer's lactate, 10
RMS *Lancastria* (ocean liner), 37
Royal Air Force (RAF), the, 1, 6, 7, 27, 33, 36, 39, 58, 59, 66, 87, 90; RAF Honington, 90; Squadrons: 30 Sqn, 77; 116 Sqn, 88
Royal Army Medical Corps (RAMC), the, 1, 2, 7, 23, 28, 34, 36, 40, 46, 47, 54, 57, 59, 75, 77, 80, 81
Royal College of Physicians in Ireland (RCPI), the, 6, 75; Kirkpatrick Archive, 6
Royal College of Surgeons in Ireland (RCSI), the, 6, 7, 21, 43, 54, 62, 77
Royal Navy (RN), the, 1, 6, 7, 9, 27, 33, 38, 43 51; ships: HMS *Acasta* (destroyer), 52; HMS *Ardent* (destroyer), 52; HMS *Ark Royal* (carrier), 51; HMS *Courageous* (carrier), 51; HMS *Gloucester* (carrier), 52; HMS *Hermes* (carrier), 54; HMS *Hermione* (cruiser), **50**; HMS *Hood* (battle cruiser), 9, 27, 51, 52–4; HMS *Mackay*, 77; HMS *Prince of Wales* (battleship), 62; HMS *Repulse* (battle cruiser), 62–3; HMS *Royal Oak* (battleship), 51; HMS *Theseus* (carrier), 98
Rommel, General Erwin, 44, 47
Roosevelt, Franklin D., 62
Rosehill, Flt Offr Sydney, 33
Royal Army Corps, the, 6
Russian Army, the, 56, 80

Samuels, Capt. Leslie, 93
sea rescues, 52
Second Battle of El Alamein, the, 46, 47
Sheill, Capt. Gordon, 57
shell dressing, **63**
Shiba, Dr Tsutomi, 86, 87
siege of Tobruk, the, 44, 72
Singapore War Memorial, the, 65
skeletal traction and leg placement operation, **92**
Smyth, Capt. Ernest Albert, 63
Solomon, Capt. Louis, 43
Sonne, Lt, 88–9 South African Medical Corps (SAMC), the, 6
St Patrick Dun's Hospital, Dublin, 40
St Stephen's College, Hong Kong, 64
Stewart, Capt. William Muir, 34
Stewart, Maj. R.R., 84
Stringer, Brig. Charles Herbert, 63
Summ, Maj. Julius, 94
supply convoys and merchant shipping, 50, 52
surrender of Japan, the, 67, 68
Suttle, Pvt, 84
suturing and stitching, 10
Swiss Repatriation Commission, the, 79

tank warfare, 8–9, 56
tanks: Churchill (UK), 9; Sherman (US), 9, **42**; T-34 (USSR), 9; Tiger I (Germany), 9
Taylor, Maj. Robert, 34, 57
technological advancements in warfare, 8–9
Thomson, Capt. Humphrey Barron, 65
Tomlinson, Dr Sterling, 64
Trinity College Dublin (TCD), 6, 7, 21, 34, 36, 39, 47, 57, 65, 75
Tripartite Pact, the, 16
Tyndall, A/Col. William, 34

United States Medical Corps (USMC), the, 6
University College Cork (UCC), 6, 7, 21, 33, 68, 87
University College Dublin (UCD), 6, 7, 21, 46
University College Galway (UCG), 6, 7, 21, 38
urban warfare, 9
US Army, the, 5, 48; Second Army, 80
US entry into the war, 62
US Navy, the, 9, 89; USS Tang (submarine), 89

Vichy government, the, 51
voluntary enlistment of Irish doctors, 3–4

Waldron, T/Maj. Francis, 59
Walker, Lt Col. Robert, 98
Walmsley, Capt. George, 34
Walsh, Surg. Lt Stanley, 98
Walsh, Surg. Rear Adm. Dermot, 27, 28, 29
war campaign medals, 25
war crimes trials, 87, 89
Whyte, Maj. Desmond, 23
Wilcock, Dr Edith Florence, 39, 40
Wilson, Capt. Terence, 95
Wilson, Lt Col. Joseph Andrew, 31
wound cleaning, 10